Manual of Exercise Testing

Manual of Exercise Testing

Third Edition

Victor F. Froelicher, M.D.

Professor of Medicine
Director, ECG/Exercise Laboratory
VA Palo Alto Health Care System
Stanford University
Palo Alto, California

Jonathan Myers, Ph.D.

Clinical Associate Professor of Medicine
VA Palo Alto Health Care System
Stanford University
Palo Alto, California

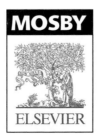

MOSBY

ELSEVIER

1600 John F. Kennedy Blvd., Suite 1800
Philadelphia, PA 19103-2899

MANUAL OF EXERCISE TESTING, THIRD EDITION ISBN-13: 978-0-323-03302-2

Notice

Knowledge and best practice in this field are constantly changing. As new research and experience broaden our knowledge, changes in practice, treatment, and drug therapy may become necessary or appropriate. Readers are advised to check the most current information provided (i) on procedures featured or (ii) by the manufacturer of each product to be administered, to verify the recommended dose of formula, the method and duration of administration, and contraindications. It is the responsibility of the practitioner, relying on their own experience and knowledge of the patient, and to make diagnoses, to determine dosages and the best treatment for each individual patient, and to take all appropriate safety precautions. To the fullest extent of the law, neither the Publisher nor the Editors assume any liability for any injury and/or damage to persons or property arising out of or related to any use of the material contained in this book.

The Publisher

Previous editions copyrighted 1989, 1994

Library of Congress Cataloging-in-Publication Data
Froelicher, Victor F.
    Manual of exercise testing / Victor F. Froelicher, Jonathan Myers.--3rd ed.
        p. cm.
    ISBN 0-323-03302-4
        1. Treadmill exercise tests--Handbooks, manuals, etc. I. Myers, Jonathan, 1957- II. Title.

    RC683.5.E94F77 2007
    616.1'207547--dc22   2006044993

Executive Publisher: Natasha Andjelkovic
Project Manager: Mary Stermel
Design Direction: Steve Stave
Marketing Manager: Dana Butler

Printed in United States of America

Last digit is the print number: 9 8 7 6 5 4 3 2 1

To my daughter Beth

Victor Froelicher, M.D.

To my parents, for their unwavering support, the sacrifices, and all the things they taught me

Jonathan Myers, Ph.D.

Preface

Welcome to the third edition of our *Manual of Exercise Testing*. As before, this manual is designed to complement our textbook, *Exercise and the Heart*, recently published in its fifth edition. The writing and references have been skimmed down for readability, and we have added many case examples of both common and interesting or rare exercise ECGs for teaching purposes. We hope that this manual provides a good instructional tool for fellows, residents, students, and clinicians who are interested in the clinical applications of the exercise test.

Since the second edition, there have been numerous important documents published, including an update of the AHA/ACC guidelines on exercise testing, the American Thoracic Society/American College of Chest Physicians Statement on Cardiopulmonary Exercise Testing, an AHA Scientific Statement on Exercise and Heart Failure, an AHA Scientific Statement on Physical Activity in the Prevention of Cardiovascular Disease, new editions of the American Association of Cardiovascular and Pulmonary Rehabilitation Guidelines, and the American College of Sports Medicine Guidelines on Exercise Testing and Prescription. Relevant information from these updated documents has been incorporated into this third edition. The necessity of practicing evidence-based medicine makes it critical that all of us defer to the panels of experts who write these guidelines. In rare cases in which the guidelines are inconsistent or we offer an opinion or recommendation that differs from the guidelines, we alert the reader.

As the field of cardiology has continued to evolve, it is important to note some of the new or changed acronyms in medicine:

- HF has been recommended as the acronym to replace CHF, because CHF has confusingly represented either chronic or congestive (acute) heart failure.

- PCI (percutaneous coronary intervention) has replaced PTCA because many techniques in addition to balloon angioplasty are currently performed by interventionalists.
- AED (automated external defibrillator) and ICD (implantable cardiac defibrillator) are used for the new biphasic defibrillator products.
- CRT (cardiac resynchronization therapy) is an implantable pacemaker for improving cardiac function that is often combined with an ICD.
- ACS (acute coronary syndrome) is the term now widely used to describe the spectrum of conditions associated with acute myocardial ischemia, including unstable angina pectoris and non–Q-wave MIs.

In this edition, we've tried to incorporate the influence of the remarkable advances in cardiology throughout the book. These advances are listed below (not in order of impact), because each advance by itself has strongly influenced exercise testing, exercise training, and clinical exercise physiology:

1. Designation of acute coronary syndromes (ACS)
2. Biomarkers for ischemia and volume overload/left ventricular dysfunction at point of contact (troponin and brain natriuretic peptide [BNP])
3. Advances in percutaneous coronary interventions (PCI), culminating in drug-eluting stents that have greatly reduced stent failure
4. Evidence-based recommendations that PCI is better than thrombolysis for acute myocardial infarction
5. Medications that convincingly improve survival in patients with heart disease
6. Pacemakers for cardiac resynchronization therapy (CRT)
7. Consideration of the exercise test as an opportunity to evaluate the complex interaction of the CV and autonomic systems

These advances have actually interacted with one another, so it is best to address them in groupings that impact health care in a similar fashion. We will address those that impact the diagnostic use of exercise testing first. Many patients who required diagnostic exercise testing after the first appearance of symptoms now have the diagnosis made by an elevation of troponin. They often go straight to cardiac catheterization. Many cardiologists feel that advances in PCI make the noninvasive diagnosis of ischemic chest pain moot because angiography can make the diagnosis and treat the problem by averting all the steps in between. The lowered restenosis rate associated with drug-eluting stents has removed, in their minds, all the reasons not to diagnose and fix the problem all in one relatively low-risk procedure. However, it is important to keep in mind that health care costs continue to rise and fewer people are insured or able to afford this invasive approach. As clinicians continue to deal with the problems of cost-efficacy, we contend that the exercise test remains the most logical gatekeeper to more expensive and/or invasive diagnostic tests. When a biomarker that can be measured at point of contact becomes validated as a way to increase the sensitivity of the test along with multivariate scores, reasonable clinicians will apply the exercise test first. Although some would disagree, we contend that the "art" of medical decision-making and the use of noninvasive tests are currently more important than ever.

Next, let us consider the advances in health care that affect the prognostic use of exercise testing. PCI for acute myocardial infarction has been shown to be better than thrombolysis for improving prognosis and lessening myocardial damage. The reason is that it is more effective than thrombolytic drugs in opening coronary arteries blocked by thrombosis. Improved patency rates mean that follow-up exercise testing is less likely to be needed routinely after MI to determine who needs coronary angiography. However, when the patient and physician want or need individualized prognostic information, there is no test more valuable than the standard exercise test. Many recent studies have confirmed that exercise capacity alone has independent and significant prognostic power, regardless of the patient's clinical history.

Surprisingly, the next two items, which relate to patients with HF, have resulted in new ideas regarding cardiovascular physiology. First, HF results in major metabolic and cellular changes that can be improved by an exercise program. These alterations have provided interesting insights into the exercise response because a major contributor to these improvements appears to be change in endothelial function. Second, implanted synchronous pacemakers have been shown to improve both ventricular function and exercise capacity. This is somewhat surprising because previously it was thought that myocyte damage was the primary event leading to LV dysfunction and that conduction disturbances were a result of this. However, improvement in function resulting from correction of dysynchrony suggests that damage to the conduction system can be the cause of LV dysfunction and impaired exercise capacity.

The following is our strongest variance from the guidelines: Exercise testing, along with risk factor assessment, should be used for screening healthy, asymptomatic individuals. We are lobbying our colleagues on this point for the following reasons:

- A number of contemporary studies have demonstrated remarkable risk ratios for the combination of the standard exercise test responses and traditional risk factors.
- Other modalities, without the favorable test characteristics of the exercise test, are being promoted for screening.
- Physical inactivity has reached epidemic proportions, and the exercise test provides an ideal way to make patients conscious of their deconditioning and to make physical activity recommendations.
- Adjusting for age and other risk factors, each MET increase in exercise capacity equates to a 10% to 25% improvement in survival.

We feel it is important to provide the following precepts in the preface regarding exercise testing methodology even though the details are in the chapters:

- The exercise protocol should be adjusted to the patient; one protocol is not appropriate for all patients.
- Exercise capacity should be reported in METs, not minutes of exercise.

- Hyperventilation prior to testing is not indicated but can be utilized at another time if a false-positive test is suspected.
- ST measurements should be made at ST0 (J-junction), and ST depression should be considered abnormal only if horizontal or downsloping; the vast majority of the clinically important ST depression occurs in V5, particularly in patients with a normal resting ECG.
- Patients should be placed supine as soon as possible post-exercise, with a cool-down walk avoided in order for the test to have its greatest diagnostic value.
- The 2- to 4-minute recovery period is critical to include in analysis of the ST response.
- Measurement of systolic blood pressure during exercise is extremely important and exertional hypotension is ominous; at this point, only manual blood pressure measurement techniques are valid.
- Age-predicted heart rate targets are largely useless because of the wide scatter for any age; a relatively low heart rate can be maximal for a given patient and submaximal for another.
- The Duke Treadmill Score should be calculated automatically on every test except for the elderly.
- Other predictive equations and heart rate recovery should be considered a standard part of the treadmill report.

To ensure the safety of exercise testing and reassure the noncardiologist performing the test, the following list of the most dangerous circumstances in the exercise testing lab should be considered:

- Testing patients with aortic valvular disease or obstructive hypertrophic cardiomyopathy (ASH or IHSS) should be done with great care. Aortic stenosis can cause cardiovascular collapse, and these patients may be difficult to resuscitate because of the outflow obstruction; IHSS can become unstable due to arrhythmia. Because of these conditions, a physical exam, including assessment of systolic murmurs, should be done before all exercise tests. If a significant murmur, is heard, an echocardiogram should be considered before performing the test.
- When patients without diagnostic Q waves on their resting ECG exhibit exercise-induced ST-segment elevation (i.e., transmural ischemia), the test should be stopped; this can be associated with dangerous arrhythmias and infarction. Exercise-induced elevation without Q waves occurs in about 1 out of 1000 clinical tests.
- A cool-down walk is advisable in the following instances:
  1. When a patient with an ischemic cardiomyopathy exhibits significant chest pain due to ischemia, because the ischemia can worsen in recovery
  2. When a patient develops exertional hypotension accompanied by ischemia (angina or ST depression), or when it occurs in a patient with a history of HF, cardiomyopathy, or recent MI
  3. When a patient with a history of collapse during exercise develops PVCs that become frequent

4. Appreciation of these circumstances can help avoid any complications in the exercise lab

Given this background, we are targeting this manual as a basic reference for the clinical aspects of exercise testing. More detailed information and references are covered in our textbook. This manual is meant for any health care provider interested in performing exercise tests so that the most valuable clinical information is obtained. It is our hope that physicians, physicians in training, and nonphysicians, including technologists involved in exercise testing, find this text helpful.

Contents

1 The Physiologic Response to the Exercise Test

Introduction

Exercise physiology is the study of the physiologic responses and adaptations that occur as a result of acute or chronic exercise. Exercise is the body's most common physiologic stress, and it places major demands on the cardiopulmonary system. For this reason, exercise can be considered the most practical test of cardiac perfusion and function. Exercise testing is a noninvasive tool to evaluate the cardiovascular system's response to exercise under carefully controlled conditions. The adaptations that occur during an exercise test allow the body to increase its resting metabolic rate up to 20 times, during which time cardiac output may increase as much as six times. The magnitude of these adjustments depends on age, gender, body size, type of exercise, fitness, and the presence or absence of heart disease. The major central and peripheral adaptations that occur from rest to maximal exercise are illustrated in Figure 1-1. Although major adaptations are also required of the endocrine, neuromotor, and thermoregulatory systems, the major focus of this chapter is on the cardiovascular response and adaptations of the heart to acute exercise.

Because of the recent interest in the use of the exercise test to evaluate the interaction of the autonomic nervous system (ANS) and the cardiovascular (CV) system, this chapter reviews this subject as well.

Basic Principles

Two basic principles of exercise physiology are important for understanding exercise testing. The first is a physiologic principle: total body oxygen uptake and myocardial oxygen uptake are distinct in their determinants and in the way they are measured or estimated (Table 1-1). Total body or ventilatory oxygen uptake (VO_2) is the amount of oxygen that is

Cardiovascular effects of exercise

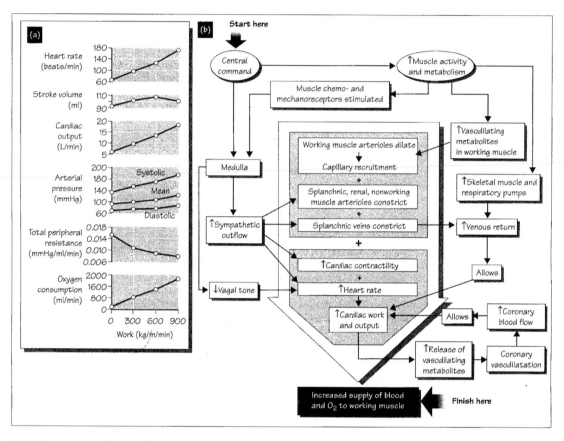

FIGURE 1-1   (a) Graphs of the hemodynamic responses to dynamic exercise. (b) Sequence of physiologic responses to dynamic exercise. (From Aaronson P, Ward J, and Wiener CM: Cardiovascular Physiology at a Glance with permission of Blackwell Publishers, Oxford, UK, 2004).

TABLE 1-1   Two Basic Principles of Exercise Physiology

Myocardial oxygen consumption	≈ Heart rate × systolic blood pressure (determinants include wall tension, approximately equal to left ventricular pressure × volume; contractility; and heart rate)
Ventilatory oxygen consumption (VO$_2$)	≈ External work performed, or cardiac output × a-VO$_2$ difference

*The arteriovenous O$_2$ difference is approximately 15 to 17 vol% at maximal exercise in most individuals; therefore VO$_2$ max generally reflects the extent to which cardiac output increases.

extracted from inspired air as the body performs work. Myocardial oxygen uptake is the amount of oxygen consumed by the heart muscle. The determinants of myocardial oxygen uptake include intramyocardial wall tension (left ventricular pressure and end-diastolic volume), contractility, and heart rate. It has been shown that myocardial oxygen uptake can be reasonably estimated by the product of heart rate and systolic blood pressure (double product). This information is valuable clinically because exercise-induced angina often occurs at the same myocardial oxygen demand (double product), and the higher the double product achieved, the better the myocardial perfusion and prognosis. When such is not the case, the influence of other factors should be suspected, such as a recent meal, abnormal ambient temperature, or coronary artery spasm.

The second principle of exercise physiology is one of pathophysiology: considerable interaction takes place between the exercise test manifestations of abnormalities in myocardial perfusion and function. The electrocardiographic (ECG) response and angina are closely related to myocardial ischemia (and coronary artery disease), whereas exercise capacity, systolic blood pressure, and heart rate responses to exercise can be determined by the presence of myocardial ischemia, myocardial dysfunction, or responses in the periphery. Exercise-induced ischemia can cause cardiac dysfunction that results in exercise impairment and an abnormal systolic blood pressure response.

The severity of ischemia or the amount of myocardium in jeopardy is known clinically to be inversely related to the heart rate, blood pressure, and exercise level achieved. However, neither resting nor exercise ejection fraction, or a change in ejection fraction during exercise, correlates well with measured or estimated maximal oxygen uptake, even in patients without signs or symptoms of ischemia.[1,2] Moreover, exercise-induced markers of ischemia do not correlate well with one another. Silent ischemia (i.e., markers of ischemia presenting without angina) does not appear to affect exercise capacity in patients with coronary heart disease.[3] Cardiac output is generally considered the most important determinant of exercise capacity, but studies suggest that in some patients with heart disease, the periphery also plays an important role in limiting exercise capacity.[4]

Concepts of Work

Because exercise testing fundamentally involves the measurement of work, several concepts regarding work are important to understand.

Work is defined as force moving through a given distance ($W = F \times D$).

If muscle contraction results in mechanical movement, work has been accomplished. **Force is equal to mass times acceleration ($F = M \times A$).**

Any weight, for example, is a force that is undergoing the resistance provided by gravity. A great deal of any work that is performed involves overcoming the resistance provided by gravity.

The basic unit of force is the newton (N). It is the force that, when applied to a 1 kg mass, gives it an acceleration of 1 m multiplied by sec^{-2}. Since work is equal to force (in newtons) times distance (in meters), another unit for work is the newton meter (Nm). One Nm is equal to one joule (J), which is another common expression of work.

Power and energy. Because work is nearly always expressed per unit of time (i.e., as a rate), an additional unit that becomes important is **power,** the rate at which work is performed. The body's metabolic equivalent (MET) of power is **energy.** Therefore it is easy to think of work as anything with weight moving at some rate across time (which is often analogous to distance).

The MET. The common biologic measure of total body work is the oxygen uptake, which is usually expressed as a rate (making it a measure of power) in liters per minute. The MET is a term commonly used clinically to express the oxygen requirement of the work rate during an exercise test on a treadmill or cycle ergometer. One MET is equated with the resting metabolic rate (approximately 3.5 ml of O_2/kg/min), and a MET value achieved from an exercise test is a multiple of the resting metabolic rate, either measured directly (as oxygen uptake) or estimated from the maximal workload achieved using standardized equations.[5]

Energy and Muscular Contraction

Muscular contraction is a complex mechanism involving the interaction of the contractile proteins actin and myosin in the presence of calcium. The myosin and actin filaments in the muscle slide past one another as the muscle fibers shorten during contraction. The source of energy for this contraction is supplied by adenosine triphosphate (ATP), which is produced in the mitochondria. ATP is stored as two products, adenosine diphosphate (ADP) and phosphate, at specific binding sites on the myosin heads.

The sequence of events that occurs when a muscle contracts depends on three other factors: calcium and two inhibitory proteins, troponin and tropomyosin. Voluntary muscle contraction begins with electrical impulses at the myoneural junction, initiating the release of calcium ions. Calcium is released into the sarcoplasmic reticulum that surrounds the muscle filaments; it binds to a special protein, troponin-C, which is attached to tropomyosin (another protein that inhibits the binding of actin and myosin), and actin. When calcium binds to troponin-C, the tropomyosin molecule is removed from its blocking position between actin and myosin, the myosin head attaches to actin, and muscular contraction occurs.

The main source of energy for muscular contraction, ATP, is produced by oxidative phosphorylation. The major fuels for this process are carbohydrates (glycogen and glucose) and free fatty acids. At rest, roughly equal amounts of energy are derived from carbohydrates and fats. Free fatty acids contribute greatly to the energy supply during low levels of exercise, but greater amounts of energy are derived from carbohydrates as exercise progresses. Maximal work relies virtually entirely on carbohydrates. Oxidative phosphorylation initially involves a series of events that take place in the cytoplasm. Glycogen and glucose are metabolized to pyruvate through glycolysis. If oxygen is available, pyruvate enters the mitochondria from the sarcoplasm and is oxidized to a compound known as acetyl coenzyme

A (acetyl CoA), which then enters a cyclical series of reactions known as the Krebs cycle. By-products of the Krebs cycle are CO_2 and hydrogen. Electrons from hydrogen enter the electron transport chain, yielding energy for the binding of phosphate (phosphorylation) from ADP to ATP. This process, oxidative phosphorylation, is the greatest source of ATP for muscle contraction. A total of 36 ATP molecules per molecule of glucose are formed in the mitochondria during this process.

The mitochondria can produce ATP for muscle contraction only if oxygen is present. At higher levels of exercise, total body oxygen demand may exceed the capacity of the cardiovascular system to deliver oxygen. However, glycolysis progresses in the cytoplasm much the same way as aerobic metabolism until pyruvate is formed. Electrons released during glycolysis are taken up by pyruvate to form lactic acid. Rapid diffusion of lactate from the cell inhibits any further steps in glycolysis. Thus oxygen-independent glycolysis is quite inefficient; two ATP molecules per molecule of glucose is the total yield from this process.

The relative exercise intensity in which lactate accumulation occurs is an important determinant of endurance performance. The degree to which lactate accumulates in the blood is related to exercise intensity and the extent to which fast-twitch (Type IIB) fibers are recruited. Although lactate can contribute to fatigue by increasing ventilation and inhibiting other enzymes of glycolysis, it can also serve as an important energy source in muscles other than those in which it was formed, and it serves as an important precursor for liver glycogen during exercise.[6,7]

Muscle Fiber Types

The body's muscle fiber types are classified on the basis of the speed with which they contract, their color, and their mitochondrial content. Type I muscle fibers, or slow-twitch muscle fibers, are red in color and contain high concentrations of mitochondria. Type II muscle fibers, or fast-twitch muscle fibers, are white in color and have low concentrations of mitochondria. Fiber color is related to the degree of myoglobin, which is a protein that both stores oxygen in the muscle and carries oxygen in the blood to the mitochondria. Not surprisingly, slow-twitch fibers, with their high myoglobin content, are more resistant to fatigue; thus a muscle with a high percentage of slow-twitch fibers is well suited for endurance exercise. However, slow-twitch fibers tend to be smaller and produce less overall force than fast-twitch fibers. Fast-twitch fibers are generally larger and tend to produce more force, although they fatigue more easily. The speed of contraction for each fiber type is based largely on the activity of the enzyme myosin ATPase, which sits in the myosin head and to which ATP combines.

Although the two fiber types can be separated by distinct characteristics, both fibers function effectively for virtually all physical activities. Myosin ATPase activity and speed of contraction of some slow-twitch fibers approximate those of fast-twitch fibers. Moreover, Type II (fast-twitch) fibers have been further divided into three subcategories: Type IIA, Type IIB, and Type IIC. The Type IIA fiber mimics the Type I fiber in that it has a high capacity for oxidative metabolism. It has been suggested that the Type IIA fiber actually is a Type II fiber that has been adapted for endurance exercise, and endurance athletes are known to have a relatively large number of these fibers.[8] The Type IIB fiber is a "true" Type II fiber in that it contains few mitochondria and is better adapted for short bursts of activity. The Type IIC fiber appears to represent an "uncommitted" fiber, capable of adapting into one of the other fiber types. Endurance athletes are genetically endowed with larger percentages of Type I fibers, and the opposite is true of sprinters and jumpers as demonstrated by muscle biopsy.

Acute Cardiopulmonary Response to Exercise

The cardiovascular system responds to acute exercise with a series of adjustments that ensure the following: active muscles receive blood supply appropriate to their metabolic needs, heat generated by the muscles is dissipated, and blood supply to the brain and heart is maintained.

This response requires a major redistribution of cardiac output along with a number of local metabolic changes. The usual measure of the capacity of the body to deliver and utilize oxygen is the maximal oxygen uptake (VO_2 max). Thus the limits of the cardiopulmonary system are historically defined by VO_2 max, which can be expressed by the Fick principle:

$$VO_2 \text{ max} = \text{Maximal cardiac output} \times \text{Maximal arteriovenous oxygen difference}$$

Cardiac output must closely match ventilation in the lung in order to deliver oxygen to the working muscle. VO_2 max is determined by the maximal amount of ventilation (VE) moving into and out of the lung and by the fraction of this ventilation that is extracted by the tissues:

$$VO_2 = VE \times (FiO_2 - FeO_2)$$

where VE is minute ventilation and FiO_2 and FeO_2 are the fractional amounts of oxygen in the inspired and expired air, respectively. To measure VO_2 accurately, CO_2 in the expired air (VCO_2) must also be measured; the major purpose of VCO_2 in this equation is to correct for the difference in ventilation between inspired and expired air. VCO_2 is also a valuable measurement clinically because the rate of increase in VCO_2 relative to the work rate or ventilation parallels the severity of heart failure and is a powerful prognostic marker.

The cardiopulmonary limits (VO_2 max) are therefore defined by the following: a central component (cardiac output) that describes the capacity of the heart to function as a pump, and peripheral factors (arteriovenous oxygen difference) that describe the capacity of the lung to oxygenate the blood delivered to it, as well as the capacity of the working muscle to extract this oxygen from the blood.

Figures 1-2 and 1-3 outline the many factors affecting cardiac output and arteriovenous oxygen difference, respectively. An abnormality in one or more of these components often characterizes the presence and extent of some form of cardiovascular or pulmonary disease.

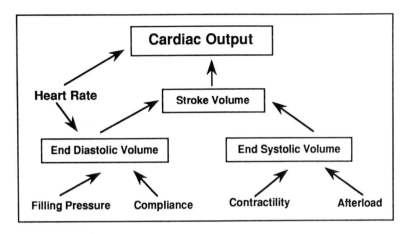

FIGURE 1-2   *Central determinants of maximal oxygen uptake. (From Myers J, Froelicher VF: Hemodynamic determinants of exercise capacity in chronic heart failure. Ann Intern Med 1991;115:377-386.)*

Central Factors

Figure 1-2 shows the central determinants of maximal ventilatory oxygen uptake.

Heart Rate

Sympathetic and parasympathetic nervous system influences underlie the cardiovascular system's first response to exercise—an increase in heart rate. Sympathetic outflow to the heart and systemic blood vessels increases while vagal outflow decreases. Vagal withdrawal is responsible for the initial change of 10 to 30 beats per minute, and the remainder is thought to be largely sympathetically mediated. Of the two major components of cardiac output, heart rate and stroke volume, heart rate is responsible for most of the increase in cardiac output during exercise, particularly at higher levels. Heart rate increases linearly with workload and oxygen uptake. Increases in heart rate occur primarily at the expense of diastolic, not systolic, time. Thus, at very high heart rates, diastolic time may be so short as to preclude adequate ventricular filling.

The heart rate response to exercise is influenced by several factors, including age, type of activity, body position, fitness, the presence of heart disease, medications, blood volume, and environment. Of these, the most important factor is age; a decline in maximal heart rate occurs with increasing age. This decline appears to be due to intrinsic cardiac changes rather than to neural influences. It should be noted that there is a great deal of variability around the regression line between maximal heart rate and age; thus age-related maximal heart rate is a relatively poor index of maximal effort (see Chapter 5). Maximal heart rate is unchanged or may be slightly reduced after a program of training. Resting heart rate is frequently reduced after training as a result of enhanced parasympathetic tone.

Stroke Volume

The product of stroke volume (the volume of blood ejected per heartbeat) and heart rate determines cardiac output. Stroke volume is equal to the difference between end-diastolic and end-systolic volume. Thus a greater diastolic filling (preload) will increase stroke volume. Alternatively, factors that increase arterial blood pressure will resist ventricular outflow (afterload) and result in a reduced stroke volume. During exercise, stroke volume increases to approximately 50% to 60% of maximal capacity, after which increases in cardiac output are due to further increases in heart rate. The extent to which increases in stroke volume during exercise reflect an increase in end-diastolic volume or a decrease in end-systolic volume, or both, is not entirely clear but appears to depend on ventricular function, body position, and intensity of exercise. In healthy subjects, stroke volume increases at rest and during exercise after a period of exercise training. Although the mechanisms have been debated, evidence suggests that this adaptation is due to increases in preload—and possibly local adaptations that reduce peripheral vascular resistance—more than increases in myocardial contractility. The end-diastolic and end-systolic responses to acute exercise have varied greatly in the literature, but depend on presence and type disease, exercise intensity, and exercise position (supine vs. upright).

In addition to heart rate, end-diastolic volume is determined by two other factors: filling pressure and ventricular compliance.

Filling Pressure The most important determinant of ventricular filling is venous pressure. The degree of venous pressure is a direct consequence of the amount of venous return. The Frank-Starling mechanism dictates that, within limits, all the blood returned to the heart will be ejected during systole. As the tissues demand greater oxygen during exercise, venous return increases, which in turn increases end-diastolic fiber length (preload), resulting in a more forceful contraction. Venous pressure increases as exercise intensity increases. Over the course of a few beats, cardiac output will equal venous return.

A number of other factors affect venous pressure and therefore filling pressure during exercise. These factors include blood volume, body position, and the pumping action of the respiratory and skeletal muscles. A greater blood volume increases venous pressure and therefore end-diastolic volume by making more blood available to the heart. Because the effects of gravity are negated, filling pressure is greatest in the supine position. In fact, stroke volume generally does not increase from rest to maximal exercise in the supine position. The intermittent mechanical constriction and relaxation in the skeletal muscles during exercise also enhance venous return. Finally, changes in intrathoracic pressure that occur with breathing during exercise facilitate the return of blood to the heart.

Ventricular Compliance Compliance is a measure of the capacity of the ventricle to stretch in response to a given volume of blood. Specifically, *compliance* is defined as the ratio of the change in volume to the change in pressure. The diastolic pressure/volume relation is curvilinear; that is, at low end-diastolic pressures, large changes in volume are accompanied by small changes in pressure, and vice versa. At the upper limits of end-diastolic pressure, ventricular compliance declines; that is, the chamber stiffness increases as it fills. Because of the difficulty in measuring end-diastolic pressure during exercise, few data are available concerning ventricular compliance during exercise in humans.

End-Systolic Volume

End-systolic volume depends on two factors: contractility and afterload.

Contractility describes the forcefulness of the heart's contraction. Increasing contractility reduces end-systolic volume, which results in a greater stroke volume and thus greater cardiac output. This process is precisely what occurs with exercise in the normal individual; the percentage of blood in the ventricle that is ejected with each beat increases, owing to an altered cross-bridge formation. Contractility is commonly quantified by the ejection fraction, the percentage of blood ejected from the ventricle during systole using radionuclide or angiographic techniques.

Afterload is a measure of the force resisting the ejection of blood by the heart. Increased afterload (or aortic pressure, as is observed with chronic hypertension) results in a reduced ejection fraction and increased end-diastolic and end-systolic volumes. During dynamic exercise, the force resisting ejection in the periphery (total peripheral resistance) is reduced by vasodilation, owing to the effect of local metabolites on the skeletal muscle vasculature. Thus, despite even a fivefold increase in cardiac output among normal subjects during exercise, mean arterial pressure increases only moderately.

Peripheral Factors (a-VO$_2$ Difference)

Figure 1-3 shows the peripheral determinants of maximal oxygen uptake. Oxygen extraction by the tissues during exercise reflects the difference between the oxygen content of the arteries (generally 18 to 20 ml O_2/100 ml at rest) and the oxygen content in the veins (generally 13 to 15 ml O_2/100 ml at rest, yielding a typical a-VO$_2$ difference at rest of 4 to 6 ml O_2/100 ml, approximately 23% extraction). During exercise, this difference widens as the working tissues extract greater amounts of oxygen; venous oxygen content reaches very low levels and a-VO$_2$ difference may be as high as 16 to 18 ml O_2/100 ml with exhaustive exercise (exceeding 85% extraction of oxygen from the blood at VO$_2$ max). Some oxygenated blood always returns to the heart, however, as smaller amounts of blood continue to flow through metabolically less active tissues that do not fully extract oxygen. Generally, a-VO$_2$ difference does not explain differences in VO$_2$ max between subjects who are relatively homogeneous. That is, a-VO$_2$ difference is generally considered to widen by a relatively "fixed" amount during exercise, and differences in VO$_2$ max have been historically explained by differences in cardiac output. Some patients with cardiovascular or pulmonary disease, however, exhibit reduced VO$_2$ max values that can be attributed to a combination of central and peripheral factors.

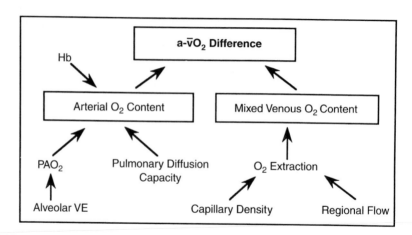

FIGURE 1-3   *Peripheral determinants of maximal oxygen uptake. The a-VO₂ difference is the difference between arterial and venous oxygen. Hb, hemoglobin; VE, minute ventilation; PAO₂, partial pressure of alveolar oxygen content. (From Myers J, Froelicher VF: Hemodynamic determinants of exercise capacity in chronic heart failure, Ann Intern Med 115:377-386, 1991.)*

Determinants of Arterial Oxygen Content

Arterial oxygen content is related to the partial pressure of arterial oxygen, which is determined in the lung by alveolar ventilation and pulmonary diffusion capacity, and in the blood by hemoglobin content. In the absence of pulmonary disease, arterial oxygen content and saturation are usually normal throughout exercise, even at very high levels. This is true even for patients with severe coronary disease or chronic heart failure. Patients with symptomatic pulmonary disease, however, often neither ventilate the alveoli adequately nor diffuse oxygen from the lung into the bloodstream normally, and a decrease in arterial oxygen saturation during exercise is one of the hallmarks of this disorder. Arterial hemoglobin content is also usually normal throughout exercise. Naturally, a condition such as anemia would reduce the oxygen-carrying capacity of the blood, along with any condition that would shift the O_2 dissociation curve leftward, such as reduced 2,3-diphosphoglycerate, reduced PCO_2, or elevated temperature.

Determinants of Venous Oxygen Content

Venous oxygen content reflects the capacity to extract oxygen from the blood as it flows through the muscle. It is determined by the amount of blood directed to the muscle (regional flow) and capillary density. Muscle blood flow increases in proportion to the increase in work rate and thus the oxygen requirement. The increase in blood flow is brought about not only by the increase in cardiac output, but also by a preferential redistribution of the cardiac output to the exercising muscle. A reduction in local vascular resistance facilitates the greater skeletal muscle flow. In turn, locally produced vasodilatory mechanisms, along with possible neurogenic dilation resulting from higher sympathetic activity, mediate the greater skeletal muscle blood flow. A marked increase in the number of open capillaries reduces diffusion distances, increases capillary blood volume, and increases mean transit time, facilitating oxygen delivery to the muscle.

Fit individuals have a greater skeletal muscle capillary density than sedentary subjects and a greater capacity to redistribute blood flow toward the working muscle and away from nonexercising tissue. The converse is true in many patients with cardiovascular disease. For example, one of the characteristics of patients with chronic heart failure is an "exaggeration" of the deconditioning response. These patients exhibit a reduced capacity to redistribute blood, a reduced capacity to vasodilate in response to exercise or following ischemia, and a reduced capillary-to-fiber ratio.

Autonomic Control

Neural Control Mechanisms

The neural control mechanisms responsible for the cardiovascular response to exercise occur through two processes that initiate and maintain this response:

Central command—neural impulses, arising from the central activity that recruits motor units, excite medullary and spinal neuronal circuits that cause the cardiovascular changes during exercise.
Muscle afferents—muscle contraction stimulates afferent endings within the skeletal muscle, which in turn reflexively evoke the cardiovascular changes.

The latter, or "exercise pressor reflex," comprises all of the cardiovascular changes reflexly induced from contracting skeletal muscle that are responsible for the increase in arterial blood pressure.

Contraction of skeletal muscle can reflexly cause changes in the efferent sympathetic and parasympathetic outputs to the cardiovascular system that are responsible for increases in arterial blood pressure, heart rate, myocardial contractility, cardiac output, and blood flow distribution. A specific subset of muscle afferents serve as ergoreceptors activated by either mechanical or metabolic perturbations. It appears that the lateral reticular nucleus may be an important site of integration, along with several other areas in the brainstem.

Both the sympathetic and parasympathetic branches of the ANS regulate heart rate during dynamic exercise. As the demand for cardiac output increases, parasympathetic activity becomes attenuated and sympathetic activity increases. The sympathetic system releases norepinephrine directly through the sympathetic trunk to the sinus node and myocardium. In addition, norepinephrine and epinephrine from the adrenal medulla act to increase heart rate and increase myocardial contractility, as well as to redirect blood flow to working muscle. By mediating peripheral vasoconstriction in relatively inactive tissues (e.g., the kidneys and hepatic-splanchnic system), the sympathetic system increases venous return while vasodilatory metabolites maintain local increased flow to active skeletal muscle. Actively contracting skeletal muscle also increases preload by acting as a venous pump and stimulating sympathetic afferent fibers within the muscle itself. Increases in heart rate, preload, and systemic vascular resistance affect increases in cardiac output and flow to metabolically active tissues while regulating blood pressure.

Pharmacologic blockade studies have helped elucidate the differential contributions of the two autonomic branches during exercise. Blockade of parasympathetic control with atropine reveals that most of the initial response to exercise, up to a heart rate of 100 to 120 beats per minute (i.e., a delta heart rate of 30 to 40 beats per minute), is attributable to the withdrawal of tonic vagal activity. Withdrawal of parasympathetic tone during mild exercise was confirmed using time and frequency domain analyses of heart rate variability. Vagal withdrawal induces a rapid increase in heart rate and cardiac output. Conversely, blockade of sympathetic control with propranolol reveals the importance of augmented sympathetic activity during moderate and heavy exercise. During light exercise, with workloads of 25% to 40% of VO_2 max or while heart rate remains within 30 beats per minute over baseline, plasma norepinephrine levels do not significantly increase, confirming that the sympathetic nervous system is more important in the latter stages of exercise.

Autonomic Modulation during Early Exercise

Controversy exists regarding the heart rate rise during early dynamic exercise. Based on the response to the 4-second exercise test developed by Claudio Araujo's group[9] and our preliminary findings, a rapid increase is normal. Individuals with the healthiest vagal tone or CV status respond to vagal withdrawal with the greatest increase. However, Falcone et al have reported excessive heart rate responses to exercise during the first minute of exercise predicts CV mortality.[10] Until this issue is resolved, clinical significance cannot be given to the early response of heart rate during the standard exercise test.

Autonomic Modulation during Immediate Recovery from Exercise

Autonomic physiology during recovery from acute bouts of exercise involves reactivation of the parasympathetic system and deactivation of sympathetic activity. The decline of heart rate after cessation of exercise is the variable most commonly analyzed to assess the underlying mechanisms. A delay in heart rate recovery has been used as a marker of autonomic dysfunction or failure of the CV system to respond to the normal autonomic responses to exercise. This delay has been shown to be a powerful prognostic marker. Time constants have been calculated by fitting heart rate decay data to a number of mathematical models, but the simple change in heart rate from peak exercise to minute 1 or 2 of recovery appears to distinguish survival as well. Early recovery after acute bouts of exercise appears to be dominated by parasympathetic reactivation, with sympathetic withdrawal becoming more important later in recovery. In a pharmacologic blockade study, Imai and colleagues[11] computed heart rate recovery decay curves using beat-to-beat data and concluded that short- and moderate-term heart rate recovery curves are vagally mediated, because heart rate decay 30 seconds and 2 minutes into recovery was prolonged with atropine and dual blockade; however, the

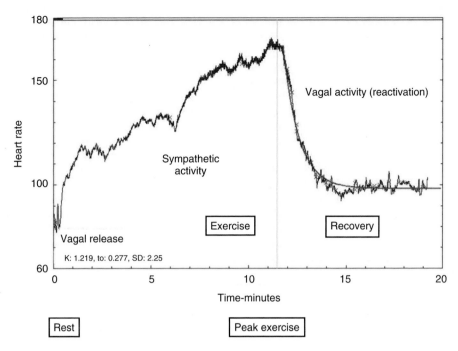

FIGURE 1-4   *An illustration of autonomic control of heart rate during the time periods of a standard graded progressive exercise test.*

heart rate decay for 2 minutes was more prolonged with dual blockade than with atropine alone, indicating that later recovery also depends on sympathetic modulation. Rather than declining, plasma norepinephrine concentrations during the first minute of recovery remain constant or even increase immediately after exercise.

Figure 1-4 illustrates the changes in autonomic control during a standard exercise test and recovery.

Summary

The major cardiopulmonary adaptations that are required of acute exercise make exercise testing a practical test of cardiac perfusion and function. The remarkable physiologic adaptations that occur with exercise have made exercise a valuable research medium not just for the study of cardiovascular disease, but also for studying physical performance in athletes and for studying the normal and abnormal physiology of other organ systems.

A major increase and redistribution of cardiac output underlies a series of adjustments that allow the body to increase its resting metabolic rate as much as 10 to 20 times with exercise. The capacity of the body to deliver and utilize oxygen is expressed as the maximal oxygen uptake. *Maximal oxygen uptake* is defined as the product of maximal cardiac output and maximal arteriovenous oxygen difference. Thus the cardiopulmonary limits are defined by (1) a central component (cardiac output) that describes the capacity of the heart to function as a pump and (2) peripheral factors (arteriovenous oxygen difference) that describe the capacity of the lung to oxygenate the blood delivered to it, as well as the capacity of the working muscle to extract this oxygen from the blood. Hemodynamic responses to exercise are greatly affected by the type of exercise being performed; by whether or not disease is present; and by the age, gender, and fitness of the individual.

Coronary artery disease is characterized by reduced myocardial oxygen supply, which, in the presence of an increased myocardial oxygen demand, can lead to myocardial ischemia and reduced cardiac performance. Despite years of study, a number of dilemmas remain in regard to the response to exercise clinically. Although myocardial perfusion and function are intuitively linked, it is often difficult to separate the impact of ischemia from that of left ventricular dysfunction on exercise responses. Indices of ventricular function and exercise capacity are poorly related. Cardiac output is considered the most important determinant of exercise capacity in normal subjects and in most patients with cardiovascular or pulmonary disease. However, among patients with disease, abnormalities in one or several of the links in the chain that defines oxygen uptake may contribute to the determination of exercise capacity.

The transport of oxygen from the air to the mitochondria of the working muscle cell requires the coupling of blood flow and ventilation to cellular metabolism. Energy for muscular contraction is provided by three sources: stored phosphates (ATP and creatine phosphate), oxygen-independent glycolysis, and oxidative metabolism. Oxidative metabolism provides the greatest source of ATP for muscular contraction. Muscular contraction is accomplished by two fiber types that differ in their contraction speed, color, and mitochondrial content. The duration and intensity of activity determine the extent to which these fuel sources and fiber types are called on.

All of the physiologic responses to exercise are mediated by the autonomic nervous system. The exercise test and the response in recovery from an exercise test are increasingly recognized as important surrogates for autonomic function. Sympathetic and parasympathetic influences on the cardiovascular system are critical in that they determine heart rate, blood pressure, cardiac output redistribution, and vascular resistance during exercise. Indirect measures of autonomic function, including heart rate variability and the rate at which heart rate increases at the onset of exercise and recovers from exercise, are important prognostic markers in patients with cardiovascular disease.

References

1. Cohn PF, Fox KM, Daly C: Silent myocardial ischemia, *Circulation* 108(10):1263-1277, 2003.
2. Myers J, Froelicher VF: Hemodynamic determinants of exercise capacity in chronic heart failure, *Ann Intern Med* 115:377-386, 1991.

3. Hammond HK, Kelley TL, Froelicher VF: Noninvasive testing in the evaluation of myocardial ischemia: agreement among tests, *J Am Coll Cardiol* 5:59-69, 1985.
4. Clark AL, Poole-Wilson PA, Coats AJ: Exercise limitation in chronic heart failure: central role of the periphery, *J Am Coll Cardiol* 28:1092-1102, 1996.
5. American College of Sports Medicine: *Guidelines for exercise testing and prescription,* ed 7, Baltimore, 2005, Lippincott Williams & Wilkins.
6. Myers J, Ashley E: Dangerous curves: a perspective on exercise, lactate, and the anaerobic threshold, *Chest* 111:787-795, 1997.
7. Brooks GA: Intra- and extra-cellular lactate shuttles, *Med Sci Sports Exerc* 32:790-799, 2000.
8. Saltin B, Henricksson J, Hugaard E, Andersen P: Fiber types and metabolic potentials of skeletal muscles in sedentary man and endurance runners, *Ann N Y Acad Sci* 301:3-29, 1977.
9. Arq Almeida MB, Ricardo DR, Araujo CG: Validation of the 4-second exercise test in the orthostatic position, *Bras Cardiol* 83(2):155-164, 2004.
10. Falcone C, Buzzi MP, Klersy C, Schwartz PJ: Rapid heart rate increase at onset of exercise predicts adverse cardiac events in patients with coronary artery disease, *Circulation* 112(13):1959-1964, 2005.
11. Imai K, Sato H, Hori M et al: Vagally mediated heart rate recovery after exercise is accelerated in athletes but blunted in patients with chronic heart failure. *J Am Coll Cardiol* 24:1529-1535.

2 Methods

Introduction

Despite technological advances in the diagnosis and treatment of cardiovascular disease, the exercise test remains an important modality. Its many applications, widespread availability, and high yield of clinically useful information make it an important gatekeeper for more expensive and invasive procedures. The numerous approaches to the exercise test, however, have been a drawback to its proper application. Excellent guidelines, which have been developed from research performed over the last 20 years (including an update of the American Heart Association/American College of Cardiology [AHA/ACC] guidelines on exercise testing, the American Thoracic Society/American College of Chest Physicians Statement on Cardiopulmonary Exercise Testing, an AHA Scientific Statement on Exercise and Heart Failure, new editions of the American Association of Cardiovascular and Pulmonary Rehabilitation Guidelines, and American College of Sports Medicine Guidelines on Exercise Testing and Prescription [www.cardiologyonline.com/guidelines.htm, www.cardiology.org]), have contributed greatly to the understanding and more uniform application of the exercise test. Relevant information from these updated documents has been incorporated into this chapter. The necessity of practicing evidence-based medicine makes it critical that all of us defer to the panels of experts who write these guidelines. Therefore we alert the reader when we suggest any practices that appear to vary from the guidelines.

Current technology, while adding both sophistication and convenience, has raised new questions about methodology. For example, all commercially available systems today use computers. Do computer-averaged exercise electrocardiograms (ECGs) improve test performance, and what should the practitioner be cautious of when considering computer measurements? What about the many computer-generated exercise scores? When should ventilatory gas exchange responses be measured during testing and what special considerations are important when using them? We hope to help the reader answer these questions.

Safety Precautions and Risks

The safety precautions outlined by the guidelines are explicit about the requirements for exercise testing. Everything necessary for cardiopulmonary resuscitation must be available, and regular drills should be performed to ascertain that personnel and equipment are ready for a cardiac emergency. The classic survey of clinical exercise facilities by Rochmis and Blackburn[1] demonstrated that exercise testing is a safe procedure, with approximately 1 death and 5 nonfatal complications per 10,000 tests. Perhaps because of an expanded knowledge concerning indications, contraindications, and endpoints, maximal exercise testing appears to be safer today than 30 years ago. In a multicenter study of patients tested for clinical reasons in the Veterans Administration (VA) Health Care System, an event rate (with "event" defined as a complication serious enough to require hospitalization) of 1.2 per 10,000 tests was reported.[2] This was similar to the widely cited findings of Gibbons and colleagues,[3] who reported the safety of exercise testing in 71,914 tests conducted over 16 years. The complication rate was 0.8 per 10,000 tests. The latter authors suggested that the low complication rate might be the result of including a cool-down walk, but low complication rates have also been observed despite laying patients supine immediately after maximal exercise and exercising higher-risk patients.[4]

It is important to note, however, that reports of acute infarctions and deaths associated with exercise testing exist. Although the test is remarkably safe, the population referred for this procedure usually is at high risk for coronary events. Irving and Bruce[5] have reported an association between exercise-induced hypotension and ventricular fibrillation. Shepard[6] has hypothesized the following risk levels for exercise testing: (1) 3 or 4 times normal mortality rates in a cross-country footrace; (2) 6 to 12 times normal mortality rates in a coronary-prone population performing unaccustomed exercise; and (3) up to 60 times normal mortality rates when exercise is performed by patients with coronary disease in a stressful environment, such as a physician's office.

Cobb and Weaver[7] estimated the risk to be over 100 times in the latter situation and pointed out the dangers of the recovery period. The risk of exercise testing in patients with coronary artery disease cannot be disregarded even with its excellent safety record.

Most problems can be avoided by having an experienced physician, nurse, or exercise physiologist standing next to the patient, measuring blood pressure, and assessing patient appearance during the test. Clinical indications for stopping (Table 2-1) should be given the highest priority. The exercise technician should operate the ECG monitor and treadmill,

TABLE 2-1   Absolute and Relative Indications for Termination of an Exercise Test

Absolute Indications

Acute myocardial infarction or suspicion of a myocardial infarction

Onset of severe angina (worse than usual)

Drop in systolic blood pressure with increasing workload accompanied by signs or symptoms, drop in systolic blood pressure below standing resting pressure, or drop in systolic blood pressure of 20 mm Hg

Serious dysrhythmias (second- or third-degree atrioventricular block, sustained ventricular tachycardia, or increasing premature ventricular contractions)

Signs of poor perfusion, including pallor, cyanosis, and cold and clammy skin

Central nervous system symptoms, including ataxia, vertigo, visual or gait problems, and confusion

Technical problems with monitoring any responses (such as with the ECG)

Patient's request

Relative Indications

Pronounced ECG changes from baseline, including more than 0.2 mV of horizontal or downsloping ST-segment depression, or 0.2 mV of ST-segment elevation (except in lead aVR)

Any chest pain that is increasing

Pronounced fatigue and shortness of breath

Wheezing

Leg cramps or intermittent claudication

Hypertensive response (systolic blood pressure > 260 mm Hg; diastolic blood pressure > 115 mm Hg)

Less serious dysrhythmias such as supraventricular tachycardia

Exercise-induced bundle branch block that cannot be distinguished from ventricular tachycardia

take the appropriate tracings, enter data on a form, and alert the physician to any abnormalities that may appear on the monitor screen.

> **Key Point:** The risk to the patient during exercise testing cannot be disregarded even with its excellent safety record. Guidelines must be followed and appropriate patient assessment and monitoring performed.

Contraindications

Table 2-2 lists the absolute and relative contraindications to performing an exercise test. Good clinical judgment should be foremost in deciding the indications and contraindications for exercise testing. In selected cases with relative contraindications, testing can provide valuable information even if the test is performed submaximally. The guidelines are highly specific for the use of the exercise test in the case of acute coronary syndrome (ACS) and as part of chest pain evaluation units.

ACS patients who are pain free, have either a normal or nondiagnostic ECG or one that is unchanged from previous tracings, and have a normal set of initial cardiac marker measurements are candidates for further evaluation to screen for nonischemic discomfort versus a low-risk ACS. If the patient is low risk and does not experience any further ischemic discomfort and a

TABLE 2-2   Absolute and Relative Contraindications to Exercise Testing

Absolute Contraindications
Acute myocardial infarction or any recent change in the resting ECG
Unstable angina
Serious cardiac dysrhythmias
Acute pericarditis or myocarditis
Endocarditis
Severe aortic stenosis
Severe left ventricular dysfunction
Acute pulmonary embolus or pulmonary infarction
Any acute or serious noncardiac disorder
Severe physical handicap

Relative Contraindications*
Any less serious noncardiac disorder
Ventricular conduction defects
Significant arterial or pulmonary hypertension
Tachydysrhythmias or bradydysrhythmias that are not serious
Moderate valvular or myocardial heart diseases
Drug effect or electrolyte abnormalities
Fixed-rate artificial pacemaker
Left main obstruction or its equivalent
Psychiatric disease or inability to cooperate

*Under certain circumstances, relative contraindications can be superseded by appropriate clinical judgement.

follow-up 12-lead ECG and cardiac marker measurements after 6 to 8 hours of observation are normal, the patient may be considered for an early stress test to provoke ischemia. This test can be performed before the discharge and should be supervised by an experienced physician. Alternatively, the patient may be discharged and return for a stress test as an outpatient within 3 days. The exact nature of the stress test may vary depending on the patient's ability to exercise on either a treadmill or bicycle and the local expertise in a given hospital setting (e.g., availability of different testing modalities at different times of the day or different days of the week). Patients who are capable of exercise and are free of confounding features on the baseline ECG, such as bundle branch block, left ventricular hypertrophy, or paced rhythms, can be evaluated with routine symptom-limited conventional exercise testing. Patients who are incapable of exercise or who have an uninterpretable baseline ECG should be considered for pharmacologic stress testing with either nuclear perfusion imaging or two-dimensional echocardiography. For sites at which such tests are not available, low-risk patients may be discharged and an exercise test scheduled within 3 days.

> **Key Point:** The risk of exercise testing can be lessened by excluding certain patients. If the guidelines for acute coronary syndrome (ACS) patients are followed, the standard exercise test can be helpful as part of a systematic approach (often in chest pain observation units).

Indications for Treadmill Test Termination

The absolute and relative indications for termination of an exercise test listed in Table 2-1 have been derived from clinical experience. Absolute indications are clear-cut, whereas relative indications can sometimes be superseded by good clinical judgment. Absolute indications include a drop in systolic blood pressure despite an increase in workload, anginal chest pain becoming worse than usual, central nervous system symptoms, signs of poor perfusion (e.g., pallor, cyanosis, and cold skin), serious dysrhythmias, technical problems with monitoring the patient, a patient's request to stop, and marked ECG changes (e.g., 2 mm or greater ST-segment elevation and 3 mm or greater horizontal or downsloping ST-segment depression). Relative indications for termination include other worrisome ST or QRS changes such as excessive junctional depression; increasing chest pain; fatigue, shortness of breath, wheezing, leg cramps, or intermittent claudication; worrisome appearance; a hypertensive response (systolic pressure > 250 mm Hg and diastolic pressure > 115 mm Hg); and less serious dysrhythmias, including supraventricular tachycardia. In some patients estimated to be at high risk by their clinical history, it may be appropriate to stop at a submaximal level, because the most severe ST-segment depression or dysrhythmias may occur only after exercise. If more information is required in a particular patient, the test can be repeated later.

> **Key Point:** The physician's judgment to stop (based on patient history and worrisome subjective responses during a test) is sufficient reason to terminate an exercise test.

Legal Concerns

Two major considerations in regard to legality are establishment of physician-patient communication before and after performance of the exercise test and adherence to the guidelines. In any procedure with a risk of complications, it is advisable to make certain that the patient understands the situation and acknowledges the risks. A test should not be performed without first obtaining the patient's informed consent, verbally and in writing. In the process of obtaining informed consent, the patient should be made aware of the potential risks and benefits of the procedure. In the absence of informed consent, a physician may be held responsible in the event of a major untoward event, even if the test is carefully performed. The argument can be made that the patient would not have undergone the procedure had he or she been made aware of the risks associated with the test. After the test, responsibility rests with the physician for prompt interpretation and consideration of the implications of the test. Communication of these results to the patient is necessary—with advice concerning adjustments in lifestyle—without delay.

The second consideration should be adherence to proper standards of care during performance of the test. Exercise testing should be carried out only by persons thoroughly trained in its administration and in the prompt recognition of possible problems. An individual trained in exercise testing and resuscitation should be readily available during the test to make judgments concerning test termination. Resuscitative equipment, especially a defibrillator, should always be available. The ACC, the AHA, and the American College of Physicians, with broad involvement from other professional organizations involved with exercise testing such as the American College of Sports Medicine, have outlined the cognitive skills needed to competently supervise exercise tests.[8] These skills include knowledge of appropriate indications and contraindications to testing, an understanding of risk assessment, the ability to recognize and treat complications, and knowledge of basic cardiovascular and exercise physiology, as well as the ability to interpret the test in different patient populations.

The need for physician presence during exercise testing has been the subject of a great deal of discussion in the past. In many cases, exercise tests can be supervised by properly trained and competent exercise physiologists, physical therapists, nurses, physician assistants, or medical technicians who are working under the direct supervision of a physician—that is, the physician must be in the immediate vicinity or on the premises or the floor and available for emergencies.[9] In situations where the patient is deemed to be at higher risk for an adverse event during exercise testing, the physician should be physically present in the exercise testing room to personally supervise the test. Such cases include, but are not limited to, patients with recent ACS or myocardial infarction (within 7 to 10 days), severe left ventricular dysfunction, severe valvular stenosis (e.g., aortic stenosis), or known complex arrhythmias. The physician's reaction to signs or symptoms should be moderated by the information the patient gives regarding his or her usual activity. If abnormal findings occur at levels of exercise that the patient usually performs, it may not be necessary to stop the test. Also, the patient's activity history should help determine appropriate work rates for testing.

> **Key Point:** Legal problems can be avoided or lessened by adhering to guidelines and communicating with the patient and family before, during, and after the test.

Patient Preparation

Preparations for exercise testing include the following:

The patient should be instructed not to eat or smoke at least 2 to 3 hours before the test and to come dressed to exercise. A brief history and physical examination should be performed to rule out any contraindications to testing (see Table 2-2). Specific questioning should determine which drugs are being taken, and potential electrolyte level abnormalities should be considered.

The physician overseeing the test should ask to see the labeled medication bottles so that they can be identified and recorded. Whether patients should stop taking beta-blocking agents before testing has been debated. Because of the potential complications associated with stopping beta blockers (including the life-threatening rebound phenomenon, in which there may be an inordinate rise in heart rate), the AHA guidelines no longer recommend that patients be removed from beta blockers routinely for testing. However, if testing is performed for diagnostic purposes, they can be gradually stopped in selected cases if a physician or nurse carefully supervises the tapering process.

If the reason for the exercise test is not apparent, the referring physician should be contacted. A 12-lead ECG should be obtained in the supine and standing positions and the supine ECG compared with previous supine ECGs. The latter is an important rule, particularly in patients with known heart disease, because an abnormality may prohibit testing. Occasionally, a patient referred for an exercise test will instead be admitted to the coronary care unit. The standing ECG is important to detect individuals who develop ST-segment depression on standing and whose test results are likely to be false positive.

Do wear comfortable clothing and shoes for the test. Athletic or walking shoes are especially good if you have them.

Do let us know if you have used any nitroglycerin or had chest pain on the day of your test.

Do bring all of your current medications in their labeled prescription bottles on your test day and take them as usual.

Do be on time for your appointment. We appreciate a phone call if you are going to be late.

Preparation for the exercise test: Please continue your normal medications on the day of the test unless you are specifically instructed to change or hold them. If you cannot keep your scheduled appointment for any reason, please call the EKG lab Monday through Friday

Do Not smoke within 3 hours of the scheduled test time.

Do Not eat solid food within 3 hours of scheduled test time.

Do Not drink alcohol or caffeinated drinks (like tea or coffee) within 3 hour of scheduled test time. Water and juice are fine.

After the test: The doctor present for the test will give you a brief report of the results. This is your opportunity to ask questions. A full report will be sent to your doctor.

Exercise Testing

YOUR DOCTOR OR NURSE

PRACTIONER HAS SCHEDULED YOU

FOR A TREADMILL EXERCISE TEST.

TIME: _____AM/PM

ON: _____

PLACE: EKG Dept./excercise lab

Please arrive at least 15 minutes early.

Patients arriving more than 20 minutes after their scheduled time may have the test cancelled and rescheduled.

FIGURE 2-1   *Patient brochure explaining the exercise test.*

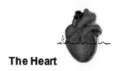

The Heart

The function of the heart is to pump blood to all the muscles, organs and tissues in your body. One way to evaluate the heart's ability to perform this function is through exercise. By exercising the heart, we may be able to find abnormalities that we could not recognize during normal daily activities. By monitoring your heart, blood pressure and breathing during an exercise test, we can gain an accurate picture of your heart's performance. This information will be used by physicians to determine the most effective treatment for keeping you healthy and active.

The Electrocardiogram

The electrocardiogram (ECG or EKG) is a recording of the electrical activity of the heart using ten electrodes attached to your skin. To gather accurate information, some light scraping of the skin may be necessary.

The Exercise Test

The exercise test is a procedure designed to help your doctor determine whether or not you have

FIGURE 2-1—Cont'd

heart disease. If you already have heart disease, the test is useful to determine the progress of your disease, the appropriateness of your current medications and to help estimate your future risk of heart problems.

During your exercise test, you will be walking on a treadmill, a motor driven belt (A stationary bicycle can also be used rather than a treadmill). The speed and incline of the treadmill will be determined by your physician. Do not worry about "passing "or "failing" the exercise test. We are just looking for your best effort. Remember, you can stop the test whenever you feel you have performed to your maximum ability.

Complications from performing an exercise test are rare. They include the possibility of dizziness, occasional changes in heart rhythm (1%) and heart attack (1 in 30,000). If you experience any chest pain, excessive shortness of breath or palpitation, let us know immediately.

For your safety, you will be monitored closely throughout the test and for at least 10 minutes afterward.

The Gas Analyzer

If the test includes analysis of the oxygen you breathe during the exercise test, you will need to wear a mask that covers your mouth and nose during the test. You will still be able to communicate with the operators regarding how you are feeling.

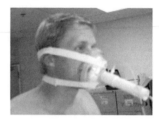

Other Information

Doctors present will ask you about your past and present medical history and also your activity levels. Please answer these questions to the best of your knowledge. You also will be asked to sign a consent form.

Thank you very much!!

There should be careful explanations of reasons for the test and the testing procedure, including its risks and possible complications, and ways to perform the test, including a demonstration of getting on and off and walking on the treadmill. Because of its effect on estimating exercise capacity and the stability of the ECG tracing, holding the handrails of the treadmill should be discouraged whenever possible. We routinely call patients after sending or giving them the brochure seen in Figure 2-1 to make sure they understand all the issues and will be on time for the test and properly prepared.

Key Point: A list provided in a brochure can help ensure that patients are adequately prepared for testing.

History and Physical Examination

Exercise testing should be an extension of the history and physical examination. A physician obtains the most information by being present to talk with, observe, and examine the patient at the time of the test. A brief physical examination should always be performed to rule out contraindications (see Table 2-2). Not only is the clinical and historical information important to optimize the diagnostic and prognostic yield of the test, but patient safety is optimized. The need for physician presence during exercise testing has been debated extensively.[9] In some instances, such as when asymptomatic, apparently healthy subjects are being screened or a repeat treadmill test is being done on a patient whose condition is stable, a physician may not need to be present but should be in close proximity and prepared to respond promptly. The physician's reaction to signs or symptoms should be moderated by the information the patient gives regarding usual activity. If abnormal findings occur at levels of exercise that the patient usually performs, it may not be necessary to stop the test. Also, the patient's activity history should help determine appropriate work rates for testing. A loud systolic murmur or other findings of concern should lead to an ECG before exercise. Recent chest pain that could possibly be due to ischemia should lead to a troponin level before testing.

> **Key Point:** When a loud systolic murmur, ECG abnormalities, or a worrisome history is present, it may be appropriate to postpone a test to first obtain biomarker results (troponin) or an echocardiogram.

Blood Pressure Measurement

Although numerous clever devices have been developed to automate blood pressure measurement during exercise, none are recommended. The time-proven method of the physician holding the patient's arm with a stethoscope placed over the brachial artery remains most reliable. The patient's arm should be free of the handrails so that noise is not transmitted up the arm. It sometimes helps to mark the brachial artery. An anesthesiologist's auscultatory piece or an electronic microphone can be fastened to the arm. A device that inflates and deflates the cuff with the push of a button can be helpful. If systolic blood pressure fails to increase or appears to be decreasing, it should be taken again immediately. If a drop in systolic blood pressure of 10 mm Hg or more occurs or if it drops below the value obtained in the standing position before testing, the test should be stopped. An increase in systolic blood pressure to 250 mm Hg or an increase in diastolic blood pressure to 115 mm Hg is also an indication to stop the test.

> **Key Point:** A dropping or flat systolic blood pressure response during exercise is ominous and can be the most important indicator of adverse events occurring during testing.

ECG Recording

Skin Preparation

Proper skin preparation is essential for the performance of an exercise test. During exercise, because noise increases with the square of resistance, it is extremely important to lower the resistance at the skin-electrode interface and thereby improve the signal-to-noise ratio. Nevertheless, it is often difficult to consistently prepare the skin properly because doing so may cause the patient discomfort and minor skin irritation. However, the performance of an exercise test with an ECG signal that cannot be continuously monitored and accurately interpreted because of artifact is worthless and can even be dangerous.

The general areas for electrode placement should be shaved if they have hair and should be cleansed with an alcohol-saturated gauze pad; it can then be helpful to mark the exact areas for electrode application with a felt-tip pen. The mark serves as a guide for removing enough of the superficial layer of skin. The placements are determined using anatomic landmarks found with the patient supine because some individuals with loose skin can have a considerable shift of electrode positions when they assume an upright position. After the placements are marked, the next step is to remove the superficial layer of skin by light abrasion with fine-grain emery paper. Skin resistance should be reduced to 5000 ohms or less, which can be verified before the exercise test with an inexpensive alternating-current impedance meter driven at 10 Hz. A direct-current meter should not be used because it can polarize the electrodes. Each electrode is tested against a common electrode with an ohm meter, and when 5000 ohms or less is not achieved, the electrode must be removed and skin preparation repeated. This maneuver saves time by obviating the need to interrupt a test because of noisy tracings. Some systems have this feature built in and automatically check skin impedance.

> **Key Point:** No amount of signal processing can overcome the noise caused by poor skin preparation. Skin preparation can be a greater problem with aging because the elderly have a higher skin resistance and tendency toward contact noise.

Electrodes and Cables

Many disposable electrodes perform adequately for exercise testing. The disposable electrodes have the advantages of quick application and no need for cleansing for reuse. A disposable electrode that has an abrasive center spun by an applicator after the electrode is attached to the skin (Quickprep) is available from Quinton Instrument Co. This approach does not require skin preparation. A clever feature of the applicator is a built-in impedance meter that stops it from spinning when the skin impedance has been appropriately lowered. Buffer amplifiers or digitizers carried by the patient are no longer advantageous. Cables develop continuity problems with use and require replacement rather than repair. We often find that replacement is necessary after roughly 500 tests. Some systems have used analog-to-digital converters in the electrode junction box carried by the patient. Because digital signals are relatively impervious to noise, the patient cable can be unshielded and is therefore very light.

Careful skin preparation and close attention to the electrode-cable interface are important for a safe and successful exercise test and are necessary no matter how elaborate or expensive the ECG recording device.

> **Key Point:** All exercise testing cables break down with use, causing electrical discontinuity noise eliminated only by cable replacement.

Lead Systems

Bipolar Lead Systems

Bipolar leads have been used in the past because of the relatively short time required for placement, the relative freedom from motion artifact, and the ease with which noise problems can be located. Figure 2-2 illustrates the electrode placements for most of the bipolar lead systems.[10] The usual

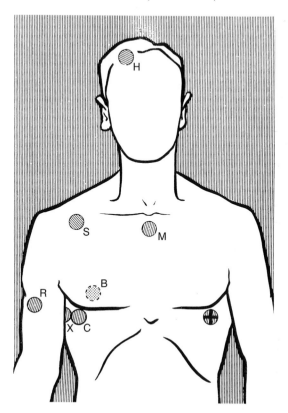

FIGURE 2-2 *Lead placement for the bipolar leads used for exercise testing.*

positive reference is an electrode placed the same as the positive reference for V5. The negative reference for V5 is Wilson's central terminal, which consists of connecting the limb electrodes to the right arm, left arm, and left leg. Virtually all current ECG systems, however, use the modified 12-lead system first described by Mason and Likar.[11]

Mason-Likar Electrode Placement

Because a 12-lead ECG cannot be obtained accurately during exercise with electrodes placed on the wrists and ankles, the electrodes are placed at the base of the limbs for exercise testing. In addition to lessening noise for exercise testing, the Mason-Likar modified placement has been demonstrated by some investigators to show no differences in ECG configuration when compared with the standard limb lead placement. However, this finding has been disputed by others who have found that the Mason-Likar placement causes amplitude changes and axis shifts when compared with standard placement. Because these could lead to diagnostic changes, it has been recommended that the modified exercise electrode placement not be used for recording a resting ECG. The preexercise ECG has been further complicated by the recommendation that it should be obtained standing, because that is the same position maintained during exercise. This situation is worsened by the common practice of moving the limb electrodes onto the chest to minimize motion artifact.

Figure 2-3 illustrates the Mason-Likar torso-mounted limb lead system. The conventional ankle and wrist electrodes are replaced by electrodes

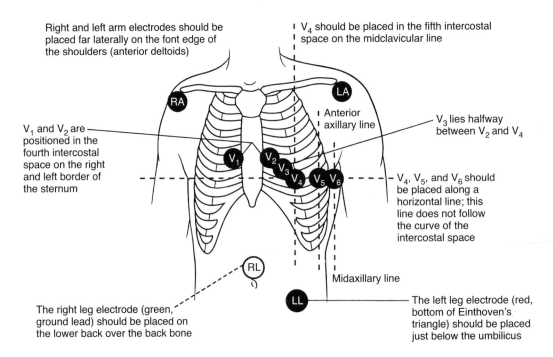

Right and left arm electrodes should be placed far laterally on the font edge of the shoulders (anterior deltoids)

V_4 should be placed in the fifth intercostal space on the midclavicular line

V_1 and V_2 are positioned in the fourth intercostal space on the right and left border of the sternum

Anterior axillary line

V_3 lies halfway between V_2 and V_4

V_4, V_5, and V_6 should be placed along a horizontal line; this line does not follow the curve of the intercostal space

Midaxillary line

The right leg electrode (green, ground lead) should be placed on the lower back over the back bone

The left leg electrode (red, bottom of Einthoven's triangle) should be placed just below the umbilicus

FIGURE 2-3   *Mason-Likar 12-lead placement used for exercise testing.*

mounted on the torso at the base of the limbs. In this way, the artifact introduced by movement of the limbs is avoided. The standard precordial leads use Wilson's central terminal as their negative reference, which is formed by connecting the right arm, left arm, and left leg. This triangular configuration around the heart results in a zero voltage reference through the cardiac cycle. The use of Wilson's central terminal for the precordial leads (V leads) requires the negative reference to be a combination of three additional electrodes rather than the single electrode used as the negative reference for bipolar leads.

The modified exercise electrode placement should not be used for routine resting ECGs. However, the changes caused by the exercise electrode placement can be kept to a minimum by keeping the arm electrodes off the chest and putting them on the anterior deltoid and by having the patient supine. In this situation, the modified exercise limb lead placement of Mason-Likar can serve well as the resting ECG reference before an exercise test.

Key Point: For exercise testing, limb electrodes should be placed as far from the heart as possible but not on the limbs; the ground electrode (right leg) can be on the back out of the cardiac field, and the left leg electrode should be below the umbilicus. The V_1, V_2, and V_4 precordial electrodes should be placed in the appropriate interspaces and V_3, V_5, and V_6 aligned according to them (see Figure 2-3).

Inferior Lead ST-Segment Depression

Miranda and colleagues[12] studied 178 men who had undergone exercise testing and coronary angiography to evaluate the diagnostic value of ST-segment depression occurring in the inferior leads. The area under the curve in lead II was not significantly greater than 0.50, suggesting that for the identification of coronary artery disease, isolated ST-segment depression in lead II appears to be unreliable.

The inferior leads may have more false-positive results and may require different criteria. This apparent lack of specificity may result from the effect of atrial repolarization in the inferior leads, which causes depression of the ST- segment. With adequate experience, atrial repolarization may be recognized as causing ST-segment depression. The end of the PR segment is depressed in a curved fashion to the same level that the ST segment begins.

Key Point: ST depression occurring in the inferior leads alone (II, aVF) can sometimes represent a false-positive response, but ST elevation in these leads suggests transmural ischemia in the area of the right coronary artery blood distribution.

Number of Leads to Record

In patients with normal resting ECGs, a V5 or similar bipolar lead along the long axis of the heart is usually adequate. In patients with ECG evidence of myocardial infarction or with a history suggesting coronary spasm, additional leads are needed. As a minimal approach, it is advisable to record three leads: a V5 type of lead, an anterior V2 type of lead, and an inferior lead such as aVF. Alternatively, Frank X, Y, and Z leads may be used. Either of these approaches is also helpful for the detection and identification of dysrhythmias. It is also advisable to record a second three-lead grouping consisting of V4, V5, and V6. Occasionally, abnormalities may be seen as borderline in V5, whereas they will be clearly abnormal in V4 or V6.

Because most meaningful ST-segment depression occurs in the lateral leads (V4, V5, and V6) when the resting ECG is normal, other leads are only necessary in patients who had a myocardial infarction, those with a history consistent with coronary spasm or variant angina, or those who have exercise-induced dysrhythmias of an uncertain type.

> **Key Point:** As much as 90% of abnormal ST depression occurs in V5 or the two adjacent precordial leads. This does not mean that other leads should be ignored, particularly in patients being evaluated for chest pain, since elevation localizes ischemia to the area beneath the electrodes. Also, arrhythmias are best diagnosed with inferior and anterior leads where the P waves are best seen.

ECG Recording Instruments

Many technologic advances in ECG recorders have taken place. The medical instrumentation industry has promptly complied with specifications set forth by various professional groups. Machines with a high-input impedance ensure that the voltage recorded graphically is equivalent to that on the surface of the body despite the high natural impedance of the skin. Optically isolated buffer amplifiers have ensured patient safety, and machines with a frequency response up to 100 Hz are commercially available. The lower end is possible because direct-current coupling is technically feasible.

Waveform Processing

Analog and digital averaging techniques have made it possible to filter and average ECG signals to remove noise. There is a need for consumer awareness in these areas because most manufacturers do not specify how the use of such procedures modifies the ECG. Both filtering and signal averaging can, in fact, distort the ECG signal. Averaging techniques are nevertheless attractive because they can produce a clean tracing when the raw data are noisy. However, the clean-looking ECG signal produced may not be a true representation of the waveform and in fact may be dangerously misleading. Also, the instruments that make computer ST-segment measurements are not entirely reliable because they are based on imperfect algorithms.

> **Key Point:** Filtering and averaging can cause false ST depression due to distortion of the raw data.

Computerization

The advantages of digital versus analog data processing include more precise and more accurate measurements, less distortion in recording, and direct accessibility to digital computer analysis and storage techniques.

Other advantages include rapid mathematical manipulation (averaging), avoidance of the drift inherent in analog components, digital algorithm control permitting changes with ease in analysis schema (software rather than hardware changes), and no degradation with repetitive playback. The advantages of digital processing when outputting data include higher plotting resolution and easy repetitive manipulation.

Computerization also helps meet the two critical needs of exercise ECG testing: the reduction of the amount of ECG data collected during testing and the elimination of electrical noise and movement artifact associated with exercise. Because an exercise test can exceed 30 minutes (including data acquisition during rest and recovery) and many physicians want to analyze all 12 leads during and after testing, the resulting quantity of ECG data and measurements can quickly become excessive. The three-lead vectorcardiographic (or three-dimensional, i.e., aVF, V2, V5) approach would reduce the amount of data; however, clinicians favor the 12-lead ECG. The exercise ECG often includes random and periodic noise of high and low frequency that can be caused by respiration, muscle artifact, electrical interference, wire continuity, and electrode-skin contact problems. In addition to reducing noise and facilitating data collection, computer processing techniques may also make precise and accurate measurements, separate and capture dysrhythmic beats, perform spatial analysis, and apply optimal diagnostic criteria for ischemia.

Although most clinicians agree that computerized analysis simplifies the evaluation of the exercise ECG, there has been disagreement about whether accuracy is enhanced.[13] A comparison of computerized resting ECG analysis programs with each other and with the analyses of expert readers led to the conclusion that physician review of any reading is necessary.[14] Although computers can record very clean representative ECG complexes and neatly print a wide variety of measurements, the algorithms they use are far from perfect and can result in serious differences from the raw signal. The physician who uses commercially available computer-aided systems to analyze the results of exercise tests should be aware of the problems and always review the raw analog recordings to see whether they are consistent with the processed output.

Even if computerization of the original raw analog ECG data could be accomplished without distortion, the problem of interpretation still remains. Numerous algorithms have been recommended for obtaining the optimal diagnostic value from the exercise ECG. These algorithms have been shown to provide improved sensitivity and specificity compared with standard visual interpretation. Often, however, this improvement has been demonstrated only by the investigator who proposed the new measurement. Furthermore, the ST measurements made by a computer can be erroneous. It is advisable to have the devices mark both the isoelectric level and the point of ST0. Even if the latter is chosen correctly, misplacement of the isoelectric line outside of the PR segment can result in incorrect ST level measurements.

Key Point: Computerized ST measurements require physician review of any reading; errors can be made both in the choice of the isoelectric line and the beginning of the ST segment.

Causes of Noise

Many of the causes of noise in the exercise ECG signal cannot be corrected, even by meticulous skin preparation. Noise is defined in this context as any electrical signal that is foreign to or distorts the true ECG waveform. Based on this definition, the types of noise that may be present can be caused by any combination of line-frequency (60 Hz), muscle, motion, respiration, contact, or continuity artifact. Line-frequency noise is generated by the interference of the 60 Hz electrical energy with the ECG. This noise can be reduced by using shielded patient cables. If in spite of these precautions this noise is still present, the simplest way to remove it is to design a 60 Hz notch filter and apply it in series with the ECG amplifier. A notch filter removes only the line frequency; that is, it attenuates all frequencies in a narrow band around 60 Hz. This noise can also be removed by attenuating all frequencies above 59 Hz; however, this method of removing line-frequency noise is not recommended because it causes waveform distortion and results in a system that does not meet AHA specifications. The most obvious manifestation of distortion caused by such filters is a decrease in R-wave amplitude; therefore a true notch filter is advisable.

Muscle noise is generated by the activation of muscle groups and is usually of high frequency. This noise, with other types of high-frequency noise, can be reduced by signal averaging. Motion noise, another form of high-frequency noise, is caused by the movement of skin and the electrodes, which causes a change in the contact resistance. Respiration causes an undulation of the waveform amplitude, so the baseline varies with the respiratory cycle. Baseline wander can be reduced by low-frequency filtering; however, this results in distortion of the ST segment and can cause artifactual ST-segment depression and slope changes. Other baseline removal approaches have been used, including linear interpolation between isoelectric regions, high-order polynomial estimates, and cubic-spline techniques, which can each smooth the baseline to various degrees.

Contact noise appears as low-frequency noise or sometimes as step discontinuity baseline drift. It can be caused by poor skin preparation resulting in high skin impedance or by air bubble entrapment in the electrode gel. It is reduced by meticulous skin preparation and by rejecting beats that show large baseline drift. Also, by using the median rather than the mean for signal averaging, this type of drift can be reduced. Continuity noise caused by intermittent breaks in the cables is rarely a problem because of technological advances in cable construction, except, of course, when cables are abused or overused.

Most of the sources of noise can be effectively reduced by beat averaging. However, two types of artifact can actually be caused in the signal-averaging process by the introduction of beats that are morphologically different from others in the average and the misalignment of beats during averaging. As the number of beats included in the average increases, the level of noise reduction is greater. The averaging time and the number of beats to be included in the average have to be compromised, though, because the morphology of ECG waveforms changes over time.

For exercise testing, the raw ECG data should be considered first, and then the averages and filtered data may be used to aid interpretation if no distortion is obvious.

> **Key Point:** The old computer adage of "garbage in, garbage out" holds for computerized ECG processing.

ECG Paper Recording

For some patients, it is advantageous to have a recorder with a slow paper speed option of 5 mm/sec. This speed makes it possible to record an entire exercise test and reduces the likelihood of missing any dysrhythmias when specifically evaluating patients with these problems. Some exercise systems allow for a "total disclosure" printout option similar to that provided with many Holter monitors. In rare instances, a faster paper speed of 50 mm/sec can be helpful for making particular evaluations, such as accurate ST-segment slope measurements.

Thermal head printers have effectively replaced all other types of printers. These recorders are remarkable in that they can use blank thermal paper and write out the grid and ECG, vector loops, and alphanumerics. They can record graphs, figures, tables, and typed reports. They are digitally driven and can produce very-high-resolution records. The paper price is comparable with that of other paper, and these devices have a reasonable cost and are very durable, particularly because a stylus is not needed.

Z-fold paper has the advantage over roll paper in that it is easily folded, and the study can be read in a manner similar to paging through a book. Exercise ECGs can be microfilmed on rolls, cartridges, or fiche cards for storage. They can also be stored in digital or analog format on magnetic media or optical disks. The latest technology involves magnetic optical disks that are erasable and have fast access and transfer times. These devices can be easily interfaced with microcomputers and can store megabytes of digital information. Lasers and inkjet printers have a delay, making them unsuitable for medical emergencies, but they offer the advantages of the inexpensiveness of standard paper and long-lived images.

> **Key Points:**
> 1. Many available recording systems have both thermal head and laser or inkjet printers; the cheaper, slower printers are used for final reports and summaries, and the thermal head printers are used for live ECG tracings (i.e., real time).
> 2. The standard "three lead by four lead groups" printout leaves only 2.5 seconds to assess ST changes or arrhythmias.
>   a. V5 should be continuously recorded when making paper records for interpretation of ischemia.
>   b. Lead II or aVF should be continuously recorded when making paper records for interpretation of arrhythmias.
>   c. Ideally, every 10 second paper recording should include continuous three-dimensional leads (II/aVF, V2, and V5).

Exercise Test Modalities

Types of Exercise

Three types of exercise can be used to stress the cardiovascular system: isometric, dynamic, and a combination of the two. Isometric exercise, which involves constant muscular contraction with minimal movement (such as a handgrip), imposes a disproportionate pressure load on the left ventricle relative to the body's ability to supply oxygen. Dynamic exercise, or rhythmic muscular activity resulting in movement, initiates a more appropriate balance between cardiac output, blood supply, and oxygen exchange. Because a delivered workload can be accurately calibrated and the physiologic response easily measured, dynamic exercise is preferred for clinical testing. In addition, dynamic exercise is preferred to isometric exercise for testing because it can be more easily graduated and controlled. Using gradual, progressive workloads of dynamic exercise, patients with coronary artery disease can be protected from rapidly increasing myocardial oxygen demand. Although bicycling is also a dynamic exercise, most individuals perform more work on a treadmill because a greater muscle mass is involved and most subjects are more familiar with walking than cycling.

Numerous modalities have been used to provide dynamic exercise for exercise testing, including steps, escalators, ladder mills, and arm ergometers. Today, however, the bicycle ergometer and the treadmill are the most commonly used dynamic exercise devices. The bicycle ergometer is usually cheaper, takes up less space, and makes less noise. Upper body motion is usually reduced, but care must be taken so that isometric exercise is not performed by the arms. The workload administered by the simple, manually braked cycle ergometers is not well calibrated and depends on pedaling speed. It can be easy for a patient to slow pedaling speed during exercise testing and decrease the administered workload, making the estimation of exercise capacity unreliable. More expensive electronically braked bicycle ergometers keep the workload at a specified level over a wide range of pedaling speeds, and have become the standard for cycle ergometer testing today.

> **Key Point:** Dynamic exercise, using a treadmill or a cycle ergometer, is a better measure of cardiovascular function and a better method of testing than isometric exercise.

Arm Ergometry

Alternative methods of exercise testing are needed for patients with vascular, orthopedic, or neurologic conditions who cannot perform leg exercise. Arm ergometry can be used in such patients.[15] However, nonexercise techniques (such as pharmacologic stress testing) are currently more popular.

Bicycle Ergometer

The bicycle ergometer is usually cheaper, takes up less space, and makes less noise than a treadmill. Upper body motion is usually reduced, but care must be taken that the arms do not perform isometric exercise. The workload administered by the simple bicycle ergometers is not well calibrated and depends on pedaling speed. It can be easy for a patient to slow pedaling speed during exercise testing and decrease the administered workload. More modern electronically braked bicycle ergometers keep the workload at a specified level over a wide range of pedaling speeds and are recommended.

Treadmill

The treadmill should have front and side rails so that patients can steady themselves, and some patients may benefit from the help of the person administering the test. The treadmill should be calibrated at least monthly. Some models can be greatly affected by the weight of the patient and will not deliver the appropriate workload to heavy patients. An emergency stop button should be readily available to the staff only. A small platform or stepping area at the level of the belt is advisable so that the patient can start the test by pedaling the belt with one foot before stepping on. Patients should not grasp the front or side rails because this decreases the work performed and the oxygen uptake and, in turn, increases exercise time, resulting in an overestimation of exercise capacity. Gripping the handrails also increases ECG muscle artifact. When patients have difficulty maintaining balance while walking, it helps to have them take their hands off the rails, close their fists, and extend one finger to touch the rails after they are accustomed to the treadmill. Some patients may require a few moments to feel comfortable enough to let go of the handrails, but grasping the handrails after the first minute of exercise should be strongly discouraged.

Bicycle Ergometer versus Treadmill

In most studies comparing upright cycle ergometer with treadmill exercise, maximum heart rate values have been roughly similar, whereas maximum oxygen uptake has been 6% to 25% greater during treadmill exercise.[16] Some studies have reported similar ECG changes with treadmill testing as compared with bicycle testing,[17] whereas others have reported more significant ischemic changes with treadmill testing.[18] However, the treadmill is the most commonly used dynamic testing modality in the United States, and the treadmill may be advantageous because patients are more familiar with walking than they are with bicycling. Patients are more likely to give the muscular effort necessary to adequately increase myocardial oxygen demand by walking than by bicycling.

> **Key Point:** Treadmills usually result in higher MET values, but maximal heart rate is usually similar to that of a bicycle. Thus bicycle testing can result in a lower prognosis estimate but has similar ability to predict ischemic disease.

Exercise Protocols

The many different exercise protocols in use have led to some confusion regarding how physicians compare tests between patients and serial tests in the same patient. The most common protocols, their stages, and the predicted oxygen cost of each stage are illustrated in Figure 2-4. When treadmill and cycle ergometer testing were first introduced into clinical practice, practitioners adopted protocols used by major researchers, such as Balke and Ware,[19] Astrand and Rodahl,[20] Bruce,[21] and Ellestad and colleagues.[22] In 1980, Stuart and Ellestad[23] surveyed 1375 exercise laboratories in North America and reported that of those performing treadmill testing, 65% used the Bruce protocol for routine clinical testing. A recent survey performed among VA exercise laboratories confirmed that the Bruce protocol remains the most commonly used; 83% of laboratories reported using the Bruce test for routine testing.[2] This protocol uses relatively large and unequal increments in work (2 to 3 MET) every 3 minutes. Large and uneven work increments such as these have been shown to result in a tendency to overestimate exercise capacity, and the lack of uniform increases in work rate can complicate the interpretation of some ST segment measurements and ventilatory gas exchange responses.[24,25] Thus exercise testing guidelines have recommended protocols with smaller and more equal increments. It is also important to individualize the test to target duration in the range of 8 to 12 minutes.

> **Key Point:** Individualized protocols with small and equal increments lasting 8 to 12 minutes are recommended for clinical use.

Ramp Testing

An approach to exercise testing that has gained interest in recent years is the ramp protocol, in which work increases constantly and continuously (Figure 2-5). The recent call for optimizing exercise testing would appear to be facilitated by the ramp approach. Because work increments are small and because it allows for increases in work to be individualized, a given test duration can be targeted. To investigate this approach, we compared ramp treadmill and bicycle tests to protocols more commonly used clinically. Ten patients with chronic heart failure, 10 with coronary artery disease who were limited by angina during exercise, 10 with coronary artery disease who were asymptomatic during exercise, and 10 age-matched normal subjects performed three bicycle tests (25 watts/2-minute stage, 50 watts/2-minute stage, and ramp) and three treadmill tests (Bruce, Balke, and ramp) in randomized order on different days. For the ramp tests, ramp rates on the bicycle and treadmill were individualized to yield test duration of approximately 10 minutes for each subject. Collectively, maximum oxygen uptake was significantly higher (18%) on the treadmill protocols than on the bicycle protocols, confirming previous observations. However, only minor differences in maximum oxygen uptake were observed between the treadmill protocols themselves or between the cycle ergometer protocols themselves.

Treadmill protocols

Functional class	Clinical status	O₂ cost ml/kg/min	METS	Bicycle ergometer (For 70 kg body weight) Kpm/min	Bruce (3 min stages) MPH	Bruce %GR	Balke-Ware % grade at 3.3 MPH 1 min stages	USAFSAM MPH	USAFSAM %GR	"Slow" USAFSAM MPH	"Slow" USAFSAM %GR	McHenry MPH	McHenry %GR	Stanford % grade at 3 MPH	Stanford % grade at 2 MPH	ACIP MPH	ACIP %GR	CHF MPH	CHF %GR	METS
Normal and I (Healthy, dependent on age, activity)		56.0	16		5.5	20										3.4	24.0			16
		52.5	15		5.0	18														15
		49.0	14	1500	4.2	16		3.3	25							3.1	24.0			14
		45.5	13																	13
		42.0	12	1350				3.3	20			3.3	21			3.0	21.0			12
	(Sedentary health)	38.5	11	1200	3.4	14				2	25	3.3	18	22.5		3.0	17.5	3.4	14.0	11
		35.0	10	1050				3.3	15			3.3	15	20.0		3.0	14.0	3.0	15.0	10
		31.5	9	900						2	20	3.3	12	17.5		3.0	10.5	3.0	12.5	9
	(Limited)	28.0	8	750	2.5	12		3.3	10			3.3	9	15.0		3.0	7.0	3.0	10.0	8
		24.5	7	600						2	15	3.3	6	12.5				3.0	7.5	7
II		21.0	6	450	1.7	10		3.3	5	2	10			10.0	17.5	3.0	3.0	2.0	10.5	6
		17.5	5							2	5	2.0	3	7.5	14.0			2.0	7.0	5
III	(Symptomatic)	14.0	4	300	1.7	5		3.3	0	2	0			5.0	10.5	2.5	2.0	2.0	3.5	4
		10.5	3		1.7	0		2.0	0					2.5	7.0	2.0	0.0			3
		7.0	2	150										0	3.5			1.5	0.0	2
IV		3.5	1															1.0	0.0	1

FIGURE 2-4 *Commonly used protocols for graded, progressive exercise testing.*

USAFSAM = United States Air Force School of Aerospace Medicine
ACIP = asymptomatic cardiac ischemia pilot
CHF = congestive heart failure (modified Naughton)
Kpm/min = Kilopond meters/minute
%GR = percent grade
MPH = miles per hour

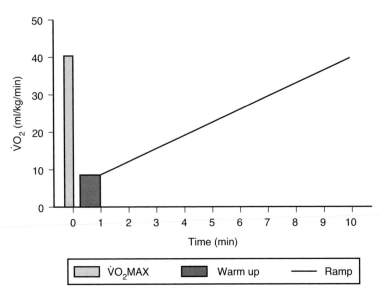

FIGURE 2-5   *Ramp protocol for graded exercise testing.*

The relationships between oxygen uptake and work rate (predicted oxygen uptake) suggest that oxygen uptake is overestimated from tests containing large work increments, and the variability in estimating oxygen uptake from work rate is markedly greater for these tests than for a ramp test. Because the ramp approach appears to offer several advantages in accordance with the exercise testing guidelines, we presently perform all our clinical and research testing using the ramp. If available equipment does not permit ramping, a gradual protocol such as the modified Balke or the United States Air Force School of Aerospace Medicine (USAFSAM) is usually appropriate when testing patients with suspected coronary disease.

The exercise protocol should be targeted for the patient rather than the reverse. Treadmill speed should be targeted to the individual's capabilities. Work increments should be even, and total time should be 8 to 12 minutes. METs, not minutes, should be reported.

> **Key Point:** A ramp test permits more accurate estimation of aerobic exercise capacity and has other advantages, including patient acceptance and an anticipated duration; ramp protocols represent the evolution from previous methods and are the preferred protocol for exercise testing today.

Questionnaires

The key to appropriately targeting a ramp is accurately predicting the individual's maximal work capacity. If a previous test is not available, a pretest estimation of an individual's exercise capacity is helpful to set the appropriate ramp rate. Functional classifications are too limited and poorly reproducible. One problem is that "usual activities" can decrease, so an individual can become greatly limited without having a change in functional class. A better approach is to use the specific activity scale of Goldman and colleagues[26] (Table 2-3), the Duke Activity Status Index (Table 2-4), or the Veterans Specific Activity Questionnaire (VSAQ) (Table 2-5). Alternatively, the patient may be questioned regarding usual activities that have a known MET cost.

> **Key Point:** Activity questionnaires enable targeting a ramp rate or another protocol to the appropriate maximal level to be reached in 8 to 12 minutes.

Borg Scale

Rather than using heart rate to clinically determine the intensity of exercise, it is preferable to use the 6-to-20 Borg scale or the nonlinear 1-to-10 scale of

---

TABLE 2-3 Specific Activity Scale of Goldman

Class I ($\geq$ 7 METs)
A patient can perform any of the following activities:
Carrying 24 pounds up eight steps
Carrying an 80-pound object
Shoveling snow
Skiing
Playing basketball, touch football, squash, or handball
Jogging or walking 5 mph

Class II ($\geq$ 5 METs)
A patient does not meet class I criteria but can perform any of the following activities
  to completion without stopping:
Carrying anything up eight steps
Having sexual intercourse
Gardening, raking, weeding
Walking 4 mph

Class III ($\geq$ 2 METs)
A patient does not meet class I or class II criteria but can perform any of the following
  activities to completion without stopping:
Walking down eight steps
Taking a shower
Changing bed sheets
Mopping floors, cleaning windows
Walking 2.5 mph
Pushing a power lawn mower
Bowling
Dressing without stopping

Class IV ($<$ 2 METs)
None of the above

TABLE 2-4 Duke Activity Scale Index (DASI)

Activity	Weight
Can you...	
Take care of yourself (i.e., eating, dressing, bathing, or using the toilet)?	2.75
Walk indoors, such as around your house?	1.75
Walk a block or two on level ground?	2.75
Climb a flight of stairs or walk up a hill?	5.50
Run a short distance?	8.00
Do light work around the house such as dusting or washing dishes?	2.70
Do moderate work around the house such as vacuuming, sweeping floors, or carrying in groceries?	3.50
Do heavy work around the house such as scrubbing floors or lifting or moving heavy furniture?	8.00
Do yard work such as raking leaves, weeding, or pushing a power mower?	4.50
Have sexual relations?	5.25
Participate in moderate recreational activities such as golf, bowling, dancing, or doubles tennis or throw a basketball or football?	6.00
Participate in strenuous sports such as swimming, singles tennis, football, basketball, or skiing?	7.50

The index equals the sum of weights for "yes" replies. VO_2 (oxygen uptake) $= 0.43 \times DASI + 9.6$

TABLE 2-5 VA Activity Questionnaire

Draw one line below the activities you are able to do routinely with minimal or no symptoms such as shortness of breath, chest discomfort, fatigue.
1 MET: Eating, getting dressed, working at a desk
2 METs: Taking a shower, walking down eight steps
3 METs: Walking slowly on a flat surface for one or two blocks, doing a moderate amount of work around the house such as vacuuming, sweeping the floors, or carrying groceries
4 METs: Doing light yard work (e.g., raking leaves, weeding, or pushing a power mower), painting or doing light carpentry
5 METs: Walking briskly (i.e., 4 mph), dancing, washing the car
6 METs: Playing nine holes of golf carrying clubs, doing heavy carpentry, mowing lawn with a push mower
7 METs: Performing heavy outdoor work (e.g., digging, spading soil), playing tennis (singles), carrying 60 pounds
8 METs: Moving heavy furniture, jogging slowly, climbing stairs quickly, carrying 20 pounds upstairs
9 METs: Bicycling at a moderate pace, sawing wood, jumping rope (slowly)
10 METs: Swimming briskly, bicycling up a hill, walking briskly uphill, jogging 6 mph
11 METs: Skiing cross-country, playing basketball (full court)
12 METs: Running briskly and continuously (level ground, 8 min/mile)
13 METs: Doing any competitive activity, including those that involve intermittent sprinting, running competitively, rowing, backpacking

TABLE 2-6   Borg 20-Point Scale of Perceived Exertion

6	
7	Very, very light
8	
9	Very light
10	
11	Fairly light
12	
13	Somewhat hard
14	
15	Hard
16	
17	Very hard
18	
19	Very, very hard
20	

perceived exertion.[27] The 6-to-20 scale was developed by noting that young men could approximate their exercise heart rate if a scale ranging from 60 to 200 was aligned with labels of "very, very light" for 60 to "very, very hard" for 200. One zero was then dropped, and the scale was used for all ages (Table 2-6). Because sensory perception of pain or exertion is nonlinear, Borg proposed the 1-to-10 scale (Table 2-7).

The Borg scale is a simple, valuable way of assessing the relative effort a patient exerts during exercise. Because no single response is adequate in determining whether a patients' effort is maximal, the perceived exertion scale response should be considered along with other physiologic responses associated with increasing effort and clinical criteria in determining the test endpoint. In our laboratory we always tell patients that they are in control; we then encourage them to reach a Borg scale rating between 17 and 20.

Key Point: Though subjective, the Borg scale is a very useful method of assessing patient effort during exercise testing.

TABLE 2-7   Borg Nonlinear 10-Point Scale of Perceived Exertion

0	Nothing at all
0.5	Extremely light (just noticeable)
1	Very light
2	Light (weak)
3	Moderate
4	Somewhat heavy
5	Heavy (strong)
6	
7	Very heavy
8	
9	
10	Extremely heavy (almost maximal)
•	Maximal

Postexercise Period

If maximal sensitivity is to be achieved with an exercise test, patients should be supine during the postexercise period. It is advisable to record about 10 seconds of ECG data while the patient is motionless but still experiencing near maximal heart rate, and then have the patient lie down. Some patients must be allowed to lie down immediately to avoid hypotension. Having the patient perform a cool-down walk after the test can delay or eliminate the appearance of ST-segment depression.[28] According to the law of La Place, the increase in venous return and thus ventricular volume in the supine position increases myocardial oxygen demand. Data from our laboratory suggest that having patients lie down may enhance ST-segment abnormalities in recovery.[29] However, a cool-down walk has been suggested to minimize the postexercise chances of dysrhythmic events in this high-risk time when catecholamine levels are high. The supine position after exercise is not as important when the test is not being performed for diagnostic purposes (e.g., fitness testing). When testing is not performed for diagnostic purposes, it may be preferable to walk slowly (1 to 1.5 mph) or continue cycling against zero or minimal resistance (up to 25 watts when testing with a cycle ergometer) for several minutes after the test.

Monitoring should continue for at least 6 to 8 minutes after exercise or until changes stabilize. An abnormal response occurring only in the recovery period is not unusual. Such responses are not false positives. Experiments confirm mechanical dysfunction and electrophysiologic abnormalities in the ischemic ventricle after exercise. A cool-down walk can be helpful when testing patients with an established diagnosis undergoing testing for other than diagnostic reasons, when testing athletes, or when testing patients with dangerous dysrhythmias.

The recovery period is extremely important for observing ST shifts and should not be interrupted by a cool-down walk or failure to monitor for at least 5 minutes. Changes isolated to the recovery period are not more likely to be false positives.

> **Key Point:** The recovery period, particularly minutes 2 to 4, is critical for ST analysis. Noise should not be a problem, and ST depression at that time has important implications regarding the presence and severity of coronary artery disease. A cool-down walk can delay or reduce recovery ST depression.

Add-Ons

Several ancillary imaging techniques, or add-ons, have been shown to provide a valuable complement to exercise electrocardiography for the evaluation of patients with known or suspected coronary artery disease. They can localize ischemia and thus guide interventions. These techniques are particularly helpful among patients with equivocal exercise electrocardiograms or those likely to exhibit false-positive or false-negative responses.

The guidelines call for their use when testing patients with more than 1 mm of ST depression at rest, left bundle branch block (LBBB), Wolf-Parkinson-White (WPW), and paced rhythms. They are frequently used to clarify abnormal ST-segment responses in asymptomatic people or those in whom the cause of chest discomfort remains uncertain, often avoiding angiography. When exercise electrocardiography and an imaging technique are combined, the diagnostic and prognostic accuracy is enhanced. The major imaging procedures are myocardial perfusion and ventricular function studies using radionuclide techniques, and exercise echocardiography. Some of the newer add-ons or substitutes for the exercise test have the advantage of being able to localize ischemia, as well as diagnose coronary disease when the baseline ECG exhibits the aforementioned abnormalities, which negate the usefulness of ST analysis. Although the newer technologies are often suggested to have better diagnostic characteristics, this is not always the case, particularly when more than the ST segments from the exercise test are used in scores. Pharmacologic stress testing is used in place of the standard exercise test for patients unable to walk or cycle or unable to give a good effort. These nonexercise stress techniques (persantine or adenosine with nuclear perfusion, dobutamine or arbutamine with echocardiography) permit diagnostic assessment of patients unable to exercise.

Key Point: The imaging add-ons are indicated when the ECG exhibits more than 1 mm of ST depression at rest, LBBB, WPW, and paced rhythms or when localization of ischemia is important.

Ventilatory Gas Exchange Responses

Because of the inaccuracies associated with estimating METs (ventilatory oxygen uptake) from workload (i.e., treadmill speed and grade), it can be important for many patients to measure physiologic work directly using ventilatory gas exchange responses, commonly referred to as *cardiopulmonary exercise testing*. Although this requires metabolic equipment, a facemask or mouthpiece, and other equipment, advances in technology have made these measurements widely available. Cardiopulmonary exercise testing adds precision to the measurement of work and also permits the assessment of other parameters, including the respiratory exchange ratio, efficiency of ventilation, and the ventilatory anaerobic threshold. The latter measurement is helpful because it usually represents a comfortable submaximal exercise limit and can be used for setting an optimal exercise prescription or an upper limit for daily activities. Clinically, this technology is often used to more precisely evaluate therapy, for the assessment of disability, and to help determine whether the heart or lungs limit exercise. Computerization of equipment has also led to the widespread use of cardiopulmonary exercise testing in sports medicine. Gas exchange measurements can supplement the exercise test by increasing precision and providing additional information concerning cardiopulmonary function during exercise. They are particularly needed to evaluate therapies using serial tests, because workload changes and estimated METs can be misleading. Because of their application for assessing prognosis in patients with heart failure, their use has become a standard part of the workup for these patients.

Key Point: Cardiopulmonary testing is clearly indicated for cardiac transplantation evaluation, evaluation of athletes, and medication evaluation with serial testing and research.

Nuclear Techniques

Nuclear Ventricular Function Assessment

One of the first techniques added to exercise was radionuclear ventriculography (RNV). This involved the intravenous injection of technetium-tagged red blood cells. Using ECG gating of images obtained from a scintillation camera, images of the blood circulating within the left ventricular chamber could be obtained. Although regurgitant blood flow from valvular lesions could not be identified, ejection fraction and ventricular volumes could be estimated. The resting values could be compared with those obtained during supine exercise, and criteria were established for abnormal. The most common criteria involved a drop in ejection fraction. This procedure is now rarely performed because its test characteristics have not fulfilled their promise.

Nuclear Perfusion Imaging

Although initially popular, the blood volume techniques have come to be surpassed by perfusion techniques. The first agent used was thallium, an isotopic analog of potassium that is taken up at variable rates by metabolically active tissue. When taken up at rest, images of metabolically active muscle such as the heart are possible. With the nuclear camera placed over the heart after intravenous injection of this isotope, images were initially viewed using x-ray film. The normal complete donut-shaped images gathered in multiple views would be broken by "cold" spots where scar was present. Defects viewed after exercise could be due to either scar or ischemia. Follow-up imaging confirmed that the "cold" spots were due to ischemia if they filled in later. As computer imaging techniques were developed, three-dimensional imaging (single photon emission computed tomography [SPECT]) and subtle differences could be plotted and scored. In recent years, ventriculograms based on the imaged wall as opposed to the blood in the chambers (as with RNV) could be constructed. Because of the technical limitations of thallium (i.e., source and life span), it has largely been replaced by chemical compounds called isonitriles that can be tagged with technetium, which has many practical advantages over thallium as an imaging agent. The isonitriles are trapped in the microcirculation, permitting imaging of the heart with a scintillation camera. Rather than a single injection as for thallium, these compounds require an injection at maximal exercise and then another later in recovery.

The differences in technology over the years and the differences in expertise and software at different facilities can complicate the comparisons of the results and application of this technology. The ventriculograms obtained with gated perfusion scans do not permit the assessment of valvular lesions or as accurate an assessment of wall motion abnormalities or ejection fraction as echocardiography.

> **Key Point:** Nuclear perfusion scans can now permit an estimation of ventricular function and wall motion abnormalities. Multigated acquisition (MUGA) of blood tagged with technetium is rarely used.

Echocardiography

The impact of the echocardiogram on cardiology has been impressive. This imaging technique is second only to contrast ventriculography via cardiac catheterization for measuring ventricular volumes, wall motion, and ejection fraction. With Doppler added, regurgitant flows can be estimated as well. Echocardiographers were quick to add this imaging modality to exercise, with most studies showing that supine, posttreadmill assessments were adequate and the more difficult imaging during exercise was not necessary. The patient must be placed supine as soon as possible after treadmill or bicycle exercise and imaging begun. A problem can occur when the imaging requires removal or displacement of the important V5 electrode where as much as 90% of the important ST changes are observed.

> **Key Point:** Echocardiography permits a superior estimate of ventricular function and wall motion abnormalities compared with nuclear perfusion scans. Furthermore, it can assess valvular function.

Biomarkers

The latest add-on to exercise testing in an attempt to improve its diagnostic characteristics are biomarkers. The first and most logical biomarker evaluated to detect ischemia brought on by exercise was troponin. Unfortunately, it has been shown that even in patients who develop ischemia during exercise testing, serum elevations in cardiac-specific troponin do not occur, demonstrating that myocardial damage does not occur.[30,31] B-type natriuretic peptide (BNP) is a hormone produced by the heart that is released by both myocardial stretching and myocardial hypoxia. Armed with this knowledge, investigators have reported several studies suggesting improvement in exercise test characteristics with BNP and its isomers.[32,33] BNP is also used to assess the presence and severity of congestive heart failure and has been shown to be a powerful prognostic marker.[34,35] The point-of-contact analysis techniques available for these assays involve a handheld battery-powered unit that uses a replaceable cartridge. Finger-stick blood samples are adequate for these analyses and the results are available immediately.

If validated using appropriate study design (similar to quantitative exercise testing and angiography [QUEXTA]), biomarker measurements could greatly improve the diagnostic characteristics of the standard office/clinic exercise test.

Summary

Use of proper methodology is critical for patient safety and accurate results. Preparing the patient physically and emotionally for testing is necessary. Good skin preparation will cause some discomfort but is necessary for providing good conductance and for avoiding artifact. The use of specific criteria for exclusion and termination, physician interaction with the patient, and appropriate emergency equipment is essential. A brief physical examination is always necessary to rule out important obstructive cardiomyopathy and aortic valve disease. Pretest standard 12-lead ECGs are needed in the supine and standing positions. The changes caused by exercise electrode placement can be kept to a minimum by keeping the arm electrodes off the chest, placing them on the shoulders, placing the leg electrodes below the umbilicus, and recording the baseline ECG supine. In this situation, the Mason-Likar modified exercise limb lead placement, if recorded supine, can serve as the resting ECG reference before an exercise test.

Few studies have correctly evaluated the relative yield or sensitivity and specificity of different electrode placements for exercise-induced ST-segment shifts. Using other leads in addition to V5 will increase the sensitivity; however, the specificity is decreased. ST-segment changes isolated to the inferior leads can on occasion be false-positive responses. For clinical purposes, vectorcardiographic and body surface mapping lead systems do not appear to offer any advantage over simpler approaches.

The exercise protocol should be progressive, with even increments in speed and grade whenever possible. Smaller, even, and more frequent work increments are preferable to larger, uneven, and less frequent increases, because the former yield a more accurate estimation of exercise capacity. It is highly advantageous to individualize the exercise protocol rather than using the same protocol for every patient. The optimum test duration is from 8 to 12 minutes; therefore the protocol workloads should be adjusted to permit this duration. Because ramp testing uses small and even increments, it permits a more accurate estimation of exercise capacity and can be individualized to yield targeted test duration. An increasing number of equipment companies manufacture a controller that performs such tests using a treadmill.

Target heart rates based on age should not be used because the relationship between maximum heart rate and age is poor and scatters widely around many different recommended regression lines. Such heart rate targets result in a submaximal test for some individuals, a maximal test for others, and an unrealistic goal for some patients. Blood pressure should be measured with a standard stethoscope and sphygmomanometer; the available automated devices cannot be relied on, particularly for detection of exertional hypotension. Borg scales are an excellent means of quantifying an individual's effort. Exercise capacity should not be reported in total time but rather as the oxygen uptake or MET equivalent of the workload achieved. This method permits the comparison of the results of many different exercise testing protocols. Hyperventilation should be avoided before testing. Subjects with and without disease may exhibit ST-segment changes with hyperventilation; thus hyperventilation to identify false-positive responders is no longer considered useful by most researchers. The postexercise period is a critical period diagnostically; therefore the patient should be placed in the supine position immediately after testing.

Key Points:

Exercise is only one of many stresses to which an organism can be exposed; therefore it is more appropriate to call an exercise test exactly that and not a stress test. Exercise capacity is the primary predictor of prognosis in all categories of patients.

The risk of exercise testing cannot be disregarded even with its excellent safety record. Guidelines must be observed and appropriate patient assessment and monitoring performed.

The risk of exercise testing can be lessened by not testing certain patients. If the guidelines for ACS patients are followed, the standard exercise test can be helpful as part of a systematic approach in chest pain observation units.

Physician judgment (based on history and subjective responses) is sufficient reason to terminate an exercise test.

Legal problems can be avoided or lessened by adhering to guidelines and communicating with the patient and family before, during, and after the test.

A list provided in a brochure can help ensure that patients are adequately prepared for testing.

A loud systolic murmur, ECG abnormalities, or a worrisome history may lead to postponing a test to first obtain biomarker results or an echocardiogram.

A dropping or flat systolic blood pressure response during exercise is ominous and can be the most important indicator of adverse events occurring during testing.

No amount of signal processing can overcome the noise caused by poor skin preparation. Skin preparation is increasingly more a problem with aging. The elderly have a higher skin resistance and a tendency toward contact noise.

All exercise testing cables break down with use, causing electrical discontinuity noise eliminated only by cable replacement.

For exercise testing, limb electrodes should be placed as far from the heart as possible but not on the limbs; the ground electrode (right leg) can be on the back out of the cardiac field, and the left leg electrode should be below the umbilicus. The precordial electrodes should be placed in the appropriate intercostal spaces.

ST depression occurring in the inferior leads alone (II, aVF) can represent a false-positive response, but ST elevation in these leads suggests transmural ischemia in the area of right coronary artery blood distribution.

Approximately 95% of the abnormal ST depression occurs in V5 or the two adjacent precordial leads. This does not mean that other leads should not be recorded, particularly in patients being evaluated for chest pain, because elevation localizes ischemia to the area beneath the electrodes.

Filtering and averaging can cause false ST depression due to distortion of the raw data.

Computerized ST measurements require physician review of any reading; errors can be made both in the choice of the isoelectric line and in the beginning of the ST segment.

The old computer adage of "garbage in, garbage out" holds for computerized ECG processing.

Many available recording systems have both thermal head and laser or inkjet printers; the cheaper, slower printers are used for final reports and summaries, and the thermal head printers are used for live ECG tracings (i.e., real time).

Dynamic exercise is a better marker of cardiovascular function and a better method of testing than isometric exercise.

Treadmills usually result in a higher MET measurement, but maximal heart rate is usually the same as with a bicycle.

Individualized protocols with small and equal increments lasting 8 to 10 minutes are recommended for clinical use.

A ramp test permits more accurate estimation of aerobic exercise capacity and has other advantages, including patient acceptance and an anticipated duration; ramp protocols represent the evolution from previous methods and are the preferred protocol today.

Activity questionnaires enable targeting a ramp to the appropriate maximal level to be reached in 9 or 10 minutes.

Though subjective, the Borg scale is a useful method of assessing patient effort during exercise testing.

The recovery period, particularly 2 to 4 minutes, are critical for ST analysis. Noise should not be a problem, and ST depression at that time has important implications regarding the presence and severity of coronary artery disease. A cool-down walk can delay or reduce recovery ST depression.

The imaging add-ons are particularly helpful when the ECG exhibits more than 1 mm of ST depression at rest, LBBB, WPW, and paced rhythms or when localization of ischemia is important.

Nuclear perfusion scans can now permit an estimation of ventricular function and wall motion abnormalities. MUGA is rarely used.

References

1. Rochmis P, Blackburn H: Exercise tests: a survey of procedures, safety, and litigation experience in approximately 170,000 tests, *JAMA* 217:1061-1066, 1971.
2. Myers J, Voodi L, Umann T, Froelicher VF: A survey of exercise testing: methods, utilization, interpretation, and safety in the VAHCS, *J Cardiopulm Rehabil* 20(4):251-258, 2000.
3. Gibbons L et al: The safety of maximal exercise testing, *Circulation* 80:846-852, 1989.
4. Yang JC, Wesley RC, Froelicher VF: Ventricular tachycardia during routine treadmill testing, *Arch Intern Med* 151:349-353, 1991.

5. Irving JB, Bruce RA: Exertional hypotension and post exertional ventricular fibrillation in stress testing, *Am J Cardiol* 39:849-851, 1977.

6. Shepard RJ: Do risks of exercise justify costly caution? *Physician Sports Med* 5:58, 1977.

7. Cobb LA, Weaver WD: Exercise: a risk for sudden death in patients with coronary heart disease, *J Am Coll Cardiol* 7:215-219, 1986.

8. Rodgers GP et al: American College of Cardiology/American Heart Association clinical competance statement on stress testing, *Circulation* 102:1726-1738, 2000.

9. American College of Sports Medicine: *Guidelines for exercise testing and prescription,* ed 7, Baltimore, 2006, Lippincott Williams & Wilkins.

10. Froelicher VF et al: A comparison of two-bipolar electrocardiographic leads to lead V5, *Chest* 70:611, 1976.

11. Gamble P et al: A comparison of the standard 12-lead electrocardiogram to exercise electrode placements, *Chest* 85:616-622, 1984.

12. Miranda CP et al: Usefulness of exercise-induced ST-segment depression in the inferior leads during exercise testing as a marker for coronary artery disease, *Am J Cardiol* 69:303-307, 1992.

13. Milliken JA, Abdollah H, Burggraf GW: False-positive treadmill exercise tests due to computer signal averaging, *Am J Cardiol* 65:946-948, 1990.

14. Willems J et al: The diagnostic performance of computer programs for the interpretation of ECGs, *N Engl J Med* 325:1767-1773, 1991.

15. Balady GJ et al: Value of arm exercise testing in detecting coronary artery disease, *Am J Cardiol* 55:37-39, 1985.

16. Myers J et al: Comparison of the ramp versus standard exercise protocols, *J Am Coll Cardiol* 17:1334-1342, 1991.

17. Wickes JR et al: Comparison of the electrocardiographic changes induced by maximum exercise testing with treadmill and cycle ergometer, *Circulation* 57:1066-1069, 1978.

18. Hambrecht RP et al: Greater diagnostic sensitivity of treadmill versus cycle exercise testing of asymptomatic men with coronary artery disease, *Am J Cardiol* 70(2):141-146, 1992.

19. Balke B, Ware R: An experimental study of physical fitness of air force personnel, *US Armed Forces Med J* 10:675-688, 1959.

20. Astrand PO, Rodahl K: *Textbook of work physiology,* New York, 1986, McGraw-Hill.

21. Bruce RA: Exercise testing of patients with coronary heart disease, *Ann Clin Res* 3:323-330, 1971.

22. Ellestad MH et al: Maximal treadmill stress testing for cardiovascular evaluation, *Circulation* 39:517-522, 1969.

23. Stuart RJ, Ellestad MH: National survey of exercise stress testing facilities, *Chest* 77:94-97, 1980.

24. Sullivan M, McKirnan MD: Errors in predicting functional capacity for postmyocardial infarction patients using a modified Bruce protocol, *Am Heart J* 107:486-491, 1984.

25. Webster MWI, Sharpe DN: Exercise testing in angina pectoris: the importance of protocol design in clinical trials, *Am Heart J* 117:505-508, 1989.

26. Goldman L et al: Comparative reproducibility and validity of systems for assessing cardiovascular function class: advantages of a new specific activity scale, *Circulation* 64:1227-1234, 1981.

27. Borg GAV: Borg's perceived exertion and pain scales. Champaign, Ill, Human Kinetics, 1998.

28. Gutman RA et al: Delay of ST depression after maximal exercise by walking for two minutes, *Circulation* 42:229-233, 1970.

29. Lachterman B et al: "Recovery only" ST segment depression and the predictive accuracy of the exercise test, *Ann Intern Med* 112:11-16, 1990.

30. Ashmaig ME et al: Changes in serum concentrations of markers of myocardial injury following treadmill exercise testing in patients with suspected ischaemic heart disease, *Med Sci Monit* 7:54-57, 2001.

31. Akdemir I et al: Does exercise-induced severe ischaemia result in elevation of plasma troponin-T level in patients with chronic coronary artery disease? *Acta Cardiol* 57:13-18, 2002.

32. Sabatine MS et al: TIMI Study Group. Acute changes in circulating natriuretic peptide levels in relation to myocardial ischemia, *J Am Coll Cardiol* 44(10):1988-1995, 2004.

33. Foote RS et al: Detection of exercise-induced ischemia by changes in B-type natriuretic peptides, *J Am Coll Cardiol* 44(10):1980-1987, 2004.

34. Wang TJ et al: Plasma natriuretic peptide levels and the risk of cardiovascular events and death, *N Engl J Med* 350(7):655-663, 2004.

35. Kragelund C et al: N-terminal pro-B-type natriuretic peptide and long-term mortality in stable coronary heart disease, *N Engl J Med* 352(7):666-675, 2005.

3   Interpretation of Hemodynamic Responses to Exercise Testing

Introduction

Hemodynamics not only includes normal and abnormal heart rate and blood pressure responses to exercise, but also cardiac output and its determinants and the influence of cardiovascular disease on cardiac output. Because exercise capacity is such an important measurement clinically and is influenced so strongly by exercise hemodynamics, this chapter also includes factors affecting exercise capacity, as well as the important issue of how normal standards for exercise capacity are expressed.

When interpreting the exercise test, it is important to consider each of its responses separately. Each type of response has a different impact on making a diagnostic or prognostic decision and must be considered along with an individual patient's clinical information. A test should not be called abnormal (or positive) or normal (or negative), but rather the interpretation should specify which responses were abnormal or normal, and each particular response should be recorded. The physician who ordered the test should receive the report. It should contain clear information that helps in patient management rather than vague "med-speak." Interpretation of the test is highly dependent on the application for which the test is used and on the population tested.

Exercise Capacity Versus Functional Classification

The functional status of patients with heart disease can be classified by symptoms during daily activities (New York Heart Association, Canadian, or Weber classifications). However, there is no validated substitute for directly measured maximal oxygen uptake (VO_2 max). Table 3-1 illustrates correlation coefficients between various functional measures, including symptom

TABLE 3-1   Correlations between Functional and Health Status Measures in 41 Patients with Heart Failure

	Age	Resting HR	EF	FVC	FEV_1	Estimated METs	VSAQ	VO_2 Peak	VO_2@VT	PE@VT	DASI	NYHA	6MWT	KC Phys Lim	KCQL	KC Sym Tot
Age	1															
Resting HR	-0.04	1														
EF	-0.19	-0.03	1													
FVC	-0.51†	-0.09	0.06	1												
FEV_1	-0.48†	-0.11	0.07	0.87‡	1											
Estimated METs	-0.53‡	-0.21	0.18	0.33	0.25	1										
VSAQ	-0.41*	-0.09	0.08	0.25	0.23	0.73‡	1									
VO_2 peak	-0.58‡	-0.04	0.46†	0.32	0.29	0.72‡	0.37*	1								
VO_2@VT	-0.35	-0.15	0.56†	0.45*	0.39*	0.46†	0.36	0.76‡	1							
PE@VT	-0.01	0.34	-0.08	-0.06	0.01	-0.68‡	-0.59†	-0.53*	-0.26	1						
DASI	-0.15	-0.04	-0.03	0.35	0.22	0.46†	0.30	0.26	0.40	-0.18	1					
NYHA	-0.14	-0.06	0.04	-0.11	-0.12	-0.31	-0.31	-0.14	-0.33	0.26	-0.64‡	1				
6MWT	-0.46†	0.10	0.28	0.28	0.17	0.59‡	0.45†	0.49†	0.39*	-0.29	0.44†	-0.32	1			
KC Phys Lim	-0.01	-0.08	0.24	0.12	0.20	0.42*	0.28*	0.25	0.24	-0.63†	0.68‡	-0.36	0.53†	1		
KCQL	-0.15	0.28	0.54†	-0.02	0.05	0.34*	0.17	0.46*	0.26	-0.25	0.24	-0.11	0.28	0.49†	1	
KC Symp Tot	-0.03	0.23	0.31	-0.27	-0.16	0.32	0.15	0.30	0.21	-0.24	0.41*	-0.33	0.27	0.62‡	0.80‡	1
KC Clin Sum	-0.02	0.08	0.30	-0.08	0.02	0.41*	0.24	0.30	0.25	-0.52*	0.60‡	-0.38*	0.44*	0.90‡	0.71‡	0.90‡

*$p < 0.05$.
†$p < 0.01$.
‡$p > 0.001$.

DASI, Duke activity status index; *EF*, ejection fraction; *Estimated METs*, METs calculated from peak treadmill speed and grade; *FEV_1*, forced expiratory volume in 1 sec; *FVC*, forced vital capacity; *HR*, heart rate; *KC Clin Sum*, Kansas City Clinical Summary score; *KC Phys Lim*, Kansas City Physical Limitation score; *KCQL*, Kansas City Quality of Life score; *KC Symp Tot*, Kansas City Total Symptom score; *6MWT*, 6-minute walk test; *NYHA*, New York Heart Association functional class; *PE*, perceived exertion; *VSAQ*, Veterans Specific Activity Questionnaire; *VT*, ventilatory threshold.

From Myers J: Association of functional and health status measures in heart failure. *J Cardiac Failure*, in press, 2006.

questionnaires, and maximal oxygen uptake in a group of patients with chronic heart failure. Note that although these functional measures are widely used as estimates of exercise capacity, their association with VO_2 max is only modest, with correlation coefficients ranging in the order of 0.25 to 0.50.

VO_2 max is the greatest amount of oxygen that a person can extract from the inspired air while performing dynamic exercise involving a large portion of the total body muscle mass. Since maximal ventilatory oxygen uptake is equal to the product of cardiac output and arteriovenous oxygen (a-VO_2) difference, it is a measure of the functional limits of the cardiovascular system. In general, maximal a-VO_2 difference is physiologically limited to roughly 15 to 17 ml/dl. Thus in many individuals maximal a-VO_2 difference widens up to fixed limit, making maximal oxygen uptake an indirect estimate of maximal cardiac output. VO_2 max depends on many factors, including natural physical endowment, activity status, age, and gender, but it is the best index of exercise capacity and maximal cardiovascular function. As a rough reference, the maximal oxygen uptake of the normal sedentary adult typically falls within the range of 25 to 45 ml O_2/kg/min, but a "normal" reference is relative to age and gender. Aerobic training can generally increase maximal oxygen uptake up to 25%. The degree of increase depends on the initial level of fitness and age, as well as the intensity, frequency, and duration of training. Individuals performing aerobic training such as distance running can have maximal oxygen uptake values as high as 60 to 80 ml O_2/kg/min.
For convenience, oxygen uptake is expressed in multiples of basal resting requirements (METs). The MET is a unit of basal oxygen uptake equal to approximately 3.5 ml O_2/kg/min. This value is the oxygen requirement to maintain life in the resting state.

Figure 3-1 illustrates the relationship between maximal oxygen uptake, exercise habits, and age.[1,2] Although the three activity levels have different regression lines that fit the data as one would expect, there is a great deal of scatter around the lines, and the correlation coefficients are relatively poor. This shows the inaccuracy associated with predicting maximal oxygen uptake from age and habitual physical activity. It is preferable to estimate an individual's maximal oxygen uptake from the workload reached while performing an exercise test. Maximal oxygen uptake is most precisely determined by direct measurement using ventilatory gas exchange techniques.

Key Point: Many different functional measures are used to classify patients with cardiovascular disease. All of them have limitations, and none is a valid substitute for directly measured oxygen uptake. This is one reason why oxygen uptake from expired gas analysis is increasingly appreciated for functional assessment and its prognostic power in various patient groups.

Questionnaire Assessment

Functional classifications are relatively limited and poorly reproducible. One problem is that "usual activities" can decrease so that an individual can become greatly limited without having a change in functional class.

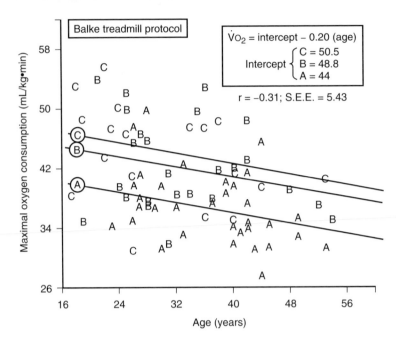

FIGURE 3-1 *Relationship between maximal oxygen uptake and current exercise status and age.* **A,** *sedentary subjects;* **B,** *moderate exercise;* **C,** *heavy exercise.*

An alternative approach is to use specific activity scales such as that of Goldman and colleagues,[3] shown in Table 2-3, and the Duke Activity Status Index (DASI), shown in Table 2-4, or to question a patient regarding usual activities that have a known MET cost. The DASI was developed at Duke; it is a brief, self-administered questionnaire that estimates functional capacity and assesses aspects of quality of life.[4] Fifty subjects undergoing exercise testing with measurement of peak oxygen uptake were studied. All subjects were questioned about their ability to perform a variety of common activities by an interviewer blinded to exercise test findings. A 12-item scale was then developed that correlated well with peak oxygen uptake. We use a similar approach to estimate a patient's exercise capacity before undergoing exercise testing in order to individualize the test and target test duration.[5] The Veterans Specific Activity Questionnaire (VSAQ) is shown in Table 2-5.

Exercise Capacity and Cardiac Function

Exercise capacity determined by exercise testing has been proposed as a means to estimate ventricular function. A direct relationship between the two is supported by the following:

1. Cardiac output is the major determinant of peak VO_2 in most individuals.
2. Resting ejection fraction (EF) and exercise capacity have prognostic value in patients with cardiovascular disease.

However, a poor relationship between resting ventricular function and exercise performance has been reported by many investigators, both among patients with coronary artery disease (CAD) and those with reduced ventricular function. Exercise-induced ischemia could limit exercise even in the presence of normal resting ventricular function; thus patients with angina would have to be excluded when assessing this relationship.

At the University of California–San Diego, the relationship between resting ventricular function and exercise performance in patients with a wide range of resting EF values who were able to exercise to volitional fatigue was investigated.[6] We compared radionuclide measurements of left ventricular perfusion and EF with treadmill responses in 88 patients who had coronary heart disease but were free of angina pectoris. Resting and exercise EF were highly correlated with nuclear perfusion scan score but not with maximal oxygen uptake. Fifty-five percent of the variability in predicting treadmill time was explained by the combination of change in heart rate (39%), thallium ischemia score (12%), and resting cardiac output (4%). The change in heart rate induced by the treadmill test explained only 27% of the variability in measured maximal oxygen uptake. The ability to increase heart rate with treadmill exercise was the most important determinant of exercise capacity. Exercise capacity was only minimally affected by asymptomatic ischemia and was relatively independent of ventricular function. A plot of resting EF versus measured maximal oxygen uptake is shown in Figure 3-2. This poor relationship ($r = 0.25$) confirms many other studies among patients with chronic heart failure and coronary heart disease. Among cardiac parameters used to predict treadmill time or VO_2 max, it was found that ischemia, resting cardiac output, and maximal end-diastolic volume, sequentially, explained 19% of the variability. When treadmill parameters were added, the change in heart rate during treadmill exercise was the most important predictor of VO_2 max, explaining 39% of the variability, followed by the ischemia score (12%)

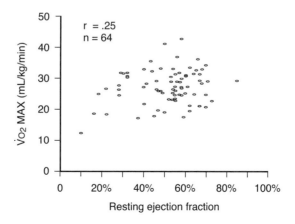

FIGURE 3-2   *A plot of resting ejection fraction versus measured maximal oxygen uptake illustrating the poor relationship even in patients not limited by angina.*

and resting cardiac output (4%), to account for a total of 55% of the variability in exercise capacity. With treadmill parameters alone considered, the change in heart rate with exercise alone explained 38% of the variance in exercise capacity.

In a similar study,[7] extensive measurements of systolic ventricular function were considered, but none of these was found to be a good predictor of maximal oxygen uptake. In a seminal study among patients with heart failure,[8] 62 patients with chronic stable heart failure were classified into functional classes based on peak VO_2. Pulmonary capillary wedge pressure and direct Fick measurements of cardiac output were made at rest and during upright exercise. The most limited patients increased cardiac output by heart rate alone and had lower maximal heart rates, lower oxygen pulse values, and a lesser change in oxygen pulse from rest to maximal exercise. Patients were symptom-limited by exercise cardiac output rather than high filling pressures. A normal exercise capacity was achieved by increasing both heart rate and stroke volume and tolerating a very high filling pressure during upright exercise. These findings were supported by those of Litchfield and colleagues[9] in a study of six patients with severe ventricular dysfunction. They observed that other compensatory mechanisms included an increase in end-diastolic volume and elevated circulating catecholamines. Higginbotham and co-workers[10] also examined determinants of upright exercise performance in 12 patients with severe left ventricular dysfunction using radionuclide angiography and invasive measurements. Multivariate analysis identified changes in heart rate, cardiac output, and a-VO_2 difference with exercise to be important predictors of VO_2. Resting EF did not correlate with VO_2 max, nor did changes in EF. Wilson and associates[11] observed that despite widely varying wedge pressure and cardiac output responses to exercise, patients with chronic heart failure had similar levels of fatigue and dyspnea responses at comparable workloads, as well as similar quality-of-life measurements.

Together these observations demonstrate that (1) exercise capacity is largely explained by the extent to which cardiac output increases (this appears to be true among both normal subjects and patients with cardiovascular disease, even those with widely ranging measures of ventricular function); and (2) the relation between exercise capacity, symptoms, and ventricular function is poor, and with the exception of maximal cardiac output, hemodynamic data contribute minimally to the explanation of variance in exercise capacity.

The discrepancy between ventricular function and exercise capacity is now well known. Studies have employed radionuclide, angiographic, and echocardiographic measures of ventricular size and function to document this finding in patients with heart disease. Correlations between exercise capacity and various indices of ventricular function have generally ranged from −0.10 to 0.25.[12] Increasing heart rate and increasing cardiac index appear to be the most important determinants of exercise capacity, but they often leave more than 50% of the variance in exercise capacity unexplained. The change in EF from rest to maximal supine exercise has no predictive power, probably because of the complex nature of this response. The established clinical impression today is that good ventricular function does not guarantee normal exercise capacity, and vice versa.

> **Key Point:** Even in patients free of angina, exercise limitations or expectations are not determined by ventricular function but rather by the patient's symptomatic response to an exercise test.

Myocardial Oxygen Demands

Although heart rate and stroke volume are important determinants of both maximal oxygen uptake and myocardial oxygen consumption, myocardial oxygen consumption has other independent determinants. The relative metabolic demands of the entire body and those of the heart are determined separately and may not change in parallel with a given intervention. The heart receives only 4% of cardiac output at rest, but it uses 10% of systemic oxygen uptake. In the myocardium, the wide arteriovenous oxygen difference of 10 to 20 vol% at rest reflects the fact that oxygen in the blood passing through the coronary artery circulation is nearly maximally extracted. This value can be compared with the 4 to 6 vol% difference across the systemic circulation. When the myocardium requires a greater oxygen supply, coronary blood flow must increase by coronary artery dilation. During exercise, coronary blood flow can increase through normal coronary arteries up to five times the normal resting flow. For clinical purposes, myocardial oxygen demand is reasonably estimated by the product of heart rate and systolic blood pressure.

Use of Nomograms to Express Exercise Capacity

One of the most important results of the exercise test is to determine an individual's exercise capacity relative to a "normal" value. This is particularly important in light of the many recent studies demonstrating the prognostic power of exercise capacity. Determining what constitutes normal can be a difficult undertaking. For example, many protocols have been developed to assess various patient populations. Rapidly advanced protocols may be suited to screening younger or more active individuals (e.g., Bruce, Ellestad), whereas more moderate ones are appropriate for older or deconditioned patients (e.g., Ramp, Naughton, Balke-Ware, United States Air Force School of Aerospace Medicine [USAFSAM]). The main disadvantage to having so many techniques has been determining equivalent workloads between them (e.g., what does 5 minutes on a modified Bruce protocol mean relative to a Balke-Ware protocol or in terms of real-life activities such as hiking or grocery shopping?).

It has been well established that maximal oxygen uptake (VO_2) can be reasonably estimated from the workload achieved on a given protocol, although there are notable limitations in doing so. The widely used equations to estimate METs come from the American College of Sports Medicine guidelines:

- Estimated METs based on *treadmill/speed and grade:* METs = (mph × 26.8) [0.1 + (grade × .018) + 3.5]/3.5
- Estimated METs based on *cycle ergometer workload:* METs = [(Watts × 12/Body weight in Kg) + 7]/3.5

As mentioned earlier, the term *metabolic equivalent* (MET) has been commonly used to describe the quantity of oxygen consumed by the body from inspired air under basal conditions. The MET is equal on average to 3.5 ml O_2kg/min.[13] A multiple of the basal metabolic rate, or MET, is a useful clinical expression of a patient's exercise capacity. Directly measured VO_2 is translated into METs by dividing by 3.5, thus providing a unitless and convenient method for expressing a patient's exercise capacity.

Because VO_2 depends on age, gender, activity status, and disease states, tables that consider these factors must be referred to in order to accurately categorize a certain MET value as either normal or abnormal. We developed a nomogram in order to make it more convenient for physicians to translate an MET level into a percentage of normal exercise capacity for males based on age and activity status.[14] We retrospectively reviewed the exercise test results of 3583 male patients referred to our laboratory for the evaluation of possible or probable CAD. Simple univariate linear regression was performed, with age as the independent variable and METs achieved as the dependent variable. This was done separately for the entire group, as well as for the "sedentary" and "active" groups. The nomograms derived from estimated MET levels are presented in Figures 3-3 and 3-4 for males, and a nomogram for females is presented in Figure 3-5.[15]

Note that there have been numerous regression equations developed in various populations; determining a "normal" value for exercise capacity relative to age is population specific. Some of the different regression equations from the literature are presented in Table 3-2. For example, the greater slope in the Veterans Administration (VA) population is consistent with a faster decline in exercise capacity with age than that found in previous studies. Regression equations can vary because of population differences, including age, activity status, state of health, definition of normal or healthy individuals, and gender. The decline in maximal heart rate with age is also steeper in our referrals, paralleling that for the slope in VO_2. Thus maximal heart rate decreased with age at a greater rate than in prior studies,[16] which could be attributed to a submaximal effort or complicating illnesses in older patients, or it may simply be due to the wide scatter that has been observed for this measurement in past studies.

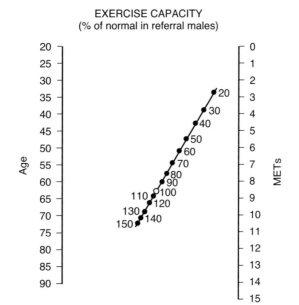

FIGURE 3-3　*Nomogram of percent normal exercise capacity for age in total population of referral males.*

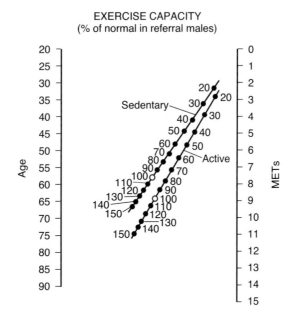

FIGURE 3-4　*Nomogram of percent normal exercise capacity in sedentary and active referral males.*

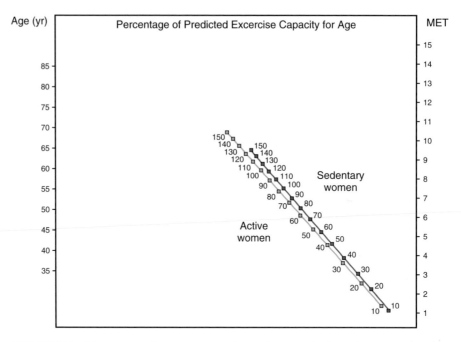

FIGURE 3-5   *Nomogram of percent normal exercise capacity in sedentary and active females. (From Gulati M et al: N Engl J Med 353[5]:468-475, 2005.)*

One must also consider differences in methodology when examining divergent results. Few such studies have used measured VO_2 in developing normal values. Additionally, the treadmill protocols were quite different, and it has been demonstrated that some protocols are more accurate than others when estimating METs. For instance, more gradual protocols may favor the elderly and thus alter the regression line. Nevertheless, the mean MET levels for age in our study agree quite well with those of prior investigations (Table 3-3). It would be difficult to sort out which study has produced the most "universal" regression equations, because all have weaknesses in either population selection or methodology.

The upward shift in the slope of the nomogram scale among volunteers whose oxygen uptake was determined directly from ventilatory gas exchange analysis is because estimating MET levels from treadmill work results in an overestimation of exercise capacity.[17] Thus the approximately 1 to 1.5 higher predicted MET values for any given age among referred patients whose exercise capacity was estimated from treadmill workload is expected.

TABLE 3-2   Equations for Predicting Maximal METs from Age

Investigator	Equation	No. Patients	Mean Age (Range)	Assessment of Activity	Definition of Normal	Oxygen Uptake	Protocol
Morris[14]	METs = 18−0.15(age)	1388	57 (21-89)	Simple questionnaire	No history of CABS, CHF, BB, digoxin, COPD, claudication, angina, prior MI, arrhythmias, or >1 Q wave on ECG	Estimated	USAFSAM
Morris[14]	METs = 18.7−0.15(age)	346 (Active)	N/A	Simple questionnaire	As above	Estimated	USAFSAM
Morris[14]	METs = 16.6−0.16(age)	479 (sedentary)	N/A	Simple questionnaire	As above	Estimated	USAFSAM
Morris[14]	METs = 14.7−0.11(age)	244	45 (20-72)	Simple questionnaire	Apparently healthy	Measured	Ramp
Froelicher[23]	METs = 13.1−0.08(age)	710	N/A (20-53)	None	Normal examination, normal resting and exercise ECG, no HTN	Measured	3.3 mph 1% grade increment per minute
Bruce[54]	METs = 13.7−0.08(age)	2092	44.4 (N/A)	None	Cardiac screening examination	Estimated	Bruce
Wolthius[20]	METs = 13−0.05(age)	704	37 (25-54)	Questionnaire interview	Normal history and physical examination, chest x-ray, resting and exercise ECG, and Holter; no arrhythmias, HTN, or medications	Measured	Balke (long) 3.3 mph 1% grade increment per minute
Dehn[55]	METs = 16.2−0.11(age)	700	52.2 (40-72)	—	—	Mixed	Mixed

BB, beta-blockers; CABS, coronary artery bypass surgery; CHF, congestive heart failure; COPD, chronic obstructive pulmonary disease; ECG, electrocardiogram; HTN, hypertension; MI, myocardial infarction; USAFSAM, United States Air Force School of Aerospace Medicine.

TABLE 3-3   MET Levels for Age Decades from Previous Studies

	Froelicher[23]	Hossack[19]	Pollock[56]	Morris (Referrals)[14]
20-29	11 ± 2	13 ± 1	12 ± 2	—
30-39	10 ± 2	12 ± 2	12 ± 2	—
40-49	10 ± 2	11 ± 2	11 ± 2	11 ± 4
50-59	—	10 ± 2	10 ± 2	9 ± 4
60-69	—	8 ± 2	8 ± 2	8 ± 3
70-79	—	5 ± 1	8 ± 2	7 ± 3
80-89	—	—	—	5 ± 3

Key Points:
1. Establishing a patient's exercise capacity relative to a normal standard is an important result of the exercise test and should be included in the test report.
2. Normal exercise capacity tables/graphs/scales are population specific.
3. Although measured oxygen uptake is the more precise measure of work, normal standards are also specific to whether oxygen uptake was measured or estimated.
4. An estimation of maximal ventilatory oxygen uptake from treadmill or cycle ergometer workload during dynamic exercise (expressed as METs) has been the common language with which investigators and clinicians communicate when assessing these widely different exercise protocols and everyday physical activities of their patients (Table 3-4).

Maximal Cardiac Output

Maximal cardiac output is the major factor limiting maximal oxygen uptake; numerous studies have demonstrated a linear relation between cardiac output and oxygen uptake during exercise. The rate of increase in cardiac output is approximately 6 liters per 1 liter increase in oxygen uptake. However, there is a wide biologic scatter between maximal cardiac output and VO_2 max in healthy persons, even when age, gender, and activity status are considered. Because both maximal cardiac output and maximal oxygen uptake decline with age, the effects of age and disease are usually difficult to separate.

McDonough and colleagues[18] measured maximal cardiac output in a group of patients and found a decline in maximal cardiac output to be the major hemodynamic consequence of symptomatic CAD and one that resulted in exercise impairment. Reductions in left ventricular performance at high levels of exercise, manifested by decreasing stroke volume and increasing pulmonary artery pressure, appeared to be the mechanism limiting cardiac output. Hossack and co-workers[19] studied 100 patients with coronary disease to characterize their aerobic and hemodynamic profiles at rest and during upright treadmill exercise. The mean maximal cardiac output, measured using the direct Fick equation, was 57% ± 14% of average normal values. The reduction in maximal heart rate (63% ± 13% of normal) was a greater factor

TABLE 3-4　MET Demands for Common Daily Activities

Activity	METs
Mild	
Baking	2.0
Billiards	2.4
Bookbinding	2.2
Canoeing (leisurely)	2.5
Conducting an orchestra	2.2
Dancing, ballroom (slow)	2.9
Golfing (with cart)	2.5
Horseback riding (walking)	2.3
Playing a musical instrument	2.0
Volleyball (noncompetitive)	2.9
Walking (2 mph)	2.5
Writing	1.7
Moderate	
Calisthenics (no weights)	4.0
Croquet	3.0
Cycling (leisurely)	3.5
Gardening (no lifting)	4.4
Golfing (without cart)	4.9
Mowing lawn (power mower)	3.0
Playing drums	3.8
Sailing	3.0
Swimming (slowly)	4.5
Walking (3 mph)	3.3
Walking (4 mph)	4.5
Vigorous	
Badminton	5.5
Chopping wood	4.9
Climbing hills	7.0
Cycling (moderate)	5.7
Dancing	6.0
Field hockey	7.7
Ice skating	5.5
Jogging (10-minute mile)	10.0
Karate or judo	6.5
Roller skating	6.5
Rope skipping	12.0
Skiing (water or downhill)	6.8
Squash	12.0
Surfing	6.0
Swimming (fast)	7.0
Tennis (doubles)	6.0

From Fletcher GF et al: *Circulation* 104:1694–1740, 2001.
NOTE: These activities can often be done at variable intensities if one assumes that the intensity is not excessive and that the courses are flat (no hills) unless so specified.

influencing the reduction in cardiac output than stroke volume (88% ± 16% of normal). Peak VO_2 was 48% ± 15% of normal, and the greater reduction in peak VO_2 compared with cardiac output was due to lower peripheral extraction in the patients with CAD. Variables that correlated with maximal cardiac output in a univariate analysis included angina severity ($r = -0.45$), peak VO_2 ($r = 0.67$), maximal heart rate ($r = -0.31$), left ventricular dysfunction ($r = -0.45$), maximal systolic blood pressure ($r = -0.31$), and number of vessels with CAD ($r = -0.30$). Resting ejection fraction did not correlate with maximal cardiac output using a multivariate analysis, but four variables correlated significantly ($r = 0.77$) with maximal cardiac output in the following order: VO_2 max, number of occluded vessels, ST depression, and gender. These data were used to estimate limits of maximal cardiac output and stroke volume in normal subjects, and these normal standards were then used to evaluate the results in the patients. Patients with an ejection fraction of less than 50% had significantly impaired age-adjusted cardiac output and stroke volume.

> **Key Point:** Cardiac output is the major hemodynamic factor influencing exercise capacity; a disruption in any of the factors that determine cardiac output (e.g., maximal heart rate, stroke volume, filling pressure, ventricular compliance, contractility, or afterload) will limit exercise capacity.

Normal Heart Rate and Blood Pressure Values

Heart rates, blood pressures, and functional responses to submaximal, maximal, and postexertional treadmill testing were collected in a group of 704 healthy, asymptomatic aircrewmen referred to the United States Air Force School of Aerospace Medicine.[20] The indicated measurements are individually described by the use of percentiles. These data provide the practicing clinician with an accurate and complete description of the response of healthy men to treadmill exercise. The reference values presented in Figure 3-6 should help determine discriminant values for separating patient groups.

Maximal Heart Rate

Methods of Recording

Maximal heart rate is the most important determinant of cardiac output during exercise, particularly at high levels. One issue of concern in the past was the method of maximal heart rate measurement. Although measuring a patient's maximal heart rate should be a simple matter, the different ways of recording it and differences in the type of exercise used can pose problems. The best way to measure maximal heart rate is to use a standard electrocardiogram (ECG) recorder and calculate instantaneous heart rate from the RR intervals. Methods using the arterial pulse or capillary blush

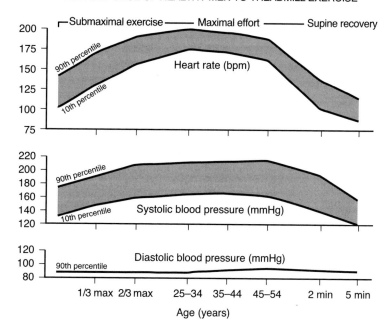

THE RESPONSE OF HEALTHY MEN TO TREADMILL EXERCISE

FIGURE 3-6   *The hemodynamic responses of over 700 healthy men to maximal treadmill exercise. Bands represent 80% of the population; 10% had values above the band, and 10% had values below the band.*

techniques are much more affected by artifact than ECG techniques. Some investigators have used averaging over the last minute of exercise or in immediate recovery; both of these averaging methods are inaccurate. Heart rate drops quickly in recovery and can climb steeply even in the last seconds of exercise. Premature beats can affect averaging and must be excluded in order to obtain the actual heart rate. Cardiotachometers are available but may fail to trigger or may trigger inappropriately on T waves, artifact, or aberrant beats, thus yielding inaccurate results. Not all cardiotachometers have the accuracy of the ECG paper technique. From a study of heart rate measurement during exercise testing, it was concluded that the number of RR intervals from a 6-second rhythm strip at the end of each minute multiplied by 10 represented a reasonable balance between convenience and precision for measuring heart rate during exercise, both in patients in normal sinus rhythm[21] and in those with an irregular ventricular response (atrial fibrillation).

Factors Limiting Maximal Heart Rate

Several factors may affect maximal heart rate during dynamic exercise (Table 3-5). Maximal heart rate declines with advancing years and is affected only minimally by gender, height, weight, and lean body mass.

TABLE 3-5   Factors Affecting Maximal Heart Rate in Response to Dynamic Exercise

Age	Bed rest
Gender	Altitude
Level of fitness	Type of exercise
Cardiovascular disease	Extent of effort exerted
Cigarette smoking	Medications

Age, Fitness, and Cardiovascular Disease

Many studies have reported maximal heart rate during treadmill testing in a variety of subjects, with and without cardiovascular disease. Regressions with age have varied depending on the population studied and other factors. Table 3-6 and Figure 3-7 summarize these studies of maximal heart rate; note the wide variation among the regression equations based on age.

A consistent finding in these studies has been a relatively poor relationship between maximal heart rate and age. Correlation coefficients in the order of −0.40 are typical, with standard deviations in the range of 10 to 15 beats per minute. In general, this relationship has not been "tightened" by considering activity status, weight, cardiac size, maximal respiratory exchange ratio, or perceived exertion. An exercise program most likely has divergent effects on this relationship at the age extremes. Younger individuals may be able to achieve larger changes in cardiac dimensions than older subjects, and those larger changes may affect maximal heart rate. Among older individuals, there may be a significant learning effect, whereby individuals are less afraid to exert themselves maximally and therefore a higher maximal heart rate is achieved on later testing when they are less apprehensive. Given the inconsistencies associated with age-related maximal heart rate, indiscriminant use of age-predicted maximal heart rate in developing an exercise prescription or in setting goals for treadmill performance should be avoided.

In an effort to clarify the relationship between maximal heart rate and age, Londeree and Moeschberger[22] performed a comprehensive review of the literature, compiling information on more than 23,000 subjects ages 5 to 81 years. Stepwise multiple regression analysis revealed that age alone accounted for 75% of the variability in maximal heart rate; other factors added only an additional 5% and included mode of exercise, level of fitness, and continent of origin, but not gender. The 95% confidence intervals, even when accounting for these factors, ranged 45 beats per minute. Heart rates at maximal exercise were lower during bicycle ergometry than on the treadmill and even lower with swimming. In addition, trained individuals had significantly lower maximal heart rates than untrained subjects did.

At USAFSAM, the cardiovascular responses to maximal treadmill testing were compared using three different popular treadmill protocols to evaluate reproducibility among tests.[23] The Bruce, Balke, and Taylor protocols were used in the evaluation of healthy men; each subject performed one test per

TABLE 3-6   Summary of Studies Assessing Maximal Heart Rate in 100 or More Subjects

Investigator	No. Subjects	Population Studied	Mean Age ± SD (Range)	Mean HR Max (SD)	Regression Line	Correlation Coefficient	Standard Error of the Estimate (Beats/Min)
Astrand[57]*	100	Asymptomatic men	50 (20-69)	166 ± 22	y = 211−0.922 (age)	NA	NA
Bruce[54]	2091	Asymptomatic men	44 ± 8	181 ± 12	y = 210−0.662 (age)	−0.44	14
Cooper[58]	2535	Asymptomatic men	43 (11-79)	181 ± 16	y = 217−0.845 (age)	NA	NA
Ellestad[29]†	2583	Asymptomatic men	42 ± 7 (10-60)	173 ± 11	y = 197−0.556 (age)	NA	NA
Warthius[20]	1317	Asymptomatic men	38 ± 8 (28-54)	183	y = 207−0.64 (age)	−0.43	10
Lester[59]	148	Asymptomatic men	43 (15-75)	187	y = 205−0.411 (age)	−0.58	NA
Bruce[54]	1295	Men with CHD	52 ± 8	148 ± 23	y = 204−1.07 (age)	−0.36	25‡
Hammond[16]	156	Men with CHD	53 ± 9	157 ± 20	y = 209−1.0 (age)	−0.30	19
Morris[14]	244	Asymptomatic men	45 (20-72)	167 ± 19	y = 200−0.72 (age)	−0.55	15
Graettinger[24]	114	Asymptomatic men	46 ± 13 (19-73)	168 ± 18	y = 199−0.63 (age)	−0.47	NA
Morris[14]	1388	Men referred for evaluation for CHD, normals only	57 (21-89)	144 ± 20	y = 196−0.9 (age)	−0.43	21

*Astrand used bicycle ergometry; all other studies were performed utilizing a treadmill.
†Data compiled from graphs in reference cited.
‡Calculated from available data.
CHD, coronary heart disease; HR Max, maximal heart rate; NA, not able to calculate from available data; SD, standard deviation.

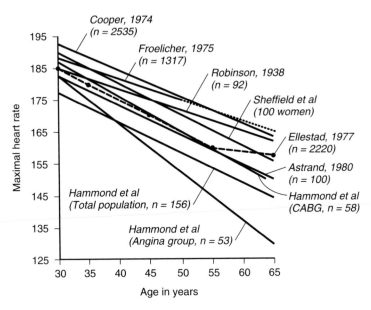

FIGURE 3-7 *Regression lines from studies in the literature assessing maximal heart rate versus age during dynamic exercise, including population size.[16] See Table 3-6 for additional details.*

week for 9 weeks, repeating each protocol three times in randomized order. The maximal heart rates achieved were reproducible within each protocol, and no significant differences in heart rate were achieved among the three protocols. Figure 3-8 shows the wide scatter in the relationship between maximal heart rate and age, even among these healthy subjects. In general, these findings agree with subsequent data from our laboratory in Long Beach.[24] In the latter study, we assessed clinical, echocardiographic, and functional determinants of maximal heart rate. Despite controlling for age, activity status, gender, and hypertension, measures of cardiac size and function added little to the prediction of maximal heart rate. Most of the variance in maximal heart rate was accounted for simply by age.

> **Key Point:** Given the large degree of individual variability in cardiac size and function, as well as the variance in the relationship between maximal heart rate and age, maximal heart rate may always be a difficult variable to explain. Given the inconsistencies associated with age-related maximal heart rate, indiscriminant use of age-predicted maximal heart rate for exercise prescription or in setting goals for treadmill performance should be avoided.

Bed Rest
Another factor that affects maximal heart rate, and one that is important clinically, is bed rest. Among the many adverse physiologic effects of bed rest are substantial increases in heart rate at rest and during exercise.[25] The lack

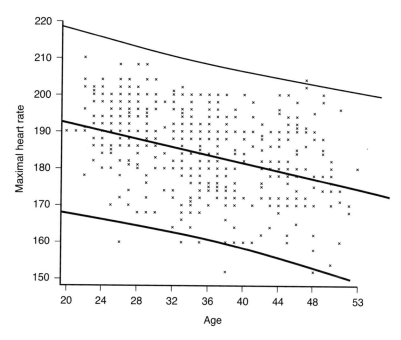

FIGURE 3-8 *United States Air Force School of Aerospace Medicine study of healthy pilots illustrating the relationship between maximal heart rate and age, along with the normal scatter.[20]*

of gravitational forces on baroreceptor mechanisms plays a role in the markedly accentuated heart rate response to exercise. Comparisons of peak VO_2 in both the supine and upright positions reveal lower values with upright exercise, but peak VO_2 during maximal supine exercise is not impaired compared with pre–bed rest measurements. Since maximal heart rates increase significantly, but VO_2 max decreases, changes in heart volume are likely involved and likely reflect changes in plasma volume during prolonged bed rest.

Altitude

Altitude affects the heart rate response to exercise. During acute exposure to altitude, heart rate increases at matched submaximal levels. Maximal heart rate decreases after prolonged exposure to altitude. At high altitude, there is a reduction in sympathetic nervous system activity, likely due to a reduction in beta-receptor sensitivity, which underlies the reduction in maximal heart rate.[26]

Motivation

Motivation to exert oneself maximally is another factor that can influence maximal heart rate. Motivation is, of course, a difficult factor to quantify.

Older patients may be restrained by poor muscle tone, pulmonary disease, claudication, orthopedic problems, and other noncardiac limitations.

Disease

The usual decline in maximal heart rate with age is not as steep in people who are free from myocardial disease and stay active, but it still occurs. We have reviewed many studies in this manual that demonstrate that maximal heart rate is inversely proportional to prognosis.

Type of Dynamic Exercise

Although steps, escalators, ladders, and other devices have been used over the years, the three predominant types of exercise testing used clinically are treadmill and supine or upright bicycle ergometry. Position and type of exercise influence the physiologic response to exercise. Maximal heart rate is consistent in a wide range of patients with various treadmill and upright cycle ergometer protocols. However, exercise capacity is typically 10% to 20% lower on a cycle ergometer than on a treadmill. Because of changes in venous return and filling pressures, the supine position results in a lower resting heart rate and higher end-diastolic volumes. When supine, there is little change in stroke volume or end-diastolic volume during exercise from values obtained at rest. Because of the unusual position and positional disadvantage, there usually is an element of isometric exercise and a lower mechanical efficiency in the supine position. In general, patients are less able to give maximal efforts in the supine position, and maximal heart rate is usually significantly lower whereas systolic blood pressure is often higher. In patients with significant CAD, angina may develop at a lower double product in the supine compared with the upright position, which may also contribute to a lower maximal heart rate.

Measures of Maximal Effort

Various objective measurements are used in efforts to confirm that a maximal effort was performed. These measurements are important because they can provide information as to whether patients have exerted themselves maximally, something that has a number of relevant diagnostic and prognostic clinical implications. Historically, a decrease or failure to increase oxygen uptake by 150 ml/min with an increase in workload has defined a plateau and was thought to accurately reflect a maximal physiologic effort when interrupted protocols were used. Although this definition remained popular for several decades, the conditions under which this criterion was developed are quite different from the way clinical exercise testing is performed. Gradually, this marker of maximal physiologic effort fell into disfavor among many physiologists.[27,28] It is infrequently seen in continuous treadmill protocols among patients with heart disease.

A plateau in VO_2 can be explained by the following:

1. The patient holding onto the handrails
2. Incomplete expired air collection
3. The criteria used for plateau
4. Differences in the gas exchange sampling interval used
5. Equipment issues

Indicators of maximal effort that have been used are listed in Table 3-7. None of the commonly used markers of maximal effort can be relied on completely. *Respiratory exchange ratio*, defined as the ratio of carbon dioxide production to oxygen utilization, increases in proportion to exercise effort. Most individuals at the point of maximal dynamic exercise reach values greater than 1.10. However, this ratio varies greatly, and its determination requires gas exchange analysis during exercise. Blood lactate levels have also been used (i.e., >7 or 8 mmol), but this requires mixed venous samples, and they also vary greatly between individuals. All objective criteria proposed are problematic because of intersubject variability and definition.

Perceived Exertion

The Borg scale subjectively grades levels of exertion. This method is best applied to match levels of perceived exertion during comparison studies. The linear scale ranges from 6 (very, very light) to 20 (very, very hard); the nonlinear scale ranges from 0 to 10, and both correlate with the percentage of maximal heart rate and other physiologic responses during exercise (see Tables 2-6 and 2-7).

> **Key Point:** Though a subjective indicator of effort, the Borg scales are very useful clinically. In addition to closely following objective responses such as blood pressure and ECG changes, it is important to determine the individual patient's perceived level of effort during the exercise test.

Chronotropic Incompetence or Heart Rate Impairment

Chronotropic incompetence and *heart rate impairment* are terms that have been used to describe inadequate heart rate responses to exercise. In a

---

TABLE 3-7   Indicators of Maximal Effort Used in Exercise Studies

Patient appearance and breathing rate
Borg scale
Age-predicted heart rate and exercise capacity
Systolic blood pressure
Expired gas measurements: respiratory exchange ratio, plateau, and exceeding the ventilatory threshold
Venous lactate concentration

---

seminal study on this issue, Ellestad and Wan[29] analyzed the results from 2700 patients tested in their treadmill laboratory. They defined a group of patients who achieved below the 95% confidence limits for maximal heart rate regressed with age as having chronotropic incompetence (CI). Patients with no ST-segment depression who had CI had a four times greater incidence of CAD than did those without CI in the 4 years after the test. A number of recent studies performed at the Cleveland Clinic have confirmed the strong prognostic value of inadequate heart rate responses to exercise.

Lauer and colleagues[30] studied 146 men and 85 women who were not taking beta-blocking agents and exhibited CI defined as (1) failure to achieve 85% of age-predicted maximal heart rate or (2) a low chronotropic index, a measure that expresses heart rate achieved accounting for age, functional capacity, and resting heart rate. The patients were followed for a mean of 41 months. Both indices were strong predictors of cardiac events (death, myocardial infarction, unstable angina, or revascularization); the relative risks for failure to achieve 85% predicted heart rate and a low chronotropic index were > 2. Similar findings were made in the Framingham cohort;[31] during a 7-year follow-up among 1575 males, an inadequate heart rate response to exercise was associated with nearly twice the risk for total mortality and cardiac events, even after adjustments were made for age and other CAD risk factors. Because the heart rate response to exercise reflects the balance between central nervous system withdrawal of vagal tone and an increase in sympathetic tone, an abnormal heart rate response to exercise is also likely related to abnormal autonomic balance.[32]

> **Key Point:** Chronotropic incompetence (CI) is a strong prognostic marker. Patients with CI most likely represent a mixed group with a variety of explanations for the impaired heart rate response, including impaired autonomic function, angina, myocardial dysfunction, and simply normal variation.

Heart Rate Recovery

A faster recovery of heart rate after exercise is associated with higher levels of fitness. Studies in this area date back to the 1930s and the work of D. B. Dill in the Harvard fatigue laboratory.[33] Contemporary studies have suggested that the rate at which heart rate recovers from exercise is mediated by autonomic factors, particularly the rate at which vagal tone is reactivated.[34]

Several provocative studies were published between 1999 and 2004 addressing the diagnostic/prognostic utility of heart rate in recovery. Cole and colleagues[35] studied 2428 patients referred for nuclear perfusion exercise testing over a 6-year period. They found that, using a decrease of <12 beats per minute at 1 minute into recovery as the definition of an abnormal response, a relative risk of 4 for mortality was observed. These investigators then addressed this issue among 5000 subjects in the Lipid Research Clinics Prevalence study.[36] Abnormal heart rate recovery was defined in this study by a decrease of <42 beats per minute at 2 minutes after exercise. Patients with an abnormal response had 2.5 times the mortality rate of those with a normal response. In a third study, Nishime and colleagues[37] studied 9454 patients who underwent exercise testing and followed them for a median of 5.2 years. Using the original <12 beats per minute at 1 minute of recovery as the cutoff for abnormal, they observed a fourfold greater mortality rate among abnormal responders.

Our group attempted to validate heart rate recovery as a prognostic marker, addressed whether it had any diagnostic value, and tried to clarify some of the methodological issues surrounding its use (e.g., what is the optimal recovery rate and at what time point after exercise should it be measured?).[38] Among 2193 patients who underwent both treadmill testing and coronary angiography over a 13-year period, we found that a decrease in heart rate <22 beats per minute at 2 minutes into recovery best identified high-risk patients (hazard ratio of 2.6). Beta-blocker therapy had no significant impact on the prognostic value of heart rate recovery. By multivariate analysis, the combination of a low exercise capacity (<5 METs) and an abnormal heart rate recovery response yielded a particularly poor prognosis, with these patients having a fivefold risk of mortality. Kaplan-Meier survival curves from this study illustrating the combination of heart rate responses in recovery and exercise capacity are illustrated in Figure 3-9. Interestingly, heart rate recovery did not add any diagnostic value.

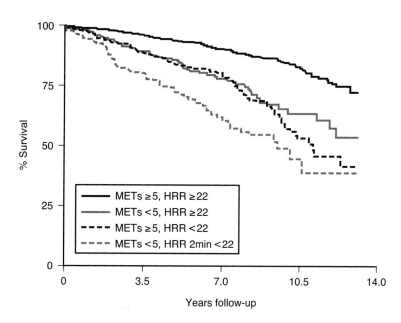

FIGURE 3-9 *Kaplan-Meier survival curves among patients exhibiting normal and abnormal heart rate recovery responses. (From Shetler K et al: J Am Coll Cardiol 38:1980-1987, 2001.)*

Given these and other recent results documenting the prognostic power of heart rate recovery, it would seem prudent to include heart rate recovery routinely as part of the test summary. Additional studies are needed, however, to clarify a number of practical issues, such as population specificity, optimal criteria, and whether or not heart rate recovery is best defined using a cool-down walk versus the supine position. Furthermore, it is highly correlated with heart rate reserve and appears to predict noncardiovascular more so than cardiovascular mortality.

> **Key Point:** Recovery heart rate should be recorded as part of every exercise test. A slow recovery of heart rate to basal levels is associated with poor prognosis. By 2 minutes after maximal exercise, heart rate should drop by at least 22 beats per minute.

Blood Pressure Response

Systolic blood pressure should rise with increasing treadmill or cycle ergometer workloads. Diastolic blood pressure usually remains about the same, but the fifth Korotkoff sound can sometimes be heard all the way to zero in healthy young subjects. Although a rising diastolic blood pressure can be associated with CAD, more likely it is a marker for labile hypertension, which leads to CAD. The highest systolic blood pressure should be achieved at maximal workload. When exercise is stopped, some individuals will experience an abrupt drop in systolic blood pressure owing to peripheral pooling. For this reason, patients should not be left standing on the treadmill when the test is terminated. The systolic blood pressure usually normalizes shortly after the patient is placed in the supine position during recovery, but it may remain below normal for several hours after the test. As mentioned earlier, the product of heart rate and systolic blood pressure (double product), determined by cuff and auscultation, correlates highly with measured myocardial oxygen uptake during exercise. Usually, an individual patient's angina symptoms are precipitated at approximately the same double product. Double product has also been used as an estimate of the maximal workload that the left ventricle can perform.

The automated devices for measuring systolic blood pressure, although popular, are not as reliable as manual methods. Though the available devices generally correlate with manual methods, they have not been adequately validated, particularly for the detection of exertional hypotension. In one study assessing the performance of many of the automated devices, it was reported that only half had acceptable accuracy and reliability.[39] Thus the major guidelines on exercise testing continue to recommend manual methods for measuring blood pressure during exercise.

In a seminal study assessing clinical correlates and the prognostic applications of blood pressure responses to exercise, Irving and colleagues[40] examined six groups of subjects. These groups included 5459 men and

749 women classified into three categories each: 2532 men and 244 women who were asymptomatic and healthy, 592 men and 158 women who were hypertensive, and 1586 men and 347 women who had clinical manifestations of CAD. Maximal systolic pressures correlated with resting systolic pressures, and this relation was independent of the diagnosis of cardiovascular disease in both men and women. The prognostic value of maximal systolic pressure for subsequent cardiovascular death was examined in the men. The annual rate of sudden cardiac death increased from 6.6 per 1000 men with maximal systolic pressures of 200 mm Hg or more to 25 and 98 per 1000, respectively, for those achieving 140 to 199 mm Hg and less than 140 mm Hg maximal systolic blood pressure. Over the last three decades, many other studies have reported that a comparatively low systolic blood pressure response to exercise is associated with a poor prognosis. This is particularly true among patients with chronic heart failure.[41]

Erikssen and colleagues[42] performed a screening exercise test on 2014 men ages 40 to 60 who experienced 300 cardiovascular deaths during 26 years of follow-up. Their average maximal heart rate was 162 beats per minute, and their average systolic blood pressure at a submaximal work rate of 100 watts was 180 mm Hg. The exercise test variables that were associated with cardiovascular death included abnormal ST changes, elevated submaximal systolic blood pressure (> 1 standard deviation [25 mm Hg]), and abnormal exercise capacity.

Key Point: The capacity to achieve an adequate systolic blood pressure requires a relatively normal-functioning left ventricle such that cardiac output increases in proportion to the increase in work rate and such that cardiac output can be sustained even when exertion is near maximal.

Exertional Hypotension

Exercise-induced hypotension (EIH) is associated with a poor prognosis, severe CAD, or both. In addition, EIH has been associated with cardiac complications during exercise testing[43-45] and is corrected by coronary artery bypass surgery.[46] Therefore monitoring of blood pressure during an exercise test is essential.

The normal blood pressure response to dynamic upright exercise is characterized by a progressive increase in systolic blood pressure, no change or a decrease in diastolic blood pressure, and a widening of the pulse pressure. Even when tested to exhaustion from prolonged exercise, normal individuals do not exhibit a reduction in systolic blood pressure. Exercise-induced decreases in systolic blood pressure can occur in patients with CAD, valvular heart disease,[47] chronic heart failure, and arrhythmias. Occasionally, patients without clinically significant heart disease exhibit EIH during exercise owing to antihypertensive therapy (including beta blockers), prolonged strenuous exercise, and vasovagal responses, and on rare occasions it been reported to occur in normal females. EIH could be due to left ventricular dysfunction, exercise-induced ischemia causing left ventricular dysfunction, or papillary muscle dysfunction and mitral regurgitation.

Numerous studies have addressed the diagnostic and prognostic implications of EIH. Their important findings regarding definition, prevalence, high-risk subgroups, intervention, and mortality rates are summarized in Table 3-8. One difficulty encountered in interpreting these studies is that although EIH is usually related to CAD and a poor prognosis, various criteria have been used to define it. This variation probably explains why the significance of EIH ranges from life threatening in some studies to benign in others. To further investigate the causes, definition, and predictive power of EIH, we analyzed patients referred for clinical reasons to the treadmill laboratory and then followed them for a 2-year period for cardiac events.[48] The population consisted of 2036 patients, 131 (6.4%) of whom exhibited a drop below standing rest. We demonstrated that the definition of "a drop below rest" was clearly a better criterion than "a drop of 20 mm Hg" for predicting increased risk for death or myocardial infarction. Therefore the odds (risk) ratio of EIH for death was calculated using only the criterion of a systolic blood pressure drop below rest. While the average prevalence of EIH in previous studies was 8% (553 of 6693) (see Table 3-8), the prevalence at Long Beach Veterans Affairs Medical Center (LBVAMC) was 5%. From previous studies, the predictive value for left main and three-vessel disease together in patients with EIH ranged from 20% to 100%, with an average of 48% for the prevalence and 68% for the predictive value. In our study, the prevalence of severe CAD in those with EIH was 45% and the predictive value was 61%. Patients with EIH clearly have an increased risk of death. In all the study subgroups, the risk of death was at least two times greater in patients with EIH than in those without EIH, with the exception of patients recovering from a recent myocardial infarction. The patients recovering from a recent myocardial infarction had the highest death rate, suggesting that the degree of left ventricular dysfunction must predominate over other predictors, including EIH.

A lower mortality rate in patients with EIH who received an intervention (coronary artery bypass surgery or percutaneous transluminal coronary angioplasty) than in those who were medically treated has been reported.[49]

Key Points:
1. The definition of EIH is of crucial importance in the evaluation of the exercise test response. A drop in systolic blood pressure below preexercise values is the most ominous criterion; a drop of 20 mm Hg or more without a fall below preexercise values has a lower predictive value. However, the exercise test should be stopped when a drop of 10 to 20 mm Hg is detected.
2. EIH can be due to either left ventricular dysfunction or ischemia. In the roughly 10% of patients in whom EIH occurs without association with either of these two factors, EIH appears to be benign. Although speculative, other potential mechanisms of EIH that deserve further investigation include exercise-induced mitral regurgitation and a (noncardiac) peripheral vasodilatory mechanism.
3. Although the mortality risk is increased in patients with EIH, two subgroups in our cohort did not show this increased risk. EIH was not associated with increased risk in those tested within 3 weeks after a myocardial infarction nor in those without a prior myocardial infarction or ischemia during the exercise test.

TABLE 3-8 Summary of Major Studies on Significance of Exercise-Induced Hypotension

Investigator	No. Subjects	Incidence of EIH* (%)	Definition of EIH	Predictive Value of EIH for LM/3VD (%)	Findings
Thomson (1975)[43]	17	—	Fall in SBP below resting levels accompanied by chest pain and ST-segment depression	100	Multivessel CAD was found in all patients with EIH. All six patients who had CABS normalized exercise BP response.
Irving (1977)[40,45]	6	—	Decrease or limited increase (<10 mm Hg) in SBP	—	EIH was associated with ventricular fibrillation after exercise in all six cases.
Levites (1978)[60]	1105	2.7	Decrease in SBP below resting level	20	Extent of CAD was not different between those with and without EIH.
Morris (1978)[44]	1020	2.5	Decrease in SBP ≥10 mm Hg	78	EIH was highly specific for multivessel CAD.
Sanmarco (1980)[61]	378	24	Failure of SBP to rise ≥ 10 mm Hg or a decrease ≥ 20 mm Hg during exercise	70	Sensitivity, specificity, and predictive value of EIH were 38.6%, 87.4%, and 70% for 3VD or LM disease, respectively; values were similar to ST-segment depression.
Weiner (1982)[49]	436	10.8	Decrease in SBP during exercise below preexercise standing level	55	EIH was not associated with exercise-induced complications, but most subjects had severe ischemic responses. EIH was reversed with CABS and has 8% 3-year mortality rate.
Hammermeister (1983)[62]	557	6.3	Decrease in exercise SBP below resting SBP	50	EIH was associated with CAD and LV dysfunction.
Hakki (1986)[63]	127	13.4	Decrease in SBP of ≥ 10 mm Hg	—	Prior MI, abnormal EF, multivessel CAD, and nuclear perfusion were defects more common with EIH.
Mazzotta (1987)[64]	224	20	Failure of BP to increase or overt decrease of BP during exercise testing	—	EIH was related to severity of LV dysfunction only when symptoms and hemodynamic decompensation existed.

Continued

TABLE 3-8   Summary of Major Studies on Significance of Exercise-Induced Hypotension—Cont'd

Investigator	No. Subjects	Incidence of EIH* (%)	Definition of EIH	Predictive Value of EIH for LM/3VD (%)	Findings
Gibbons (1987)[65]	820	3	Decrease in SBP at peak exercise ≥ 10 mm Hg from SBP at rest	—	Of 27 patients with EIH, 22 had 3VD or LM CAD; most had decreased EF and wall motion abnormalities with exercise.
Dubach (1988)[48]	2036	6.4	Decrease in SBP during exercise below standing preexercise value	61	EIH was associated with 3.2 times the risk for cardiac events during 2-year follow-up. When defined as drop in SBP of only 20 mm Hg, EIH was not associated with increased risk.
Morrow (1993)[66]	2546	3.1	Fall in SBP below standing rest	—	Degree of decrease or failure to raise SBP graded by 1-4 used as part of multivariate score to predict mortality risk.
Frenneaux (1992)[67]	129 (HCM)	33	Decrease in SBP ≥ 20 mm Hg	—	EIH due to lower systemic vascular resistance at peak exercise.
Iskandrian (1992)[68]	25 (CAD)	—	Decrease in SBP ≥ 20 mm Hg	—	Extent of CAD and thallium ischemia similar between those with and without EIH.

*Percent incidence of EIH among cohort of exercise test referrals.

BP, blood pressure; CABS, coronary artery bypass surgery; CAD, coronary artery disease; DCM, dilated cardiomyopathy; EF, ejection fraction; EIH, exercise-induced hypotension; LM, left main; LV, left ventricular; MI, myocardial infarction; SBP, systolic blood pressure; 3VD, three-vessel disease.

Excessive Rise in Systolic Blood Pressure at Peak Exercise

An excessive rise in systolic blood pressure during an exercise test, frequently termed *exercise-induced hypertension*, has received much less attention than exertional hypotension (Table 3-9). Hypertensive responses, often defined as an increase in systolic blood pressure to levels exceeding 220 to 250 mm Hg, have generally been associated with lower morality rates relative to normal blood pressure responses.[50] Exaggerated systolic blood pressure responses to exercise are more common in elderly subjects and those with hypertension, even when blood pressure is well controlled at rest, and has been suggested to be a predictor of future resting hypertension and the development of left ventricular hypertrophy.[51]

The clinical significance of exercise-induced hypertension has not been fully clarified. This response may be associated with resting hypertension, may be a normal variant, or may have another underlying cause such as a neurogenic abnormality associated with peripheral vascular regulation. The long-standing recommendation in the guidelines to stop an exercise test when systolic blood pressure reaches ≥ 250 mm Hg represents an intuitive and reasonable limit rather than one based on clinical studies.

Exercise-Recovery Ratio for Systolic Blood Pressure

The ratio of systolic blood pressure in recovery to peak exercise systolic blood pressure has been reported to be a marker of CAD. This ratio is not widely used, however, perhaps because the mechanism for this response and

TABLE 3-9 Summary of Major Studies on Significance of Excessive Blood Pressure Responses to Exercise

Investigator	No. Subjects	Incidence of EBP (%)*	Definition of EBP	Findings
Lauer (1995)[50]	9608	33	>210 mm Hg in men, >190 mm Hg in women	EBP associated with lower prevalence of severe CAD and lower mortality rate (RR = 0.2).
Chatterjee (1996)[69]	100	26	Any increase in DBP with exercise	80% of abnormal responders had CAD vs. 45% of normal responders.
Wilson (1990)[70]	35	35	≥230 mm Hg SBP, ≥100 mm Hg DBP	EBP subjects had similar cardiac output responses to exercise, but higher peripheral resistance.
Allison (1999)[71]	150	—	≥214 mm Hg systolic	Subjects with EBP were 3.6 times more likely to have a CV event, and and 2.4 times more like to have future diagnosis of hypertension.
Ha (2002)[51]	132	24	>220 mm Hg SBP in men; >190 SBP in women, or increase in DBP >10 or above 90 mm Hg	82% of those with EBP had positive exercise tests; EBP associated with wall motion abnormalities by echo even in absence of CAD.

*Usually a selected group or including only those referred for angiography. Actual overall incidence of EBP is much lower.
CAD, coronary artery disease; *DBP,* diastolic blood pressure; *EBP,* excessive blood pressure response to exercise; *RR,* relative risk; *SBP,* systolic blood pressure.

its association with disease have not been fully defined. Another problem has been differences in the criteria used and the time point in recovery used to derive the ratio. Several studies have used a ratio of systolic blood pressure at 3 minutes into recovery to peak exercise of 0.90 as a cutoff point for abnormal, and have demonstrated a diagnostic accuracy for CAD similar to that for ST depression.[52,53]

Summary

The increased demand for myocardial oxygen required by dynamic exercise is the key to the use of exercise testing as a diagnostic tool for CAD. Myocardial oxygen consumption cannot be directly measured in a practical manner, but its relative demand can be estimated from its determinants, such as heart rate, wall tension (left ventricular pressure and diastolic volume), contractility, and cardiac work. Although all of these factors increase during exercise, increased heart rate is particularly important in patients who have obstructive CAD. An increase in heart rate results in a shortening of the diastolic filling period, the time during which coronary blood flow is the greatest. In normal coronary arteries, dilation occurs. In obstructed vessels, however, dilation is limited and flow can be decreased by the shortening of the diastolic filling period. This causes inadequate blood flow and therefore insufficient oxygen supply.

Hemodynamic information, including heart rate, blood pressure, and exercise capacity, are important features of the exercise test. Because it can objectively quantify exercise capacity, exercise testing is now commonly used for disability evaluation rather than reliance on functional classifications. No questionnaire or submaximal test can provide as reliable a result as a symptom-limited exercise test. Age-predicted maximal heart rate targets are relatively useless for clinical purposes, and they should not be used for exercise testing endpoints. It is surprising how much steeper the age-related decline in maximal heart rate is in clinically referred populations as compared with age-matched normal subjects or volunteers. Nomograms greatly facilitate the description of exercise capacity relative to age and enable comparisons among patients. However, numerous different regression equations express exercise capacity relative to gender and age.

When expressing exercise capacity as a relative percentage of what is deemed normal, careful consideration should be given to population specificity. Exercise capacity is influenced by many factors other than age and gender, including health, activity level, body composition, and the exercise mode and protocol used. Additional studies are needed to develop normal standards for exercise capacity in women. Although exertional hypotension has been defined in many different ways, it has been shown to predict severe angiographic CAD and is associated with a poor prognosis. A failure of systolic blood pressure to adequately increase is particularly worrisome in patients who have sustained a myocardial infarction. The exercise test should always be stopped when a sustained reduction in systolic pressure occurs. Recent studies have documented the prognostic power of chronotropic incompetence during exercise and the rate at which heart rate recovers following an exercise test. Although many laboratories now routinely include these responses as part of the exercise test report, several methodological issues need to be standardized. The diagnostic and prognostic value of the recovery/peak exercise systolic blood pressure ratio requires further study. Until automated devices are adequately validated, we recommend that blood pressure be taken manually with a cuff and stethoscope.

References

1. Froelicher VF et al: Prediction of maximal oxygen consumption. Comparison of the Bruce and Balke treadmill protocols, *Chest* 68:331-336, 1975.
2. Patterson J et al: Treadmill exercise in assessment of the functional capacity of patients with cardiac disease, *Am J Cardiol* 30:757, 1972.
3. Goldman L, Hashimoto B, Cook EF, Loscaltzo A: Comparative reproducibility and validity of systems for assessing cardiovascular functional class: advantages of a new specific activity scale, *Circulation* 64:1227-1234, 1981.
4. Hlatky M et al: A brief, self-administered questionnaire to determine functional capacity (the Duke Activity Status Index), *Am J Cardiol* 64:651-654, 1989.
5. Myers J et al: A nomogram to predict exercise capacity from a specific activity questionnaire and clinical data, *Am J Cardiol* 73: 591-596, 1994.
6. McKirnan D, Sullivan M, Jensen D, Froelicher VF: Treadmill performance and cardiac function in selected patients with coronary heart disease, *J Am Coll Cardiol* 3:253-261, 1984.
7. Ehsani AA et al: The effects of left ventricular systolic function on maximal aerobic exercise capacity in asymptomatic patients with coronary artery disease, *Circulation* 70:552-560, 1984.
8. Weber KT, Kinasewitz GT, Janicki J, Fishman AP: Oxygen utilization and ventilation during exercise in patients with chronic cardiac failure, *Circulation* 65:1213-1222, 1982.
9. Litchfield RL et al: Normal exercise capacity in patients with severe left ventricular dysfunction: compensatory mechanisms, *Circulation* 66:129-134, 1982.
10. Higginbotham MB et al: Determinants of variable exercise performance among patients with severe left ventricular dysfunction, *Am J Cardiol* 51:52-60, 1983.
11. Wilson J et al: Dissociation between exertional symptoms and circulatory function in patients with heart failure, *Circulation* 92:47-53, 1995.
12. Myers J, Froelicher VF: Hemodynamic determinants of exercise capacity in chronic heart failure, *Ann Intern Med* 115:377-386, 1991.
13. Jette M, Sidney K, Blumchen G: Metabolic equivalents (METs) in exercise testing, exercise prescription, and evaluation of functional capacity, *Clin Cardiol* 13:555-565, 1990.

14. Morris C et al: Nomogram based on metabolic equivalents and age for assessing aerobic capacity in men, *J Am Coll Cardiol* 22:175-182, 1993.
15. Gulati M et al: The prognostic value of a nomogram for exercise capacity in women, *N Engl J Med* 353(5):468-475, 2005.
16. Hammond HK, Froelicher VF: Normal and abnormal heart rate responses to exercise, *Prog Cardiovasc Dis* 27:271-296, 1985.
17. Roberts JM et al: Predicting oxygen uptake from treadmill testing in normal subjects and coronary artery disease patients, *Am Heart J* 108:1454-1460, 1984.
18. McDonough JR, Danielson RA, Willis RE, Vine KL: Maximal cardiac output during exercise in patients with coronary artery disease, *Am J Cardiol* 33:23-29, 1974.
19. Hossack KF, Bruce RA, Kusumi F, Kannagi T: Prediction of maximal cardiac output in preoperative patients with coronary artery disease, *Am J Cardiol* 52(7):721-726, 1983.
20. Wolthuis RA, Froelicher VF Jr, Fischer J, Triebwasser JH: The response of healthy men to treadmill exercise, *Circulation* 55(1):153-157, 1977.
21. Atwood JE et al: Optimal sampling interval to estimate heart rate at rest and during exercise in atrial fibrillation, *Am J Cardiol* 63:45-48, 1989.
22. Londeree BR, Moeschberger ML: Influence of age and other factors on maximal heart rate, *J Card Rehab* 4:44-49, 1984.
23. Froelicher VF et al: A comparison of three maximal treadmill exercise protocols, *J Appl Physiol* 36:720-725, 1974.
24. Graettinger W et al: Influence of left ventricular chamber size on maximal heart rate, *Chest* 107:341-345, 1995.
25. Convertino V et al: Cardiovascular responses to exercise in middle-aged man after 10 days of bedrest, *Circulation* 65:134-140, 1982.
26. Hartley LH, Vogel JA, Cruz JC: Reduction of maximal exercise heart rate at altitude and its reversal with atropine, *J Appl Physiol* 36:362-365, 1974.
27. Noakes TD: Maximal oxygen uptake: "classical" versus "contemporary" viewpoints: a rebuttal, *Med Sci Sports Exerc* 30:1381-1398, 1998.
28. Myers J, Walsh D, Sullivan M, Froelicher VF: Effect of sampling on variability and plateau in oxygen uptake. *J Appl Physiol* 68(1): 404-410, 1990.
29. Ellestad MH, Wan MKC: Predictive implications of stress testing—follow-up of 2700 subjects after maximal treadmill stress testing, *Circulation* 51:363-369, 1975.
30. Lauer M et al: Association of chronotropic incompetence with echocardiographic ischemia and prognosis, *J Am Coll Cardiol* 32(5):1280-1286, 1998.
31. Lauer M et al: Impaired heart rate response to graded exercise: prognostic implications of chronotropic incompetence in the Framingham Heart Study, *Circulation* 93:1520-1526, 1996.
32. Hammond HK, Kelly TL, Froelicher VF: Radionuclide imaging correlates of heart rate impairment during maximal exercise testing, *J Am Coll Cardiol* 2(5):826-833, 1983.

33. Cotton FS, Dill DB: On the relation between the heart rate during exercise and that of immediate post exercise period, *Am J Physiol* 111:544-556, 1935.

34. Imai K et al: Vagally mediated heart rate recovery after exercise is accelerated in athletes but blunted in patients with chronic heart failure, *J Am Coll Cardiol* 24:1529-1535, 1994.

35. Cole CR et al: Heart-rate recovery immediately after exercise as a predictor of mortality, *N Engl J Med* 341:1351-1357, 1999.

36. Cole RC, Foody JM, Blackstone EH, Lauer MS: Heart rate recovery after submaximal exercise testing as a predictor of mortality in a cardiovascularly healthy cohort, *Ann Intern Med* 132:552-555, 2000.

37. Nishime EO et al: Heart rate recovery and treadmill exercise score as predictors of mortality in patients referred for exercise ECG, *JAMA* 284:1392-1398, 2000.

38. Shetler K et al: Heart rate recovery: validation and methodologic issues, *J Am Coll Cardiol* 38:1980-1987, 2001.

39. Bailey RH, Bauer JH: Ambulatory blood pressure measurement, *Arch Intern Med* 153:2741, 1993.

40. Irving JB, Bruce RA, DeRouen TA: Variations in and significance of systolic pressure during maximal exercise (treadmill) testing, *Am J Cardiol* 39(6):841-848, 1977.

41. Myers J et al: Clinical, hemodynamic, and cardiopulmonary exercise test determinants of survival in patients referred for evaluation of heart failure, *Ann Intern Med* 129:286-293, 1998.

42. Erikssen G et al: Exercise testing of healthy men in a new perspective: from diagnosis to prognosis, *Eur Heart J* 25(11):978-986, 2004.

43. Thomson PD, Kelemen MH: Hypotension accompanying the onset of exertional angina, *Circulation* 52:28-32, 1975.

44. Morris SN, Phillips JF, Jordan JW, McHenry PL: Incidence of significance of decreases in systolic blood pressure during graded treadmill exercise testing, *Am J Cardiol* 41:221-226, 1978.

45. Irving JB, Bruce RA: Exertional hypotension and postexertional ventricular fibrillation in stress testing, *Am J Cardiol* 39(6):849-851, 1977.

46. Li W, Riggins R, Anderson R: Reversal of exertional hypotension after coronary bypass grafting, *Am J Cardiol* 44:607-611, 1979.

47. Atwood JE, Kawanashi S, Myers J, Froelicher VF: Exercise testing in patients with aortic stenosis, *Chest* 93:1083-1087, 1988.

48. Dubach P et al: Exercise-induced hypotension in a male population—criteria, causes, and prognosis, *Circulation* 78:1380-1387, 1988.

49. Weiner DA, McCabe CH, Cutler SS, Ryan TJ: Decrease in systolic blood pressure during exercise testing: reproducibility, response to coronary bypass surgery and prognostic significance, *Am J Cardiol* 49:1627-1631, 1982.

50. Lauer MS et al: Angiographic and prognostic implications of an exaggerated exercise systolic blood pressure response and rest systolic blood pressure in adults undergoing evaluation for suspected coronary artery disease, *J Am Coll Cardiol* 26:1630-1636, 1995.

51. Ha JW et al: Hypertensive response to exercise: a potential cause for new wall motion abnormality in the absence of coronary artery disease, *J Am Coll Cardiol* 39:323-327, 2002.

52. Taylor AJ, Beller GA: Postexercise systolic blood pressure response: clinical application to the assessment of ischemic heart disease, *Am Fam Physician* 58(5):1126-1130, 1998.

53. Laukkanen JA et al: Systolic blood pressure during recovery from exercise and the risk of acute myocardial infarction in middle-aged men, *Hypertension* 44:820-825, 2004.

54. Bruce RA, Fisher LD, Hossack KF: Validation of exercise enhanced risk assessment of coronary heart disease events: longitudinal changes in incidence in Seattle community practice, *J Am Coll Cardiol* 5:875-881, 1985.

55. Dehn MM, Bruce RA: Longitudinal variations in maximal oxygen intake with age and activity, *J Appl Physiol* 33:805-807, 1972.

56. Pollock ML, Bohannon RL, Cooper KH et al: A comparative analysis of four protocols for maximal treadmill stress testing. *Am Heart J* 92:39-46, 1976.

57. Astrand PO, Bergh U, Kilborn A: A 33-yr follow-up of peak oxygen uptake and related variables of former physical education students, *J Appl Physiol* 82:1844-1852, 1997.

58. Cooper KH et al: Physical fitness leves vs selected coronary risk factors: A cross-sectional study, *JAMA* 236:166-169, 1976.

59. Lester M, Sheffield LT, Trammell P, Reeves TJ: The effect of age and athletic training on the maximal heart rate during muscular exercise, *Am Heart J* 76:370-376, 1968.

60. Levites R, Baker T, Anderson G: The significance of hypotension developing during treadmill exercise testing, *Am Heart J* 95:747-753, 1978.

61. Sanmarco M, Pontius S, Selvester R: Abnormal blood pressure response and marked ischemic ST-segment depression as predictors of severe coronary artery disease, *Circulation* 61:572-578, 1980.

62. Hammermeister KE, DeRouen TA, Dodge HT, Zia M: Prognostic and predictive value of exertional hypotension in suspected coronary heart disease, *Am J Cardiol* 51:1261-1265, 1983.

63. Hakki AH et al: Determinants of abnormal blood pressure response to exercise in coronary artery disease, *Am J Cardiol* 57:71-75, 1986.

64. Mazzotta G et al: Significance of abnormal blood pressure response during exercise induced myocardial dysfunction after recent acute myocardial infarction, *Am J Cardiol* 59:1256-1260, 1987.

65. Gibbons R, Hu D, Clements I et al: Anatomic and functional significance of a hypotensive response during supine exercise radionuclide ventriculography. *Am J Cardiol* 60:1-4, 1987.

66. Morrow K, Morris CK, Froelicher VF et al: Prediction of cardiovascular death in men undergoing noninvasive evaluation for coronary artery disease. *Ann Intern Med* 118:689-695, 1993.

67. Frenneaux MP, Counihan PJ, Caforio A et al: Abnormal blood pressure response during exercise in hypertrophic cardiomyopathy. *Circulation* 82:1995-2002, 1990.

68. Iskandrian AS, Kegel JG, Lemlek J et al: Mechanism of exercise-induced hypotension in coronary artery disease. *Am J Cardiol* 69:1517-1520, 1992.

69. Chatterjee S, Kumar S, Shetty DP, Panja M: Significance of exercise induced increase in the diastolic pressure as an indicator of severe coronary artery disease, *J Indian Med Assoc* 94:443-444, 451, 1996.

70. Wilson MF, Sung BH, Pincomb GA, Lovallo WR: Exaggerated blood pressure response to exercise in men at risk for systemic hpertension, *Am J Cardiol* 66:731-736, 1990.

71. Allison TG et al: Prognostic significance of exercise-induced systemic hypertension in healthy subjects, *Am J Cardiol* 83:371-375, 1999.

4. Interpretation of the Electrocardiogram

Introduction

This chapter presents information regarding the electrocardiographic (ECG) response to exercise. The three ST-segment responses to exercise associated with ischemia—elevation, normalization, and depression—are presented. Because of the parallel significance and interaction with chest pain, this symptomatic response to exercise testing is discussed as well. Exercise test–induced arrhythmias are the final ECG response to be considered.

Studies of the Electrocardiographic Response to Exercise

The key historical studies describing the ECG response to progressive, dynamic exercise are outlined by the year of their presentation:

1908—Einthoven reported the first attempt to evaluate the response of the electrocardiogram (ECG) to exercise. He made a number of accurate observations in a postexercise ECG, including an increase in the amplitude of the P and T waves and depression of the J junction.[1]

1928—Fiel and Siegel first noted ST depression with exercise.

1930—Masters step test introduced.

1953—Simonson reported the electrocardiographic response to treadmill testing of a wide age range of normal subjects.[2]

1965—Blomqvist reported his classic description of the response of the Frank vectorcardiographic leads to bicycle exercise using computer techniques.[3]

1973—Rautaharju and colleagues[4] analyzed P-, ST-, and T-vector functions in the Frank leads in response to exercise. They reported that all P-wave vector measurements increased during exercise and were compatible with right atrial overload, whereas T-wave vectors decreased slightly. The ST-segment vector shifted clockwise to the right and upward.

1975—Simoons and Hugenholtz[5] reported Frank lead vectorcardiographic changes during exercise in normal subjects. The direction and magnitudes of time-normalized P, QRS, and ST vectors and other QRS parameters were analyzed during and after exercise in 56 apparently healthy men, ages 23 to 62 years. The PR interval and the P-wave amplitude increased during exercise. Direction of the P vectors did not change, differing with previous reports that had noted changes consistent with right atrial overload. No significant change in QRS magnitude was observed, and the magnitude in spatial orientation and the maximum QRS vectors remained constant. QRS onset to T-wave peak shortened. The terminal QRS vectors and the initial ST vectors gradually shortened and shifted to the right and upward. The T-wave amplitude lessened during exercise. In the first minute of recovery, the P and T magnitudes markedly increased, and then all measurements gradually returned to the resting level. There was an increase in S-wave duration in leads X and Y, and right-axis shift in the QRS complex was heart rate dependent. The ST-segment shifted upward to the right and posterior, and T-wave magnitude increased markedly in the first minute of recovery. The QRS complex shortened in some young individuals during exercise.

1979—The United States Air Force Medical Corps (USAFMC) Normal Aircrewmen Study was based on digital data from 40 low-risk normal subjects, processed, and analyzed across treadmill times on the basis of waveform component and lead.[6]

USAFMC Normal Aircrewmen Study

Figure 4-1 illustrates the waveforms produced using median values of the measurements of all 40 subjects for leads V5, aVF (Y), and V2 (Z). These figures demonstrate the specific waveform alterations that occur in response to maximal treadmill exercise. Supine, exercise to a heart rate of 120 beats per minute, maximal exercise, 1-minute recovery, and 5-minute recovery were chosen as representative times. There is depression of the J junction and peaking of the T waves at maximal exercise and at 1-minute recovery. Along with the J-junction depression (QRS end or ST0), marked ST upsloping is seen. J-junction depression did not occur in the Z lead (which is equivalent to and of the same polarity as V2). As the R wave decreases in amplitude, the S wave increases in depth. The QS duration shortens minimally, but the RT duration decreases in a larger amount.

> **Key Point:** Junctional ST depression below the PR isoelectric line is normally seen with increasing heart rate, and early repolarization normally decreases to or below the isoelectric line.

Q-Wave, R-Wave, and S-Wave Amplitudes

In leads CM5, V5, CC5, and Y, the Q wave shows very small changes from the resting values; however, it does become slightly more negative at maximal exercise. Q-wave changes were not noted in the Z lead. Changes in

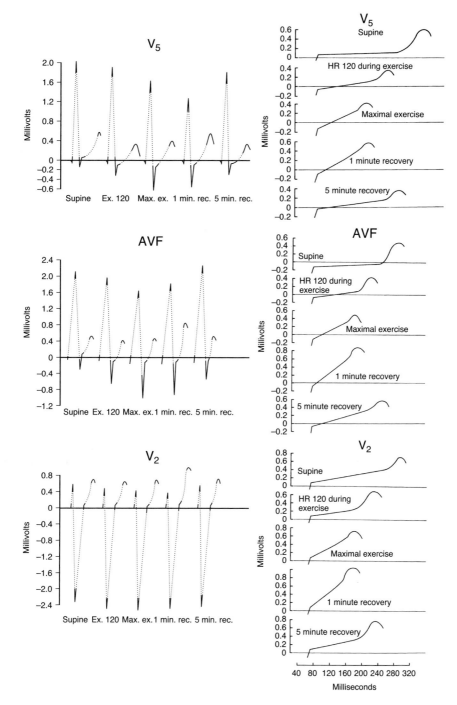

FIGURE 4-1 *The waveforms produced using median values of the measurements of all 40 subjects for leads V5, Y, and Z. These figures demonstrate the specific waveform alterations that occur in response to maximal treadmill exercise. Supine, exercise to a heart rate of 120 beats per minute, maximal exercise, 1-minute recovery, and 5-minute recovery were chosen as representative times for presentation of these median-based simulated waveforms.*

median R-wave amplitude are not detected until near-maximal and maximal effort is approached. At maximal exercise and on into 1-minute recovery, a sharp decrease in R-wave amplitude is observed in CM5, V5, and CC5. These changes are not seen in the Z lead. The lowest median R-wave value in Y occurred at maximal exercise, with R-wave amplitude increasing by 1-minute recovery. In leads CM5, V5, and CC5 the lowest R-wave amplitude was seen at 1-minute recovery. This quite different temporal response in R waves in the lateral versus inferior leads is unexplained. Although there was little change in Z, the S wave became greater in depth or more negative at maximal exercise, and then gradually returned to resting values in recovery. A decrease in the QRS duration occurred that was shortest at maximal exercise, returning to baseline at 3 minutes of recovery. A steady decrease in the duration of the RT interval occurred, with the shortest interval at maximal exercise and 1-minute recovery.

ST Slope, J-Junction Depression, and T-Wave Amplitude

The first amplitude measurement of the ST segment is made at the beginning of the ST segment, known as ST0 or the J junction, and it also is the end of the QRS complex. This measurement has the widest range of responses to changes in heart rate of any ECG waveform, and distinguishing this normal response from its response to ischemia is key to the diagnostic application of the exercise ECG. The amplitude of the J junction in lead Z changed little through exercise, but elevated slightly in recovery. It appears that the lead system affects the anterior-posterior presentation of the ST vector more than anticipated. The J junction was depressed in all other leads to a maximum depression at maximal exercise, and then it gradually returned toward preexercise values slowly in recovery. There was very little difference between the three left precordial leads. A dramatic increase in ST-segment slope was observed in all leads and was greatest at 1-minute recovery.

These changes returned toward pretest values during later recovery. The greatest or steepest slopes were seen in lead CM5, which did not show the greatest ST-segment depression. A gradual decrease in T-wave amplitude was observed in all leads during early exercise. At maximal exercise the T wave began to increase, and at 1-minute recovery the amplitude was equivalent to resting values, except in leads Y and Z where they were greater than at rest.

> **Key Point:** Considerable data are available regarding the normal ECG response to dynamic exercise. Anterior-posterior ST shifts appear to be the most variable ST measurement in normals, possibly due to anatomic differences, making their significance in disease states uncertain.

Controversial ECG Responses to Exercise

R-Wave Changes

R-wave amplitude normally decreases with exercise. It has been suggested that an increase in amplitude is diagnostic of coronary artery disease (CAD).

Data on asymptomatic normals has demonstrated that the R-wave amplitude typically increases from rest to submaximal exercise, perhaps to a heart rate of 140 beats per minute, and then decreases to the maximal exercise endpoint (see Figure 4-1). Therefore if a patient were limited by exercise intolerance, whether because of objective or subjective symptoms or signs, the R-wave amplitude would increase from rest to such an endpoint. Such patients may be demonstrating a normal R-wave response but be classified "abnormal," because the severity of disease results in a lower exercise capacity and heart rate.

> **Key Point:** Exercise-induced changes in R-wave amplitude have no independent predictive power. They are associated with CAD because patients with coronary disease are often submaximally tested, at which point R-wave amplitude normally increases from baseline. If exercised further to higher intensity, the normal decrease in R wave at maximal exercise is usually observed.

Percent R-Wave Changes

Figure 4-2 illustrates the percent change of R-wave amplitude for each individual compared with R wave at supine rest in V5 and lead Y (similar to leads II or aVF). At lower exercise heart rates, the great variability in the R-wave response was apparent, and many normal individuals had significant increases in R-wave amplitude. Though most showed a decline at maximum exercise, some normal subjects had an increase, whereas others showed very little decrease. At 1-minute recovery there was a greater tendency toward a decline in lead V5 but not in Y. Further into recovery, R-wave amplitude remained decreased in lead V5 but increased in Y.

S-Wave Changes

During exercise there is an increase in the S wave in the lateral precordial leads. It was hypothesized that this increase in the S wave reflects the normal increase in cardiac contractility during exercise and that its absence is indicative of ventricular dysfunction. It is also possible that the increase in S wave is caused by exercise-induced axis shifts and conduction alterations.

U-Wave Changes

In 1980, Gerson and co-workers[7] reported on 248 patients who underwent exercise testing with leads CC5 and VL monitored, 36 of whom had exercise-induced U-wave inversion. Of 71 patients with significant left anterior descending or left main disease and no prior myocardial infarction (MI), 35% had U-wave inversion compared with only 4% of 57 patients without left anterior descending or left main disease and only 1% of 82 patients who had no CAD. Kodama and colleagues[8] performed treadmill tests on 60 patients with angina pectoris whose culprit lesion was located only in the left anterior descending artery. They concluded that the exercise-induced U-wave inversion in patients with one-vessel disease of the left anterior descending

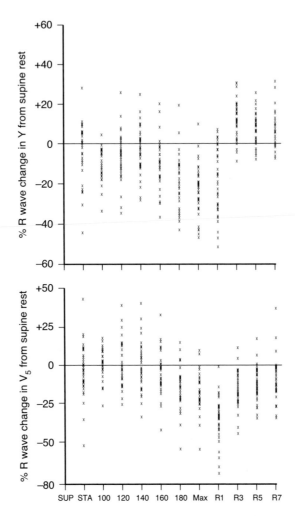

FIGURE 4-2 *R-wave changes relative to heart rate during progressive treadmill exercise in a group of low-risk normal individuals. This figure illustrates the percent change of R-wave amplitude for each individual compared with his R-wave at supine rest in V5 and Y.*

artery indicates the severe degree of myocardial ischemia induced in the territory perfused by the left anterior descending artery. However, it did not have independent significance because it closely correlates with the presence of ST-segment shift. Hayat and colleagues[9] reported exercise-induced positive U waves to be an infrequent but specific marker of significant single coronary (circumflex or right) artery stenosis that disappeared after percutaneous coronary intervention (PCI). In a study of 20 patients recovering from an anterior wall MI, Miwa and colleagues[10] concluded that exercise-induced negative U waves in precordial leads were a specific marker for the presence of viable myocardium. These authors also concluded that exercise-induced U-wave alterations were a marker for well-developed collateral circulation in patients with stable but severe effort angina.[11]

> **Key Point:** Exercise-induced U-wave inversion appears to be a rare but specific indicator for myocardial ischemia.

Abnormal ST-Segment Changes

Epicardial electrode mapping usually records ST-segment elevation over areas of severe ischemia and ST-segment depression over areas of lesser ischemia. ST-segment depression is the reciprocal of the injury effect occurring in the endocardium as viewed from an electrode overlying normal epicardium. ST-segment elevation seen from the same electrode reflects transmural injury or, less frequently, epicardial injury. On the ECG recorded from the skin, exercise-induced myocardial ischemia can result in one of three ST-segment manifestations: elevation, normalization, or depression. These are discussed in depth in the following sections.

ST-Segment Elevation

The most common ECG abnormality seen in the exercise laboratory is ST-segment depression, whereas ST elevation is relatively rare (Table 4-1). Its prevalence depends on the population tested, but it occurs more frequently in patients who have had a Q-wave MI.[12-15] Sriwattanakomen and colleagues[16] reviewed 1620 exercise tests and found 3.8% to have ST-segment elevation when all leads except aVR were evaluated. Longhurst and Kraus[17] reviewed 6040 consecutive exercise tests and found 106 patients (1.8%) without previous MIs who had exercise-induced ST-segment elevation.

Waters and colleagues[18] reported that 47 of 720 patients who underwent treadmill testing developed ST elevation. Chahine and colleagues[14] found 29 patients with ST-segment elevation among 840 patients who had an exercise test. Bruce and colleagues[19] reported a prevalence of 0.5% in the Seattle Heart Watch Study in 1974, but later Bruce and Fisher[20] reported a prevalence of 5% in 1136 patients observed in Seattle community practice. De Feyter and colleagues,[21] in their study of 680 patients, reported a prevalence of 1%, but a multilead system was not used. The Coronary Artery Surgery Study registry data were compared with the results of the Seattle Heart Watch Study, and the 6-year mortality rate for patients with ST elevation was found to be significantly higher than that for patients with ST depression (29% vs. 14%).[22] Braat and colleagues[23] found lead V4R ST elevation to be associated with stenosis of the right coronary artery.

Simoons and Withagen[24] investigated the spatial orientation of exercise-induced ST-segment changes in relation to the presence of dyskinetic areas, as demonstrated by left ventriculography. ST-segment elevation occurred over dyskinetic areas. In patients with dyskinetic areas, the direction of the ST-segment changes varied so widely that only the

TABLE 4-1   Studies of Exercise-Induced ST-Segment Elevation during Standard Clinical Testing

Study	Size of Population Tested	Type of Population	Percent Population with Prior MI	No. of Leads Measured for Elevation	Criteria for Elevation	Prevalence of Abnormal Elevation (%)	Percent Prior MI in Patients with Elevation
Bruce (1988)	3050	Angina	47	11	1 mm	4.7	83
Bruce (1974)	1136	CHD	47	CB_5	>0	0.5	57
Sriwattankomen (1980)	1620	All referred	—	11	1 mm	3.8	47
Longhurst (1979)	6040	All referred	—	12 + XYZ	0.5 mm	1.6	0
Chahine (1976)	840	VAMC	—	V_5, V_6	1 mm	3.5	80
Stiles (1980)	650	541 patients with ST-segment depression vs.109 with ST-segment elevation	10	11	1 mm	4	61
Waters (1980)	720	Mixed	1	12/CM_5	—	6.5	76

From Nostratian FJ, Froelicher VF: Exercise-induced ST elevation, *Am J Cardiol* 63:986-987, 1989. *All referred,* all patients referred to exercise lab; *CB_5,* V_5 positive electrode placement, negative electrode on the back; *CHD,* coronary heart disease; *CM_5,* V_5 positive electrode placement, negative electrode on the top of the manubrium; *MI,* myocardial infarction; *VAMC,* Veterans Affairs Medical Center.

magnitude of the changes could be used as a criterion for exercise-induced ischemia. Dunn and colleagues[25] performed exercise thallium scans on 35 patients with exercise-induced ST-segment elevation and coronary artery obstruction. Without a previous infarct, they found ST-segment elevation to indicate the site of severe transient ischemia; associated ST-segment depression was usually reciprocal. In patients with Q waves, exercise-induced ST-segment elevation may be due to ischemia around the infarct, abnormal wall motion, or both. Association ST-segment depression may be due to a second area of ischemia rather than being reciprocal. Mark and colleagues[26] studied 452 consecutive patients with one-vessel disease who underwent treadmill testing to determine if patterns of ST depression or elevation during exercise testing provide reliable information about the location of an underlying coronary lesion. They found ST elevation during exercise testing, although uncommon, to be a reliable guide to the underlying coronary lesion, whereas ST depression was not.

Methods of ST Elevation Measurement

ST-segment depression is measured from the isoelectric baseline, or when ST-segment depression is present at rest, the amount of additional depression is measured. However, ST-segment elevation is always considered from the baseline ST level. Whether the elevation occurs over or adjacent to Q waves or in non–Q-wave areas is important. Unfortunately, many of the studies do

TABLE 4-2   Some Factors in Assessing Studies of Exercise-Induced ST-Segment Elevation

Population tested (prevalence of patients with myocardial infarction, variant angina, or spasm)
Baseline (resting) ECG
ECG leads monitored
Leads in which elevation occurs relative to Q waves
Criteria for measuring elevation
Methods of ST-shift detection (visual or computerized)

not provide the methods of measurement or the condition of the underlying ECG. Table 4-2 lists some of the factors that should be considered when assessing studies of ST elevation. Figure 4-3 illustrates the points of measurement.

Is ST Elevation Caused by Ischemia or Wall Motion Abnormality?

There is controversy regarding whether ischemia[27] or wall motion abnormalities[28] are the major cause of ST-segment elevation. ST elevation can occur in patients with normal coronary arteries who develop spasm and have an excellent prognosis.[29,30] It has been reported that exercise-induced ST elevation can be abolished by coronary bypass surgery.[31]

The major studies are summarized in Table 4-1. Figure 4-4 is an example of ST elevation in a normal baseline ECG. Figure 4-5 illustrates the typical ST elevation over Q waves that occurs after an MI. This patient is unusual in that the elevation occurs in multiple areas.

> **Key Point:** In patients with ST elevation during exercise when no abnormal Q wave is seen on the baseline ECG, there is a very high likelihood of a significant proximal narrowing in the coronary artery supplying the area where it occurs. It is also more likely to be associated with serious arrhythmias. When elevation occurs in an ECG with abnormal Q waves, it is usually due to a wall motion abnormality, but the elevation can conceal ischemic ST depression.

ST-Segment Normalization or Absence of Change

Another manifestation of ischemia can be no change or normalization of the ST segment because of cancellation effects. ECG abnormalities at rest, including T-wave inversion and ST-segment depression, have been reported to return to normal during attacks of angina and during exercise in some patients with ischemic heart disease. This cancellation effect is a rare occurrence, but it should be kept in mind. The ST segment and the T wave represent the portion of ventricular repolarization that is not cancelled. Because ventricular geometry can be roughly approximated by a hollow ellipsoid open at one end, the widespread cancellation of the relatively slowly dispersing electrical forces during repolarization is understandable.

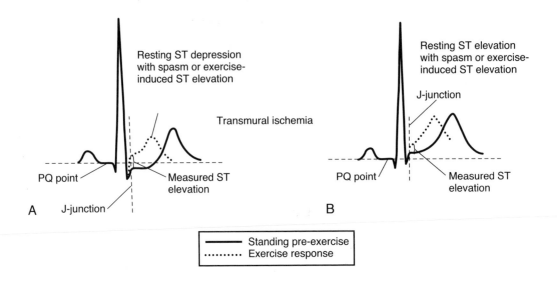

Resting ST depression
with spasm or exercise-
induced ST elevation

Transmural ischemia

PQ point

Measured ST
elevation

A   J-junction

Resting ST elevation
with spasm or exercise-
induced ST elevation

J-junction

PQ point

Measured ST
elevation

B

——— Standing pre-exercise
·········· Exercise response

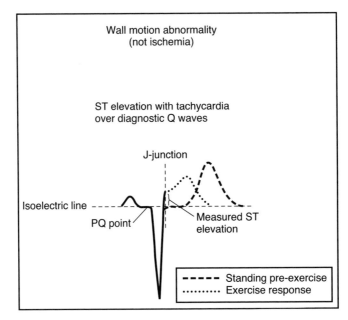

Wall motion abnormality
(not ischemia)

ST elevation with tachycardia
over diagnostic Q waves

J-junction

Isoelectric line

PQ point

Measured ST
elevation

– – – – – Standing pre-exercise
·········· Exercise response

FIGURE 4-3   *An illustration of the points of measurement of ST elevation in the presence and absence of Q waves and ST abnormalities at rest.*

Patients with severe CAD would be most likely to have cancellation occur, yet they have the highest prevalence of abnormal tests.[32,33]

Key Point: This normalization of ST-segment depression can be due to ischemic ST-segment elevation when accompanied by ischemic chest pain, an abnormal perfusion scan, or abnormal exercise echocardiography.

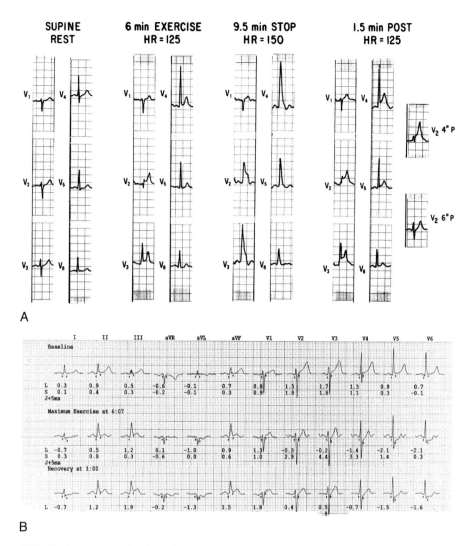

FIGURE 4-4 *Example of ST elevation in two patients with a normal resting ECG.* **A,** *The anterior ST elevation is due to transmural anterior ischemia associated with a tight proximal left anterior descending coronary artery lesion that responded to percutaneous coronary intervention (PCI).* **B,** *The inferior ST elevation with reciprocal lateral depression is due to a total right coronary artery occlusion.*

ST-Segment Depression

The most common manifestation of exercise-induced myocardial ischemia is ST-segment depression. The standard criterion for this type of abnormal response is horizontal or downward sloping ST-segment depression of 0.1 mV or more for 60 to 80 msec. It appears to be due to generalized subendocardial ischemia. A "steal" phenomenon is likely from ischemic areas because of the effect of extensive collateralization in the subendocardium. ST depression does not localize the area of ischemia, as

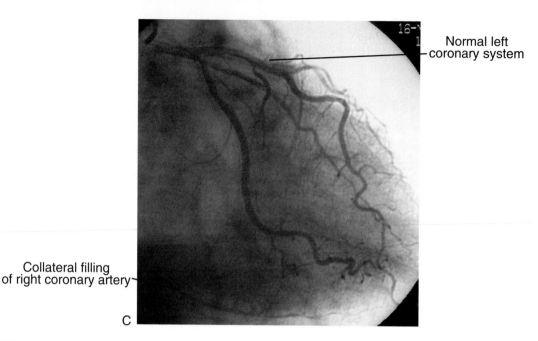

Normal left coronary system

Collateral filling of right coronary artery

C

FIGURE 4-4—Cont'd *C, The left coronary angiogram showing a normal left coronary system with collateral filling of the distal right coronary artery found in the patient in part B.*

does ST elevation, or help to indicate which coronary artery is occluded. The normal ST-segment vector response to tachycardia and to exercise is a shift rightward and upward. The degree of this shift appears to have a fair amount of biologic variation. Most normal individuals will have early repolarization at rest, which will shift to the isoelectric PR-segment line in the inferior, lateral, and anterior leads with exercise. This shift can be further influenced by ischemia and myocardial scars. When the later portions of the ST segment are affected, flattening or downward depression can be recorded. Both local effects and the direction of the spatial changes during repolarization cause the ST segment to have a different appearance at the many surface sites that can be monitored. The more leads with these apparent ischemic shifts, the more severe the disease.

The probability and severity of CAD are directly related to the amount of J-junction depression and are inversely related to the slope of the ST segment. Downsloping ST-segment depression is more serious than is horizontal depression, and both are more serious than upsloping depression. However, patients with upsloping ST-segment depression, especially when the slope is less than 1 mV/sec, probably are at increased risk. If a slowly ascending slope is used as a criterion for abnormal, the specificity of exercise testing will be decreased (more false positives), although the test may become more sensitive. One lead can show upsloping ST depression while

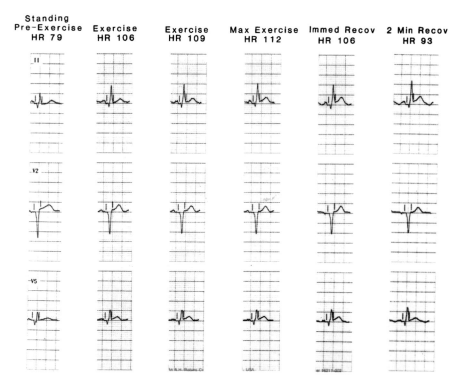

| Standing Pre-Exercise HR 79 | Exercise HR 106 | Exercise HR 109 | Max Exercise HR 112 | Immed Recov HR 106 | 2 Min Recov HR 93 |

FIGURE 4-5 *Example of ST-segment elevation in a patient with an ECG exhibiting Q waves due to an inferior-lateral MI.*

an adjacent lead shows horizontal or downsloping depression. If an apparently borderline ST segment with an inadequate slope is recorded in a single precordial lead in a patient highly suspected of having CAD, multiple precordial leads should be scanned before the exercise test is called normal. An upsloping depressed ST segment may be the precursor to abnormal ST-segment depression in the recovery period or at higher heart rates during greater workloads. It is preferable to call tests with an inadequate ST-segment slope but with ST-segment depression a borderline response, but added emphasis should be placed on other clinical and exercise responses. Examples of the various criteria for ischemic ST depression are shown in Figure 4-6.

> **Key Point:** Classic ST-segment depression criteria for ischemia is 1 mm or greater (0.1 mV, 100 μV) of horizontal or downsloping ST depression, either from the PR isoelectric line or from the ST level at rest if the ST segment is below the PR isoelectric line.

ST Depression in Recovery
Because of technical limitations, the first diagnostic use of the exercise ECG involved observations made only after exercise. After ECG techniques were developed that made accurate ECG recording possible during activity, the

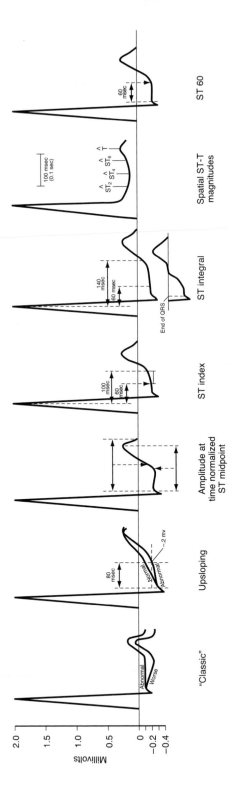

FIGURE 4-6 *Examples of the various criteria for ischemic ST-segment depression proposed by various researchers.*

emphasis in testing shifted to changes occurring during the exercise period itself. It even was proposed that such changes are more likely to represent false-positive responses[34] or are due to coronary artery spasm.[35] To facilitate imaging as soon as possible during recovery, studies including the add-on procedures of nuclear perfusion and echocardiography sometimes do not include an ECG evaluation done after exercise.[36] Though a cool-down walk is known to obscure recovery ST shifts,[37] a cool-down walk has been recommended for safety concerns.[38]

To resolve these issues, we selected patients from a group of 3351 who underwent routine clinical exercise testing.[39] Thirty percent of this group underwent coronary angiography within 3 months of testing. After excluding females, patients with an MI, individuals with prior coronary intervention, and those with left bundle branch block, 271 patients remained. Most were referred for testing because of chest pain syndromes; the remainder were tested for exercise capacity evaluation or miscellaneous other reasons.

Abnormal responders were divided into "exercise only," "recovery only," and "abnormal in both exercise and recovery" as exclusive groups. In addition, "all abnormal" included those abnormal at any time (i.e., all of the above); "abnormal in exercise" was defined as all tests that were abnormal during exercise (i.e., "exercise only" plus "exercise and recovery"), as if only the ECG was monitored during exercise; and "abnormal in recovery" was defined as all tests that were abnormal in recovery (i.e., "recovery only" plus "exercise and recovery"), as if the ECG was monitored only during recovery. This issue was addressed mainly by comparison of the "all abnormal" and "abnormal in exercise" groups.

Of the 271 patients, 107 had no coronary lesion of 75% or greater narrowing, 119 had one- or two-vessel disease, and 45 had left main or three-vessel disease. The mean age of the total population was 59 years, and more than half had typical angina pectoris. Overall, 21% were taking beta blockers and 12% were taking digoxin. Table 4-3 describes the patterns of ST responses observed. Of the 271 patients, 138 (51%) had abnormal ST responses; 20 (7%) had abnormal ST-segment responses in recovery only; 16 (6%) had abnormal ST-segment responses during "exercise only"; and 102 (38%) had abnormal ST responses both during exercise and recovery.

As shown in Table 4-3, there are few meaningful differences in the clinical features associated with the five patterns of ST depression. Those with a normal response were the youngest. As expected, angina during the test was significantly more common in those with ST depression than in those without, but over half of the patients with ST depression exhibited silent ischemia. Differences in maximal ST depression during and after exercise were consistent with the criteria for each group. In the "recovery only" group, the mean value for ST depression during exercise was 1.3 mm but the slopes were upward in those with 1 mm or more depression, and none was abnormal by standard criteria during exercise.

Other Studies Evaluating "Recovery Only" Changes

Several earlier studies considered ST-segment changes occurring in recovery only. The Program of Surgical Control of Hyperlipidemia (POSCH) data set

TABLE 4-3 Clinical and Exercise Variables in LBVAMC Study of Performance of Temporal Patterns of ST-Segment Depression for Predicting Angiographically Documented Coronary Artery Disease

	Normal ST Responses (133 Patients)	Abnormal ST Responses					
		Exercise or Recovery (138 Patients)	Exercise without Recovery Considered (188 Patients)	Recovery without Exercise Considered (122 Patients)	Exercise and Recovery (102 Patients)	Exercise Only (16 Patients)	Recovery Only (20 Patients)
Age (years)	58 ± 9	61 ± 8	61 ± 8	61 ± 7	61 ± 7	62 ± 9	62 ± 7
Drugs used (%)							
Beta blocker	19	23	22	24	23	19	30
Digoxin	14	10	12	10	12	13	0
Chest pain at presentation (%)							
Typical	42	61	63	62	63	56	50
Atypical	35	26	23	25	22	31	45
None or noncardiac	23	13	14	13	15	13	5
Chest pain during exercise (%)	21	53	53	52	53	56	50 ($p < 0.01$)
ST-segment depression (mm)							
Exercise	0.3 ± 0.7	2.1 ± 1.0	2.3 ± 0.9	2.2 ± 1.0	2.4 ± 1.0	1.7 ± 0.6	1.3 ± 0.8
Recovery	0.3 ± 0.6	1.9 ± 1.0	2.0 ± 1.0	2.1 ± 0.9	2.0 ± 0.9	0.7 ± 0.6	1.6 ± 0.6
Hemodynamic values (METs)	7 ± 3	7 ± 3	7 ± 3	7 ± 3	8 ± 3	7 ± 3	7 ± 3
Maximal heart rate (beats/min)	129 ± 24	129 ± 19	128 ± 18	129 ± 18	128 ± 17	132 ± 2	135 ± 22
Maximal systolic blood pressure (mm Hg)	171 ± 30	167 ± 28	166 ± 28	167 ± 28	165 ± 28	167 ± 30	173 ± 27
Maximal double product (×10)	22 ± 6	22 ± 5	21 ± 5	22 ± 5	21 ± 5	22 ± 6	24 ± 6
Cardiac catheterization values							
Vessels with ≥75% stenosis	1.5	1.7	1.7	1.8	1.8	1.0	1.5 ($p < 0.001$)
Ejection fraction (%)	67	66	66	65	65	72	67

was used for one such analysis and as baseline evaluation included both treadmill exercise testing and coronary angiography. Karnegis and colleagues[40] investigated hemodynamic, angiographic, and ECG variables in subjects whose diagnostic ECG changes appeared during exercise rather than during recovery. The authors concluded that the same clinical significance should be attributed to abnormal ST responses that occur during recovery, and that ECG, hemodynamic, and catheterization variables do not distinguish between subjects who exhibit these two different temporal responses. Savage and colleagues[41] evaluated 2000 exercise tests and identified 62 patients (3.2%) who developed 1 mm or more horizontal or downsloping ST-segment depression in the recovery period despite a normal ST response during exercise. They concluded that isolated postexercise ST-segment depression was usually associated with CAD, often multivessel disease.

At the School of Aerospace Medicine, we considered patterns of ST-segment depression in two groups of asymptomatic men undergoing screening exercise testing; one group underwent coronary angiography and the other group was followed for 5 years for cardiac events.[42] Maximal treadmill testing was performed with only bipolar CC5 lead monitored with patients supine after exercise. ST interpretation was the same as in the current study. As shown in Table 4-4, "recovery only" ST-segment depression had a similar predictive value as other patterns.

Ellestad[43] commented on patients who do not have ST-segment depression with or immediately after exercise, but who develop changes 3 to 8 minutes later. In a follow-up of 308 subjects, he found this response to be a definite but weak predictor of subsequent coronary events. He contrasted them with a normal group who had ST depression at rest, returned to normal with exercise, and again developed ST depression late in recovery. The Baltimore Longitudinal Study of Aging group analyzed the treadmill tests of 825 healthy volunteers who were 22 to 89 years of age.[44] Ischemic ST-segment changes

TABLE 4-4 Analysis of Predictive Value of Various Patterns of ST-Segment Depression from Screening Asymptomatic Aircrewmen

ST Depression Occurrence Time	140 Men with Abnormal ST Response in Follow-up Study			111 Men with Abnormal ST Response in Angiographic Study	
	Occurrence Rate (%)	Risk Ratio*	Predictive Value (%)	Occurrence Rate (%)	Predictive Value (%)
Exercise only	9	7	23	11	8
Recovery only	36	4	12	42	28
Exercise and recovery	55	12	25	47	39
All abnormal responders	100	14	20	100	30

*Relative risk for cardiac events during follow-up observation compared with that for normal responders.

NOTE: Recovery-only ST-segment depression had a predictive value similar to that of other patterns.

developing during recovery in these apparently healthy individuals had the same adverse prognostic significance as we found in the U.S. Air Force. At an Italian university hospital, clinical and angiographic data were compared for 574 consecutive patients who developed ST-segment depression during the exercise test and for 79 patients who developed ST-segment depression only during the recovery.[45] There were no differences between the two groups in major clinical features. Significant coronary artery stenoses were found in 488 of the 574 patients (85%) and in 62 of the 79 patients (78%). Three-vessel or left main disease was found in 29% vs.18%. After 4 years, there were no significant differences in major cardiac events between the groups.

Conclusions Regarding ST Depression during Recovery

Abnormal ST depression occurring only in recovery provides clinically useful information and is not more likely to represent a false-positive response. When considered together with changes in exercise, changes in recovery increase the sensitivity of the exercise test without a decline in predictive value. A cool-down walk should be avoided after exercise testing, and exercise test scores and nuclear testing should consider recovery ST measurements. Avoidance of a cool-down walk has not resulted in an increased complication rate. The importance of recovery measurements made by computer was consistent with previous experience from visual analysis. That is, recovery changes are not generally false positives as previously thought and they have excellent diagnostic value. Also, the receiver operating characteristic (ROC) curve values for other ST measurements in recovery tended to be greater than comparable measurements during maximal exercise. The recovery period is probably so important because the conflicting impact of increasing heart rate during exercise "pulling" up the ST segment (resulting in a trend toward a positive slope) is no longer present. It is important to have the patient lie down immediately after exercise and not perform a cool-down walk for the recovery measurement to function as it did in our studies.

> **Key Point:** Abnormal ST-segment depression occurring only in recovery and not exercise has the same association with ischemia as ST depression only during exercise.

R-Wave Amplitude Adjustment

The degree of exercise-induced ST depression can be influenced by R-wave amplitude, and perhaps should be normalized to a standard voltage. Prior studies have suggested that adjusting ST-depression measurements by R-wave amplitudes may yield greater diagnostic results than ST-depression measurements alone.[46] The reason is that patients with small R-wave amplitudes do not manifest as much ST depression with exercise despite the presence of CAD, whereas patients with large R-wave amplitudes would have exaggerated ST changes.[47] The average "gain factor" correction of R-wave amplitude should be approximately 25 mm (i.e., average R-wave voltage in V5). In the studies by Hollenberg and colleagues,[48] the magnitude of ST-segment depression was calibrated to standard R-wave amplitude of 12 mm in lead

V5 and 8 mm in lead aVF. Hakki and colleagues[49] in Finland studied the influence of exercise R-wave amplitude on ST-segment depression in 81 patients with coronary disease and found perfusion scans to be helpful to improve the sensitivity of the test in patients with low R-wave amplitude.

> **Key Point:** R-wave amplitude adjustment of any ST measurement does not improve the diagnostic performance of the exercise test.

Resting ST-Segment Displacement

ST-segment elevation on a resting ECG is a common and usually a healthy phenomenon. Although it is called "early repolarization," it most likely is late depolarization. It is usually most prominent with bradycardia and normally sinks to the isoelectric line with tachycardia. Figure 4-7 is an illustration of exercise-induced ST depression and elevation on a baseline ECG with early repolarization. Abnormal elevation is measured from the upward shift from the baseline level (normally the ST segment sinks with increasing heart rate). Abnormal depression is measured only from where it crosses the isoelectric line. The drop from baseline elevation is not counted as abnormal. Figure 4-8 illustrates how ST shifts are measured when the baseline ECG shows depression. The additional depression is measured from the baseline level of the ST segment and not from the isoelectric line. Elevation is measured from the baseline depression and can actually result in "normalization" of the ST segment.

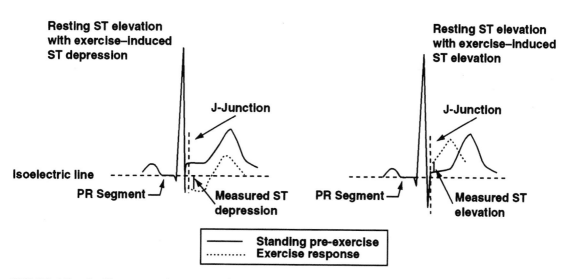

FIGURE 4-7   *An illustration of exercise-induced ST-segment depression and elevation on a baseline ECG with early repolarization.*

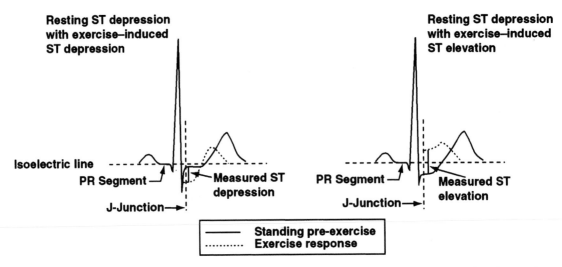

FIGURE 4-8 *An illustration of exercise-induced ST-segment depression and elevation on a baseline ECG with ST-segment depression.*

Exercise-Induced ST-Segment Depression Not Caused by Coronary Artery Disease

Table 4-5 lists some of the conditions that can possibly result in false-positive responses. In a population with a high prevalence of heart disease other than CAD, an abnormal ST response would be as diagnostic for that disease as it would be for CAD in populations with a high prevalence of CAD. Digitalis and other drugs can cause exercise-induced repolarization abnormalities in normal individuals. Patients who have had abnormal responses and who have anemia, have electrolyte abnormalities, or are on medications that affect the ST segment should be retested when these conditions are altered. Meals can alter the ST segment and T wave in the resting ECG and can potentially cause a false-positive response. To avoid this problem, all ECG studies should be performed after at least a 4-hour fast. This requirement is

TABLE 4-5   Some Conditions That Can Result in False-Positive Responses

Valvular heart disease	Left ventricular hypertrophy
Congenital heart disease	Wolff-Parkinson-White syndrome
Vasoregulatory abnormality	Preexcitation variants
Cardiomyopathies	Mitral valve prolapse syndrome
Pericardial disorders	Hyperventilation repolarization abnormality
Drug administration	Hypertension
Electrolyte abnormalities	Excessive double product
Bundle branch block	Improper lead systems
Nonfasting state	Incorrect criteria
Anemia	Improper interpretation
Sudden excessive exercise	Interventricular conduction defect with T-wave
Inadequate recording equipment	inversion

also important because of the hemodynamic stress put on the cardiovascular system by eating—after eating, exercise capacity is decreased and angina occurs at lower hemodynamic stress levels.

Women

Gender has an effect on the exercise ECG that is not explained by hormones alone. Estrogen given to men does not increase the rate of false-positive responses.[50] It has been suggested that the lower specificity of exercise-induced ST-segment depression in women is due to hemodynamic or hemoglobin concentration differences. The diagnostic characteristics of exercise-induced ST-segment depression in women are discussed in Chapter 5. It appears that exercise-induced ST depression is more common in adolescent girls than boys.[51]

Digoxin

Sundqvist and colleagues[52] reported the effect of digoxin on the ECG at rest and during and after exercise in 11 healthy subjects. Exercise was performed on a heart rate–controlled bicycle ergometer with stepwise increased loads up to a heart rate of 170 beats per minute. The subjects were studied after digoxin at two dose levels and after withdrawal of digoxin. Administration of digoxin induced significant ST-T depression at rest and during exercise even at the small dose. The ST-T changes were numerically small and dose dependent. There was usually junctional depression and no downsloping, but six individuals had as much as 1 mm of ST depression. The most pronounced ST depression occurred at a heart rate of 110 to 130 beats per minute. At higher heart rates the ST depression was less pronounced but still statistically significant. During the first minutes after exercise, no significant digitalis-induced ST-T depression was seen. This type of reaction is not usually seen in myocardial ischemia. Fourteen days after withdrawal of the drug, there were no significant digitalis-induced ST-T changes. In a subsequent study in 20 normal individuals, the authors concluded that the digoxin-induced ST depression during exercise mimics exercise-induced changes in patients with CAD, but could be discerned by the analysis of ST/HR loops.[53] This is in agreement with observations by Tonkon and associates,[54] who studied 15 normal subjects, before and after the administration of digoxin, with exercise testing. Fourteen subjects developed 0.1 to 0.5 mV of ST-segment depression with exercise, but the ST segments normalized at maximal exercise and remained normal throughout recovery. Sketch and co-workers[55] studied 98 healthy men, ages 22 to 70 years, who were administered digoxin at 0.25 mg per day for 14 days and then underwent daily exercise testing until it was interpreted as normal. Twenty-four subjects had an abnormal ST response to exercise, and in 20 of them the ST-segment depression resolved less than 4 minutes into recovery.

Key Point: Digoxin has been shown to produce abnormal ST depression in response to exercise in one third of apparently healthy individuals.[56] The prevalence of abnormal responses is directly related to age—perhaps digoxin uncovers subclinical coronary disease.

Left Bundle Branch Block

Whinnery and associates[57] reported 31 asymptomatic men who serially developed left bundle branch block (LBBB) and who were studied with both maximal treadmill testing and coronary angiography. They demonstrated that there could be a marked degree of exercise-induced ST-segment depression in addition to that found at rest in healthy men with LBBB. No difference was found between the ST-segment response to exercise in those with or those without significant CAD. Thus the ST-segment response to exercise testing cannot be used to make diagnostic decisions in patients with LBBB. Ellestad's group reported exercise testing in 41 patients with LBBB.[58] Seven were nonischemic and 34 had coronary artery obstruction. ST depression greater than 0.5 mm from baseline when measured at the J point in leads II and aVF and an increase of R-wave amplitude in lead II were associated with ischemia.

Exercise-Induced Left Bundle Branch Block   The records of 2584 consecutive patients who underwent both treadmill testing and coronary angiography were reviewed to determine the relation between exercise-induced acceleration-dependent LBBB and the presence of CAD.[59] Rate-dependent LBBB during exercise was identified in 28 patients (1.1%), who were categorized according to their symptoms: classic angina pectoris, atypical chest pain, symptomatic arrhythmias, and asymptomatic. Asymptomatic individuals were being screened for silent CAD. CAD was present in 7 of 10 patients who had classic angina pectoris, but 12 of 13 patients with atypical chest pain had normal coronary arteries. All 10 patients in whom LBBB developed at a heart rate of 125 beats per minute or higher were free of CAD, whereas 9 of 18 patients in whom LBBB developed at a heart rate of less than 125 beats per minute had CAD. Normal coronary arteries were present in three patients with angina and in whom both chest pain and LBBB developed during exercise. The authors reached the following conclusions: (1) patients with atypical chest pain and rate-dependent LBBB are significantly less likely to have CAD than patients with classic angina; (2) the onset of LBBB at a heart rate of 125 beats per minute or higher is highly associated with the presence of normal coronary arteries, regardless of patient presentation; and (3) patients with angina in whom both chest pain and LBBB develop during exercise may have normal coronary arteries.

At Mayo Clinic, the estimated prevalence of the development of transient LBBB during exercise is 0.5%.[60] In a matched control cohort study, 70 cases of exercise-induced LBBB were identified and matched with 70 controls based on age, test date, sex, prior history of CAD, hypertension, diabetes, smoking, and beta-blocker use. A total of 37 events occurred in 25 patients during a mean follow-up period of 3.7 years. There were seven deaths, of which five occurred among patients with exercise-induced LBBB. Exercise-induced LBBB independently was associated with a threefold higher risk of death and major cardiac events.

> **Key Point:** LBBB at rest or exercise-induced LBBB is an ominous finding; however, it makes the analysis of ST shifts during exercise meaningless.

Right Bundle Branch Block

We reported the response to maximal treadmill testing of 40 asymptomatic men with acquired right bundle branch block at the USAFSAM.[61] There was no exercise-induced ST-segment depression in the inferior and lateral leads but there frequently was in the anterior precordial leads. This is most apparent in the right precordial leads with an rSR' or a notched R wave; these leads often show a downsloping ST segment at rest, and such a finding is thus not indicative of myocardial ischemia. Figure 4-9 shows ST depression in the lateral leads in patients with angina, and Figure 4-10 shows no ST depression in the lateral leads in a patient without coronary heart disease, both with anterior ST depression.

Wolfe-Parkinson-White Syndrome

Wolfe-Parkinson-White syndrome (WPW) is a conduction disturbance in which atrial impulses are transmitted to the ventricle by an accessory pathway in addition to normal atrioventricular conduction. The result of depolarization reaching the ventricles by two wave fronts is the delta wave (ventricular activation due to the accessory pathway), a short PR interval, and a widened QRS complex.[62] During exercise, increases in sympathetic tone, decreases in vagal tone, and subsequent changes in the automaticity of conductive tissues may result in ECG changes. ST-segment depression simulating ischemia occurs in approximately 50% of patients.[63,64] Pappone and colleagues[65] have proposed the routine use of electrophysiologic testing to risk stratify young asymptomatic patients for sudden death. If a screening strategy of routine exercise testing were employed in asymptomatic young males, exercise testing before electrophysiologic study would potentially eliminate the need for invasive risk stratification in the 20% of asymptomatic WPW patients whose delta wave disappears.

> **Key Point:** LBBB and WPW negate ST analysis for ischemia, and right bundle branch block allows for ST analysis for ischemia in all but the anterior leads, where the T-wave inversion due to aberrant conduction.

Atrial Repolarization

In patients with atrioventricular dissociation, the duration of atrial repolarization (the atrial T wave) can play a role in the normal rate-related depression of the J junction in inferior leads (aVF, II) and can increase S-wave amplitude.[66] The effect of atrial repolarization on the ST segments in the lateral leads is less important, but it affects a bipolar lead such as CM5, which contains anterior and inferior forces. Sapin and colleagues[67] postulated that exaggerated atrial repolarization waves during exercise could produce ST-segment depression mimicking myocardial ischemia. Multivariable

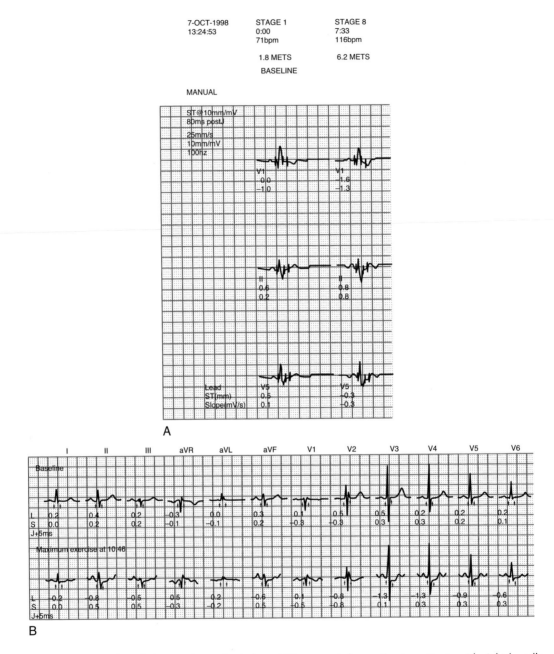

FIGURE 4-9 *Examples of abnormal exercise-induced ST-segment depression in patients with right bundle branch block with coronary artery disease and ischemia.* **A,** *Patient with abnormal ST-segment depression in the lateral leads.* **B,** *Patient with ST-segment depression in V2 that represents ischemia because the T waves are not inverted in V2 as they normally are in patients with RBBB (both are true positives).*

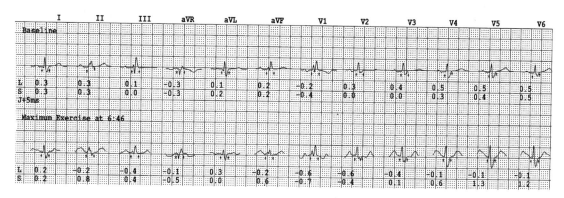

FIGURE 4-10   *Example of exercise-induced ST-segment depression in the anterior leads but not in the lateral leads in a patient with right bundle branch block without evidence for ischemia or coronary artery disease (i.e., a false positive ST response).*

analysis revealed that exercise duration and downsloping PR segments in the inferior ECG leads were independent predictors of a false-positive test. This has been validated in a larger sample.[68]

> **Key Point:** Atrial repolarization can cause false-positive ST depression, particularly in the inferior leads (where the P-wave vector is strongest) and when the PR interval is short.

Hyperventilation Abnormalities

Individuals with ST repolarization changes including classic ST depression with hyperventilation before treadmill testing can have abnormal exercise-induced ST-segment changes without CAD. Such changes are unusual and have rarely been responsible for false-positive tests.[69] Orthostatic and hyperventilation changes have been associated with the mitral valve prolapse syndrome, vasoregulatory asthenia, and vasoregulatory abnormalities. When they do occur with exercise-induced changes, the interpretation of ischemia should be avoided and the clinician must rely on other parameters to make a diagnosis. Prolonged hyperventilation should be avoided because it can induce ECG abnormalities and arrhythmias in both normal individuals and patients with heart disease. The associated tachycardia can even precipitate angina in patients with obstructive coronary disease. Shorter periods of hyperventilation (< 30 seconds) may be used to identify a small percentage of those with "false positive" abnormal exercise-induced ST responses.[70]

> **Key Point:** Hyperventilation before testing is no longer recommended as a means to detect false-positive ST responses.

Other Causes

Individuals with the left ventricular hypertrophy and strain pattern on their resting ECG are at high risk for CAD, but the ST ischemic response is less specific in them. This may be due to an imbalance between supply and the demand of the hypertrophied muscle. Individuals with WPW free of CAD can have exercise-induced ST-segment depression. Some individuals with preexcitation, a short PR interval, and a normal QRS complex may have a false-positive exercise test. Patients with mitral valve prolapse have been reported to have abnormal exercise tests but normal coronary angiograms.

It has been hypothesized that hypertension or an excessive double product (systolic blood pressure times heart rate) during exercise could have a physiologic imbalance between myocardial oxygen supply and demand, but this has not been validated. Barnard and co-workers[71] demonstrated that a sudden high workload of treadmill exercise can yield ST-segment depression in healthy individuals on this basis. Foster and associates[72] could not reproduce the ST-segment depression with sudden strenuous bicycle exercise even though ejection fraction dropped in their normal subjects. A recorder with an inadequate frequency response can either simulate ST-segment depression in normal subjects or show upsloping depression when horizontal depression is actually present. Use of the proper equipment should avoid this type of distortion. In conclusion, the conditions discussed previously can be avoided and should not be the major causes of false-positive responses in a good exercise laboratory. The most common cause of a false-positive test should be the normal variant in a patient who has a physiologic ST-segment vector that is similar to that produced by ischemia. It is interesting to hypothesize that a genomic variation might be responsible for this response.

ST Shift Location and Ischemia

Validating the localization of ischemia with coronary angiography has several limitations. First, collaterals may adequately perfuse areas of the heart served by an obstructed artery. Second, coronary angiography cannot quantify the degree to which an infarcted area of the heart remains ischemic. Finally, the validity of relating anatomic lesions visualized at rest to exercise-induced changes in the ECG is questionable. These limitations partially explain the difficulty correlating ECG alterations with the specific number or location of coronary angiographic obstructions. Precise localization of critical ischemia has assumed more than academic interest with coronary interventions so widely available. Localization could help direct surgical intervention to the site of jeopardized myocardium or the source of angina pectoris.

At the University of California–San Diego, we studied 54 patients with stable coronary heart disease, all with exercise-induced perfusion defects.[73] Their exercise ECG test results were compared with their nuclear images and also with 14 low-risk normal subjects. Exercise data were analyzed for spatial

ST-vector shifts using a computer program in order to most accurately classify ST-segment depression and elevation. None of the ischemic sites or angiographic diseased areas could be specifically identified by exercise-induced ST-vector shifts.

Fuchs and colleagues[74] evaluated the 12-lead ECG for localizing the site of CAD in 134 patients with angiographically documented single-vessel coronary disease. They reviewed 10 years of cardiac catheterization at Johns Hopkins Hospital to select those patients who had ECGs recorded during MI, spontaneous rest angina, or treadmill exercise. Q-wave location correctly identified the location of the coronary lesion in 98% of the cases, ST elevation in 91%, T-wave inversion in 84%, and ST depression in only 60%. No response could separate right from left circumflex CAD. ST-segment elevation was recorded in 20 of the 56 patients who underwent exercise testing. All 56 had angina during the test. An association was found only between elevation in limb lead III and right coronary artery disease. Simoons and colleagues[24] studied the exercise-induced spatial ST-vector shifts 30 and 80 msec after QRS end in 34 patients who had coronary angiography and nuclear perfusion exercise scans because of clinically important chest pain. They could find no systematic difference in the ST-vector direction of patients with anteroseptal compared with patients with posterolateral perfusion defects. These studies have been corroborated by the excellent angiographic studies.

> **Key Point:** ST-segment depression in II and aVF does not necessarily mean that there is inferior ischemia (or right coronary artery disease) nor does ST depression in V5 mean that there is lateral ischemia (or left coronary artery disease). However, exercise-induced ST elevation does localize to either an artery with an occlusion or spasm or to an area of dyskinesia.

Chest Pain

The reproduction of chest pain during the test is very important to classify and report. Although nonspecific chest pain is of importance to recognize, true angina pectoris has diagnostic and prognostic importance. The Duke treadmill angina score has been validated as an important qualifier of the probability and severity of CAD. All it requires is the assessment of whether or not angina occurs and if it is the reason for stopping the test (Table 4-6).

TABLE 4-6   Duke Treadmill Angina Score

Score	Definition
0	No angina
1	Angina occurred
2	Angina was the reason for stopping the test

> **Key Point:** The Duke treadmill angina score should always be recorded as part of the exercise test.

Typical angina pectoris is a pressure, tightness, or pain located in or beneath the sternum. It can radiate to the neck or down the left arm. Some patients have a shortness of breath that has been called an "angina equivalent," but this is not true angina. Patients can describe an angina that comes on at low levels of exercise and goes away as they warm up and progress to higher work levels (walk-through or warm-up angina). Some patients get angina in the recovery phase, usually within 5 minutes. True angina is not pinpoint, pleuritic, knifelike, or palpable. The exercise test is an important opportunity to reproduce the patient's symptoms and determine if they are really angina pectoris or a nonspecific chest pain.

Weiner and co-workers[75] reported 281 consecutive patients studied with treadmill testing and coronary angiography. They were grouped according to the following responses: (1) ST-segment depression and treadmill test–induced chest pain (90% prevalence CAD), (2) ST-segment depression and no chest pain (65% prevalence CAD), (3) treadmill test–induced chest pain and no ST-segment changes (70% prevalence CAD), and (4) neither chest pain nor ST-segment changes (35% prevalence CAD). Cole and Ellestad[76] followed 95 patients with abnormal treadmill tests. At 5-year follow-up, the incidence of CAD was 73% in those with both chest pain and an abnormal ST-segment response compared with 43% in those who only had an abnormal ST-segment response. Mortality rate was also twice as high in those with both ST-segment changes and chest pain induced by the treadmill test.

A fascinating study from Norway has added additional importance to angina and exercise testing. During 1972–1975, 2014 apparently healthy men ages 40 to 59 years underwent an examination including history, clinical examination, exercise ECG, and the World Health Organization (WHO) angina questionnaire.[77] Sixty-eight had possible angina, and 115 were excluded because they had definite angina or abnormal exercise ECGs. At 26 years, men with possible angina had a cardiovascular mortality rate of 25% (17 of 68) versus 14% (252 of 1831) among men without angina. They also had a higher incidence of cardiac events. Multivariate analysis including risk factors showed that possible angina was an independent risk factor (twofold relative risk). This study demonstrates that men with possible angina, even with a normal exercise test, have a greater risk of coronary heart disease. Note that the exercise test did not bring on the angina in these men with a positive angina history.

> **Key Point:** Anginal chest pain induced by the exercise test predicts the presence of CAD, and when it occurs with ST segment depression, they are even more predictive of CAD than either alone. It is important, though, that a careful description of the pain be obtained from the patient to ascertain that it is typical or atypical angina rather than nonischemic chest pain.

Do Diabetics Have a Higher Prevalence of Silent Ischemia during Treadmill Testing Than Nondiabetics?

Silent Ischemia More Common in Diabetics

Nesto and colleagues[78] studied 50 patients with diabetes and 50 patients without diabetes selected consecutively with ischemia on exercise perfusion scan. The two groups had similar clinical characteristics, treadmill test results, and extent of infarction and ischemia, but only 14 patients with diabetes compared with 34 patients without diabetes had angina during exertional ischemia. In diabetic patients the extent of retinopathy, nephropathy, or peripheral neuropathy was similar in patients with and without angina. These authors found angina to be an unreliable index of myocardial ischemia in diabetic patients and believed that periodic objective assessment of the extent of ischemia was warranted. A similar study but with angiographic endpoints found diabetics receiving insulin or with retinopathy to have twice the prevalence of silent ischemia than nondiabetics,[79] and two studies found diabetics with neuropathy to have more silent ischemia than nondiabetics.[80,81]

After PCI and then a nuclear perfusion scan, 114 diabetic patients were followed for 2 years for cardiac events.[82] Even after PCI, these now asymptomatic diabetic patients had a high frequency of persistent silent ischemia that was associated with a high risk for repeat interventional procedure, although no increase in major cardiac events was observed.

In the Detection of Ischemia in Asymptomatic Diabetics (DIAD) study, 1123 patients with type 2 diabetes, ages 50 to 75 years, with no known or suspected CAD, were randomly assigned to either stress testing and 5-year clinical follow-up or to follow-up only.[83] The prevalence of ischemia in 522 patients randomized to stress testing was assessed by adenosine myocardial perfusion imaging. A total of 113 patients (22%) had silent ischemia, including 83 with regional myocardial perfusion abnormalities and 30 with normal perfusion but other abnormalities. These investigators concluded that silent myocardial ischemia occurs in greater than one in five asymptomatic patients with type 2 diabetes. Traditional and emerging cardiac risk factors were not associated with abnormal stress tests, although cardiac autonomic dysfunction was a strong predictor of ischemia. Though suggesting a high prevalence of silent ischemia in diabetics, there was no comparison with nondiabetics using the same techniques.

Silent Ischemia Not More Common in Diabetics

In a landmark Danish study, the prevalence of ischemia was compared in diabetics and nondiabetics.[84] A random sample of 120 users of insulin and 120 users of oral hypoglycemic agents ages 40 to 75 years living in Denmark were asked to participate. Abnormal ST depression on either exercise or Holter was considered indicative of myocardial ischemia. Angina pectoris was considered present if the Rose questionnaire was positive or chest pain accompanied ECG evidence of ischemia. The observed prevalence of silent ischemia in diabetics was 13.5% and was no different in matched controls. No association was found between silent ischemia and gender or diabetes type. Hypertension was highly predictive of silent ischemia in the diabetic subjects, but other variables did not have a predictive value. In this population-based study of silent ischemia in diabetes, the frequency of silent ischemia did not differ significantly between diabetics and nondiabetics.

An analysis was performed to determine whether diabetic patients with coronary disease enrolled in the Asymptomatic Cardiac Ischemia Pilot (ACIP) had more episodes of asymptomatic ischemia during exercise testing and Holter monitoring than nondiabetic patients.[85] Angiographic findings and the prevalence and magnitude of ischemia during the qualifying Holter and exercise study were compared by the presence and absence of diabetes mellitus in 558 randomized ACIP patients. Seventy-seven patients had a history of diabetes and were taking oral hypoglycemics or insulin. Multivessel disease (87% vs. 74%) was more frequent in the diabetics. The percentages of patients without angina during the exercise test were similar in the diabetic and nondiabetic groups (about 35%). Time to onset of 1 mm ST-segment depression and time to onset of angina were similar in both groups. The percentages of patients with only asymptomatic ST-segment depression during the Holter were similar in the diabetic and nondiabetic groups (94% vs. 88%, respectively). However, total ischemic time, ischemic time per episode, and the maximum depth of ST-segment depression tended to be less in the diabetic group. Unlike the previous study, entry into the ACIP required a cardiac event, so the subjects were not truly asymptomatic.

Falcone and colleagues[86] recruited a total of 618 patients with CAD: 309 were consecutive diabetic patients and 309 were age- and gender-matched nondiabetic patients. Myocardial ischemia was evaluated both during daily life and during exercise testing. Angina pectoris during daily life was more frequent in diabetic than in nondiabetic patients (80% vs. 74%). The anginal pain intensity either during daily life or acute MI, the prevalence of a previous MI, the extent of CAD, and exercise parameters were similar in diabetics and nondiabetics. Silent ischemia during exercise occurred in 179 diabetics (58%) and in 197 nondiabetics (64%). Both diabetics and nondiabetics with silent exertional myocardial ischemia differed from symptomatic subjects in higher heart rate, systolic blood pressure, METs, and maximum ST-segment depression at peak exercise. The prevalence of silent myocardial ischemia during exercise was similar in diabetic and nondiabetic CAD patients, as has been our experience with exercise testing in veterans.[87]

Conclusions Regarding Silent Ischemia

In patients with stable CAD who have not suffered a recent MI, silent ischemia on exercise testing does not identify a high-risk population and actually predicts a better outcome than symptomatic ischemia. In this instance it may be appropriate that "only the squeaky wheel gets the grease"—that only those patients with angina and exercise-induced ST depression should be considered for interventions.[88] Furthermore, the evidence base for the common clinical axiom that diabetics have a higher prevalence of silent ischemia is far from conclusive.

> **Key Point:** Silent myocardial ischemia (ST depression without angina) during treadmill testing in patients without their diabetic status considered does not predict increased risk for death over those with both ST depression and angina. The concern that patients with silent myocardial ischemia were at higher risk than their peers with angina because of failure of their warning mechanism has not been substantiated. That silent ischemia is more common in diabetics is actually a clinical impression more than an evidence-based fact.

Interpretation of Exercise Test–Induced Arrhythmias

Definition and Historical Perspective

It has been recommended that exercise testing be used as a noninvasive method for exposing cardiac arrhythmias, particularly when the symptoms are brought on by exercise.[89] The information obtained can complement information obtained from ambulatory monitoring and electrophysiologic testing.[90] The available data indicate the following:

1. EIVA are relatively safe except in high-risk groups (i.e., cardiomyopathy and valvular patients or when excercise test induced ST elevation occurs).
2. Their independent diagnostic and prognostic characteristics are weak.
3. An adverse effect on prognosis is late in follow up (5–10 years or more).

Couplets, or nonsustained ventricular tachycardia, occur during exercise or recovery in up to a third of patients tested. Even in patients with known heart disease, there is a small risk of inducing sustained ventricular tachycardia or ventricular fibrillation during exercise. In patients in whom arrhythmias are known to be induced by exercise, exercise testing is an excellent method by which the effectiveness of antiarrhythmic drug treatment can be assessed, bearing in mind that they are often not reproducible and that certain antiarrhythmic drugs are known to be associated with exercise-induced ventricular tachycardia.[91-94]

Some studies suggest that exercise test–induced ventricular arrhythmias (ETIVAs) confer a poor prognosis,[95-97] whereas others contest this.[98-100] Fewer data are available regarding exercise test–induced supraventricular arrhythmias. The clinical significance of ETIVAs in those without documented cardiovascular disease presents another dilemma. Although a recent study found that healthy volunteers with ETIVAs had an increased mortality rate,[101] earlier studies did not produce similar results.[102,103] It is unclear if the prognosis associated with ETIVA differs based on the presence of cardiovascular disease, ischemic changes during exercise, or the presence of premature ventricular contractions at rest (i.e., an indicator of the arrhythmic substrate).

Physiologic and Pathophysiologic Basis

Exercise produces a number of important physiologic changes, namely the activation of the sympathetic nervous system and an increase in the availability of circulating catecholamines, which can predispose to arrhythmias.[104-106]

These changes interact with the three major mechanisms involved in the generation of arrhythmias: enhanced automaticity, triggered automaticity, and reentry. Other potential proarrhythmic mechanisms include electrolyte shifts, baroreceptor activation, myocardial stretch, and ischemia.[107,108] Atrial arrhythmias may reflect underlying left atrial enlargement and ventricular dysfunction.

The heart may be at greatest risk in the postexercise period when plasma potassium is low and the adrenergic tone is high. Most dangerous exercise-induced arrhythmias occur at this time, and they can be lessened or avoided by cool-down activities. Abnormal regulation of electrolyte and cardiac sympathovagal balance in recovery most likely increases the susceptibility to arrhythmias, particularly when ischemia is present.

Any alteration in the delicate chemical balance and natural pathophysiologic response to exercise may also contribute to cardiac arrhythmias. Studies have linked certain antiarrhythmic drugs with exercise-induced ventricular tachycardia. Ranger and colleagues[109] hypothesized that the sinus tachycardia seen during exercise may enhance flecainide-induced conduction slowing by increasing use-dependent sodium channel blockade, thereby facilitating the occurrence of ventricular reentry. Their study found that the best predictor of further exercise-induced QRS slowing was the change in QRS duration produced by flecainide at rest.

Other studies have delineated varying electrical patterns that may predispose patients to exercise-induced ventricular arrhythmias. A Dutch group studied the initiating mechanisms of exercise-induced ventricular tachycardia in 6000 patients.[110] One percent had 194 episodes of ventricular tachycardia during the test. Forty-two percent of these occurred during exercise and 58% during recovery. Two different initiating patterns were observed before ventricular tachycardia: a short-long-short sequence of R-R intervals (28%) or a regular RR pattern (63%).

In addition to a regular RR pattern, one of the forms of the long QT syndrome has also been linked to exercise-induced sudden death.[111] Familial catecholaminergic polymorphic ventricular tachycardia (CPVT) is a rare arrhythmogenic disease manifesting with exercise- or stress-induced ventricular arrhythmias, syncope, and even sudden death. CPVT is inherited as an autosomal dominant or autosomal recessive trait, usually with high penetrance.[112] The clinical, structural, and ECG findings in this disorder have been characterized by use of genome-wide linkage analysis, mapping the disease-causing gene to chromosome 1q42-q43. Mutations of the cardiac ryanodine receptor gene (RyR2) have been demonstrated to underlie this life-threatening disease. In addition, RyR2 mutations were identified in patients affected with a variant form of arrhythmogenic right ventricular dysplasia (ARVD2), a phenotypically distinct disease entity. Identification of the causal mutations has enabled molecular diagnosis in the affected families, which is of major importance in identifying individuals at risk of an arrhythmia. Recently, several groups have delineated the functional effects of the RyR2 mutations associated with CPVT and ARVD2. The results are slightly contradictory, and further studies are thus needed to clarify the exact molecular mechanisms leading to arrhythmia induction.

Methodology

Arrhythmia Detection Technology

The reported studies have used a number of different technologies to record and diagnose arrhythmias occurring in association with exercise testing. The earliest studies simply relied on physicians or technicians (or both) to recognize arrhythmias appearing on the monitor or recorded on the ECG output. This was dependent on the skill and attention of the observer to note the arrhythmia and record it by manually initiating an ECG recording. As the exercise devices became more sophisticated, they incorporated software algorithms that detected arrhythmias and automatically initiated an ECG recording. The noise associated with exercise represented a challenge to these algorithms, frequently triggering them. Therefore in most clinical settings they are disabled to stop from wasting ECG paper.

Because of the exercise environment, algorithms developed for monitoring patients in the hospital or during ambulatory ECG recordings could not easily be implemented or relied on. A Holter technique that has been enabled in some commercially available exercise systems has been total disclosure of all ECG complexes. Noise can make the recognition of arrhythmias difficult even using these types of printouts. More recently, exercise systems have included the capacity to record all ECG data during and after exercise. These stored, digitized signals can be subjected to sophisticated software techniques off-line employing noise reduction algorithms and Holter-like ECG analysis.

Definition

Study design and the means by which ETIAs have been captured have differed significantly enough that it has been difficult to come to a consensus regarding prevalence rates, much less extrapolating prognostic information from data available. Clearly, the methods of recording and capturing premature ventricular contractions (PVCs) greatly affect the prevalence data, and as technology advances, the multitude of options available for data collection may make standardization even more difficult. Even in studies where data have been obtained using similar equipment setups, there have been discrepancies in categorizing and defining the information acquired. These discrepancies often stem from basic controversy in deciding what data should be labeled as an exercise-induced ventricular arrhythmia. This inconsistency in the definition of ETIA has played a large role in limiting not only data collection, but also the prognostic value of much of the information available. Studies have used varying criteria to define ETIA, with some studies considering ETIA to be present if any PVC or premature atrial contractions (PAC) was recorded during exercise. Furthermore, runs defined as ventricular tachycardia or sustained ventricular tachycardia have varied from three or more. One approach has been to consider a certain threshold of complexes per minute or an absolute number of ectopy per minute.

The problems with defining ETIVA do not lie solely in differentiating how many PVCs occur, but also include the time frame and pattern in which they occur. In addition to examining ventricular arrhythmias during the actual exercise period, data from before the test and during the cool-down period should be considered, as well as how the timing affects their occurrence. Furthermore, whether or not one does a cool-down walk after exercise can affect the appearance of ectopy. To complicate things further, the importance of resting PVCs at any prior time (i.e., the arrhythmic substrate) is rarely considered.

Population Selection

Multiple factors have been shown to be associated with the prevalence of ETIVA. The problem lies in elucidating the exact relationship between these factors and ETIVA, and explaining their prognostic significance. Studies have focused on particular healthy populations such as aviators and policemen, whereas others have targeted random samples of such with or without screening for baseline heart disease (e.g., Framingham). Other studies have targeted patients referred for exercise testing for clinical reasons, including those known to have arrhythmias. Different prevalence of ETIVAs can be expected from these different populations.

Age   Many studies have demonstrated a direct relationship between age and the prevalence of ETIVAs.[113] In the healthy volunteers of the Baltimore Aging Study, 1.1% had exercise-induced arrhythmias, but only one was younger than 65.[113] We reported similar results in the U.S. Air Force (USAF) (Tables 4-7 and 4-8). What remains unresolved is whether this is due to aging itself, alterations in sympathetic tone, or the diseases that accrue with aging.

Key Point: Rest and exercise-induced PVCs increase in prevalence with age.

Ischemia   Some studies have suggested an association of ETIVAs with exercise-induced ischemia[97,114]; however, other studies refute these

TABLE 4-7   Number and Percentage of Healthy Aircrewmen with Other Than Single or Occasional PVCs

Age	Number	Percent
20-29	24	6.6
30-39	52	7.6
40-53	78	13.1

Froelicher VF et al: Advisory Group for Aerospace Research and Development. NATO AGARD Publishing, Neuilly-sur-Seine, France, 1975. $n = 1640$ healthy aviators.

TABLE 4-8   Number and Percentage of Healthy Aircrewmen with "Ominous" Patterns of PVC Occurrence

Age	Number	Percent
20-29	3	0.8%
30-39	7	1.0%
40-53	21	3.5%

Froelicher VF et al: Advisory Group for Aerospace Research and Development. NATO AGARD Publishing, Neuilly-sur-Seine, France, 1975. *n* = 1640 healthy aviators.

results.[98,100,102,115,116] It does seem apparent that ETIVAs are more common in patients with CAD. McHenry and colleagues reported that patients with documented ETIVA had a greater prevalence of abnormal ischemia and wall motion abnormalities with exercise.[115] During exercise testing up to a heart rate of 130 beats per minute, 27% of patients with angiographic CAD experienced ETIVAs, compared with only 9% of patients with normal angiograms. Reproducibility is always an issue in all studies of EIVA as discussed later.[114] Patients with three-vessel CAD and left ventricular wall motion abnormalities were found to have a significantly greater prevalence of ETIVAs. Detry and colleagues[117] reported on six patients without MI specifically referred to them for spontaneous angina known to be associated with ST elevation. During exercise testing, five of the patients exhibited elevation; three of these patients developed ventricular tachycardia and one developed ventricular fibrillation.

> **Key Point:** During exercise, transmural ischemia associated with ST-segment elevation is arrhythmogenic, whereas subendocardial ischemia associated with ST-segment depression generally is not.

Gender   Bias in many of the previously reported series has also limited their external validity. Studies comparing the prognostic value of ETIVAs in men and women have shown a lower risk in women, but this may be due to their lower CAD mortality rates.[101,118]

Reproducibility

The issue of reproducibility has complicated defining the prognostic significance of ETIVA as it relates to outcomes.[119,120] It must be concluded that the marked variability of ETIVA during repeat maximal exercise testing in a clinically normal population appears to negate the usefulness of this finding during a single test as a marker of future cardiovascular disease. However, subjects whose arrhythmias are reproducible may form a group more likely to develop clinical cardiovascular disease in long-term follow-up studies.

Prevalence of Exercise Test–Induced Ventricular Tachycardia

Three studies considering the safety of exercise testing reported the occurrence of ventricular tachycardia during the test specifically. Condini and colleagues[121] described 47 patients with exercise test–induced ventricular tachycardia (ETIVT) occurring during exercise testing (a prevalence of 0.8% in 5730 treadmill tests). Forty of the 47 patients had heart disease, mostly CAD. Ventricular tachycardia was brief and self-terminated in all but one instance. Milanes and colleagues[122] reported a 4% prevalence of ventricular tachycardia in 900 treadmill tests performed in patients with CAD compared with 0.07% prevalence in 1700 tests among patients without CAD. Of note, 79% of patients with ventricular fibrillation or tachycardia had an abnormal ST response as well. In 2000, Fujiwara and colleagues[123] examined the conditions surrounding the onset of ventricular tachycardia and ventricular fibrillation following the completion of exercise testing. From a database of 7594 patients, 60 patients (0.8%) were identified as having had ETIVT during treadmill testing. In the recovery period, within 2 minutes after exercise, nine patients experienced ventricular tachycardia.

Follow-up Issues

Completeness and length of follow-up are both important because some of the studies suggest that the risk of ETIVA appears later (> 10 years) rather than early. This makes studying ETIVA more difficult because the longer the follow-up time, the greater the risk of losing patients to follow-up. Comorbidities also are important to consider, particularly cigarette smoking and lung disease, because they are thought to be associated with ETIVA and affect outcomes.

Clinical Prognostic Studies

Exercise Test–Induced Supraventricular Arrhythmias

Few studies have evaluated if exercise test–induced supraventricular arrhythmias (ETISVAs) (supraventricular or atrial arrhythmias during exercise testing) are predictive of an increased risk of cardiac events and death. Atrial arrhythmias may reflect underlying left atrial enlargement and ventricular dysfunction, which themselves predict mortality. The following two studies are the only recent studies performed on this subject.

Bunch and colleagues[124] performed exercise echocardiography in 5375 patients (age 61 ± 12 years) with known or suspected CAD. In stepwise multivariate analysis, ETISVAs were not predictive of any endpoint when taking into account traditional clinical variables and exercise test results. The prevalence, characteristics, and prognostic significance of ETISVAs were examined in 843 male and 540 female asymptomatic volunteers ages 20 to 94 years from the Baltimore Longitudinal Study of Aging who underwent exercise testing.[125] ETISVAs occurred at a rate of one test per 51 men (6%) and 34 women (6.3%). The 85 subjects with ETISVAs were significantly older than the 1298 free from this arrhythmia (66. vs 50 years of age). The prevalence of ETISVAs increased with age in men ($p < 0.001$) but not in women. Most of the 141 discrete episodes of ETISVA were paroxysmal SVT, with heart rates varying from 105 to 290 beats per minute. Nearly half of ETISVAs occurred at peak effort. Coronary risk factors, echocardiographic left atrial size, and the prevalence of exercise-induced ischemic ST-segment depression (11% vs. 13%) were similar in 85 subjects with ETISVA and 170 control subjects matched for age and sex. During follow-up, eight subjects (10%), but only three controls (2%), developed atrial fibrillation or paroxysmal SVT a mean of 6 years (range 2 to 12) after their index exercise test. Six subjects developed atrial fibrillation; in four of these six the arrhythmia was sustained. The relative risk of developing lone atrial fibrillation during follow-up in those subjects with exercise-induced SVT was 8 times. Thus exercise-induced SVT does not appear to be a marker for latent heart disease, but 10% of those with exercise-induced SVT and only 2% of controls developed spontaneous atrial fibrillation or paroxysmal SVT during the follow-up period.

> **Key Point:** ETISVAs are relatively rare compared with ventricular arrhythmias and appear to be benign except for their association with the future development of atrial fibrillation.

Exercise Test–Induced Ventricular Arrhythmias

In examining patients without CAD, most recent studies suggest that ETIVAs are associated with increased cardiovascular morbidity or mortality rates, whereas the earlier studies are mixed. The Baltimore Aging Study reported 1160 subjects between ages 21 and 96 years who underwent treadmill testing an average of 2.4 times.[126] Eighty (6.9%) developed frequent (> 10% of beats in any 1 minute) or repetitive (more than three beats in a row) PVCs on at least one of these tests. Only age appeared to distinguish those with ETIVA, but in these predominantly older, asymptomatic individuals without apparent heart disease, ETIVA did not appear to predict increased cardiac morbidity or mortality risk.[102]

A 6-year follow-up study of 1390 male USAF aircrewmen referred to the USAF School of Aerospace Medicine was reported in 1974.[127] The ECG strips were continuously recorded and stored on 8 mm microfilm, which was replayed by a trained observer and the arrhythmias recorded retrospectively. Ominous treadmill-induced arrhythmias were defined as frequent PVCs at near-maximal or maximal exercise, or three consecutive PVCs or more occurring at any time.[128] Frequent PVCs were defined as 10 or more PVCs out of any 50 consecutive beats. Ominous arrhythmias were noted in 2.1% of this apparently healthy, select population. Coronary heart disease was defined as onset of angina pectoris, MI, or cardiovascular death. The risk of developing coronary heart disease over the follow-up period with these arrhythmias was three times greater than in those who did not develop ominous arrhythmias.

In 2000, Jouven and colleagues[101] evaluated 6101 asymptomatic French men between ages 42 and 53 years who were free of clinically detectable cardiovascular disease. Patients underwent exercise testing and were monitored for the presence of two or more consecutive PVCs. In their multivariate model, adjustments were made for age, body mass index, heart rate at rest, systolic blood pressure, tobacco use, level of physical activity, diabetes, cholesterol, and the PVCs before exercise and during recovery from exercise. The subjects were followed for 23 years for cardiovascular death. They concluded that frequent PVCs (a run of two or more making up 10% of any 30 seconds) during exercise in men without detectable cardiovascular disease is associated with a long-term increase in cardiovascular mortality risk.

The Framingham Offspring Study participants (1397 men; mean age, 43 years) who were free of cardiovascular disease and who underwent a routine exercise test were recently reported; ETIVAs were noted in 792 participants (27%) using an off-line Holter-type analysis computer system (median, 0.22 PVCs/min of exercise).[129] Age and male sex were key correlates of ETIVA. During follow-up (mean 15 years), 142 (113 men) had a first hard coronary heart disease (CHD) event and 171 participants (109 men) died. ETIVAs were not associated with hard CHD events but were associated with increased all-cause mortality rates (multivariable-adjusted hazards ratio, 1.9 for infrequent, and 1.7 for frequent ETIVAs versus none). The relations of ETIVAs to mortality risk were not influenced by ETIVA grade, presence of recovery ETIVA, left ventricular dysfunction, or an ischemic ST-segment response. ETIVAs were associated with up to a greater than two times increased risk of all-cause mortality at a much lower threshold than previously reported. Surprisingly, the risk was not isolated to those with cardiovascular endpoints, making the mechanism unsettled.

Researchers at Cleveland Clinic reported on 29,244 patients (mean 56 years of age; 70% men) who had been referred for exercise testing without heart failure, valve disease, or arrhythmia.[130] ETIVAs were defined by the presence of seven or more PVCs per minute, ventricular bigeminy or trigeminy, ventricular couplets or triplets, or ventricular tachycardia/fibrillation (VT/VF). ETIVAs occurred only during exercise in 945 patients (3%), only during recovery in 589 (2%), and during both exercise and recovery in 491 (2%). There were 1862 deaths during a mean of 5 years of follow-up. ETIVA during exercise predicted an increased risk of death (5-year death rate, 9%, vs. 5% among patients without ETIVA; hazard ratio 1:8), but ETIVA during recovery was a stronger predictor (11% vs. 5%; hazard ratio 2:4). After propensity matching for confounding variables, arrhythmias during recovery predicted an increased risk of death (adjusted hazard ratio, 1.5), but ETIVA during exercise did not.

In 1984, Sami and colleagues[131] performed a retrospective study to examine the significance of ETIVA in patients with stable CAD from the Coronary Artery Surgery Study. The population included 1486 patients selected from 1975 to 1979, followed for an average of 4.3 years. Patients with CAD and ETIVA had similar clinical and angiographic characteristics as those with CAD without ETIVA. The only difference discovered was the average ejection fraction (EF), which was 50% for those with ETIVA and 64% for those without any PVCs. The 5-year event-free survival was not influenced by the presence of ETIVA in this study. Using a stepwise Cox regression analysis, the authors concluded that only the number of coronary arteries diseased and the EF were associated with cardiac events.[131] Similar conclusions were drawn by Weiner and colleagues[132] and Nair and colleagues[133] in two separate studies that same year. In a small study by Nair and colleagues,[133] frequent or complex ETIVAs were not shown to predict 4-year mortality rate in patients with CAD. Others have also reported that in patients with documented CAD and no prior history of severe ventricular ectopy at rest, exercise-induced frequent or complex PVCs were not predictive of 2-year mortality rate.[98,134] Califf and colleagues[135] studied the prognostic value of ETIVA in 1293 consecutive nonsurgically treated patients. In the 620 patients with significant CAD, patients with paired complexes or ventricular tachycardia had a lower 3-year survival rate (75%) than did patients with simple ventricular arrhythmia (83%) and patients with no ETIVA (90%).

We performed a retrospective analysis of 6213 consecutive males referred for exercise tests and followed for 6 years.[136] ETIVAs were defined as frequent PVCs constituting greater than 10% of all ventricular depolarizations during any 30-second ECG recording, or a run of three consecutive PVCs during exercise or recovery. Twenty percent died during follow-up. ETIVA occurred in 503 patients (8%); the prevalence of ETIVA increased in older patients and in those with cardiopulmonary disease, resting PVCs, and ischemia during exercise. ETIVAs were associated with mortality rate irrespective of the presence of cardiopulmonary disease or exercise-induced ischemia. In those without cardiopulmonary disease, mortality rate differed more so later in follow-up than earlier. In those without resting PVCs, ETIVAs were also predictive of death, but in those with resting PVCs, prognosis was not worsened by the presence of ETIVA. We concluded that exercise-induced ischemia does not affect the prognostic value of ETIVA, whereas the arrhythmic substrate does, and furthermore that ETIVA and resting PVCs are both independent predictors of death after consideration of other clinical and exercise test variables. A reanalysis of this data set was performed when cardiovascular mortality rate became available.[137] From this subsequent analysis, we concluded that ETIVAs are independent predictors of cardiovascular death after adjusting for other clinical and exercise test variables; ETIVA combined with resting PVCs carries the highest risk.

Elhendy and colleagues[138] assessed the relationship between ETIVA and exercise echocardiography in patients with suspected CAD. Their study included 1460 patients (mean age 64 ± 10 years; 867 men) with intermediate pretest probability of CAD and no history of MI or revascularization. ETIVA occurred in 146 patients (10%). Compared with patients without ETIVA, those with ETIVA had a greater prevalence of abnormal exercise echocardiographic findings. During 2.7 years of follow-up, cardiac death and nonfatal MI occurred in 36 patients. Following a multivariate analysis of combined clinical and exercise test variables, they concluded that independent predictors of cardiac events were ETIVA and maximal heart rate.

Exercise-Induced Ventricular Tachycardia

On a retrospective review of 3351 veterans who had undergone routine clinical exercise testing, we identified 55 patients with exercise-induced ventricular tachycardia.[139] *Nonsustained ventricular tachycardia* was defined as three or more consecutive ventricular premature beats. *Sustained ventricular tachycardia* was defined as ventricular tachycardia longer than 30 seconds or requiring intervention. Of the 50 episodes of nonsustained ventricular tachycardia, 26 episodes occurred during exercise and 24 occurred in recovery; only 10 occurred at peak exercise and led to cessation of the exercise test. Five patients had exercise-induced sustained ventricular tachycardia; two patients had bouts of ventricular tachycardia during exercise and three during recovery. Of these five patients, only two patients required intervention: one was given lidocaine intravenously and one was cardioverted because of hypotension. The only other episode of serious ventricular arrhythmia to occur in this time period occurred in a patient without prior cardiac history who developed ventricular fibrillation during exercise that required electrical defibrillation. Of the 55 patients with exercise-induced ventricular tachycardia, 45 had clinical evidence of CAD; this included 19 with a prior MI and 14 with interventions. Two patients had cardiomyopathy, three had valvular heart disease, and five had no clinical evidence of heart disease. Our major findings were that the occurrence of nonsustained exercise-induced ventricular tachycardia during routine treadmill testing was not associated with complications during testing or with increased cardiovascular mortality rate within 2 years after testing. In our study, the prevalence and reproducibility of exercise-induced ventricular tachycardia were both low (1.2% and 6.9%, respectively). The annual mortality rate among patients with exercise-induced ventricular tachycardia was 1.7% compared with 2.4% (171 deaths in 3351 patients) in the study population. Though exercise-induced ventricular tachycardia did not portend a worsened prognosis even among our patients with CAD, this finding cannot be extended to the five patients with sustained ventricular tachycardia, because of their small number and because they were treated.

In general during exercise, transmural ischemia associated with ST-segment elevation is arrhythmogenic, whereas subendocardial ischemia associated with ST-segment depression is not. In our study, none of the patients with nonsustained ventricular tachycardia had ST elevation with their exercise test and 20 had abnormal ST depression. Of the five patients with sustained ventricular tachycardia, none had ST elevation and two patients had abnormal ST depression before the onset of ventricular tachycardia. Detry and colleagues[140] reported on six patients without MI specifically referred to them for spontaneous angina known to be associated with ST elevation. During exercise testing, five patients exhibited elevation; of these five, three developed ventricular tachycardia and one developed ventricular fibrillation. We have subsequently seen one such patient who developed ST elevation and then ventricular tachycardia (20 beats) at maximal exercise. Figure 4-11 is an example of a patient with exercise-induced ventricular tachycardia and PVCs associated with ST elevation.

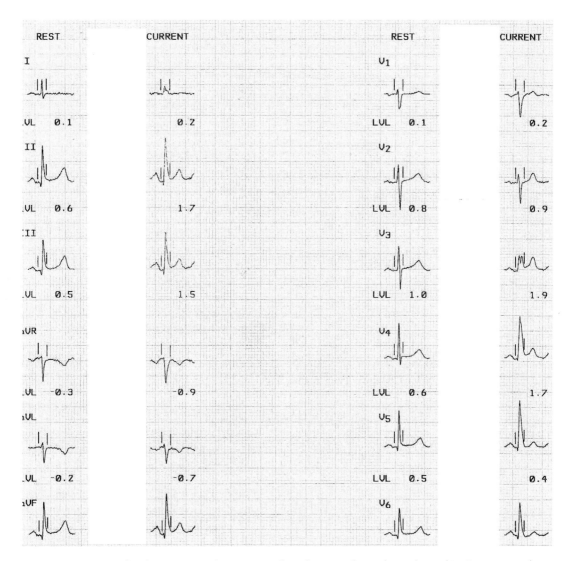

FIGURE 4-11   *Example of a patient with exercise-induced ventricular tachycardia and PVCs associated with ST elevation.*

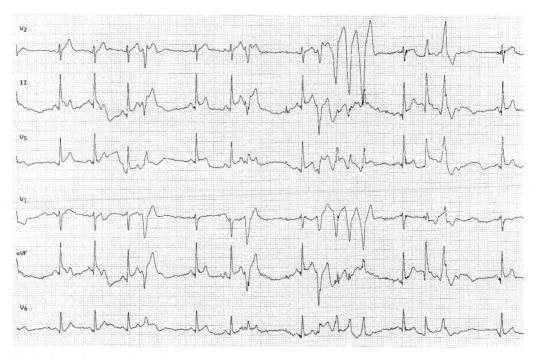

Maximal exercise recordings above.

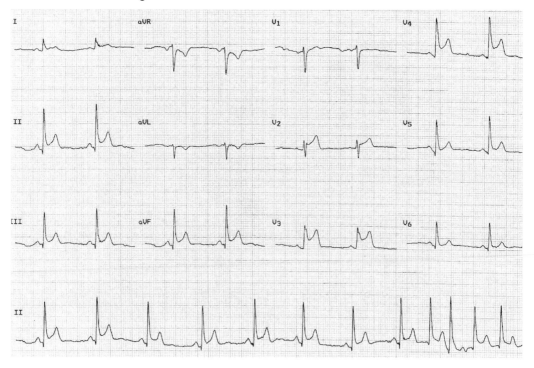

FIGURE 4-11—*Cont'd.*

Complications during exercise testing were reviewed in 25,075 consecutive patients, 14,037 men and 11,038 women, who underwent a total of 47,656 maximal treadmill or bicycle exercise tests between April 1985 and March 1999.[141] The mean age of the patients was 53 years. *Nonsustained ventricular tachycardia* was defined as eight or more consecutive ventricular ectopic beats at greater than 100 beats per minute. Patients undergoing exercise testing to evaluate the efficacy of pharmacotherapy for ventricular tachycardia were excluded. Twenty patients (0.08%) had exercise-induced ventricular tachycardia: six had ischemic heart disease, two had cardiomyopathy, five had other cardiac diseases, and seven showed no clinical evidence of heart disease.

Detry and colleagues[142] observed 6 cases of ventricular fibrillation (VF) and 40 cases of ventricular tachycardia (VT) in 7500 consecutive maximal exercise tests (0.6%); 13 patients had a sustained VT and 27 patients had a single short run of VT. No patient died immediately, but 11 patients died during the follow-up. The prognosis was determined by the underlying disease (most often CAD) and the type of arrhythmia. The 5-year survival rate was 84% in patients with a short run of VT and only 43% in patients with VF or sustained VT.

Fleg and Lakatta[113] analyzed data from the Baltimore Longitudinal Study on Aging to evaluate the prognostic impact of exercise-induced ventricular tachycardia. Of 597 male and 325 female volunteers between ages 21 and 96 years, 10 subjects (7 men and 3 women) with exercise-induced ventricular tachycardia (three PVCs in a row) were identified, representing 1.1% of those tested; only one was younger than 65 years. Exercise-induced ventricular tachycardia in these healthy subjects occurred mainly in the elderly; was limited to short, asymptomatic runs of 3 to 6 beats, usually near peak exercise; and did not predict increased cardiovascular morbidity or mortality rates over a 2-year follow-up.

The results of the studies analyzed above are summarized in Table 4-9.

ETIVA in Hypertrophic Cardiomyopathy

In addition to the research examining the prognostic value of ETIVA in patients with CAD, studies have also explored the implications of ETIVA in patients with other cardiac disorders such as hypertrophic cardiomyopathy (HCM). It had been proposed that nonsustained ventricular tachycardia (NSVT) is only of prognostic importance in patients with HCM when repetitive, prolonged, or associated with symptoms. In 2003, Monserrat and colleagues[143] examined the characteristics of NSVT episodes during Holter monitoring in patients with HCM in an attempt to determine their relationship to age and prognosis. The study included 531 patients with HCM (323 male, 39 ± 15 years). All underwent ambulatory ECG monitoring for 2 days. The team discovered that a total of 104 patients (19.6%) had NSVT and that the proportion of patients with NSVT increased with age ($p = 0.008$). Maximum left ventricular wall thickness and left atrial size were greater in patients with NSVT. Mean follow-up for this study was 70 ± 40 months. Sixty-eight patients died, 32 from sudden cardiac death. Twenty-one patients received an implantable cardioverter defibrillator (ICD). There were

TABLE 4-9 Analysis of 22 Clinical Prognostic Studies of Ventricular Ectopy during Exercise Testing

Results / Populations	Number of Studies	Does Ischemia Predict ETIVA (When Considered)?	Is Ventricular Ectopy Predictive of Mortality (Number of Studies)? Rest	Exercise	Recovery
Clinical Population					
Referred for symptoms	8	5 out of 6	1	5	1
Known CAD	7	2 out of 3	0	2	1
Healthy population					
Asymptomatic	5	1 out of 4	0	1	0
Screening study for employment	2	Not evaluated	0	2	1

NOTE: This table demonstrates that the majority of clinical studies of exercise testing and arrhythmias have included populations with clinical indications for exercise testing. In these populations, those with symptoms were more likely to have exercise-induced ventricular ectopy that was predictive of mortality. In addition, ischemia was correlated with exercise-induced ventricular arrhythmias. However, given the limited number of studies and absence of follow-up and assessment of ischemia in some reports, the data remain inconclusive.
CAD, coronary artery disease; ETIVA, exercise test–induced ventricular arrhythmias.

four appropriate ICD discharges. In patients 30 years old or younger (but not older than 30), 5-year freedom from sudden death was lower in those with NSVT (78% vs. 94%). There was no relation between the duration, frequency, or rate of NSVT runs and prognosis at any age. The odds ratio of sudden death in patients 30 years old or younger with NSVT was 4.4 compared with 2.2 in patients older than 30 years of age.

> **Key Point:** Nonsustained ventricular tachycardia is associated with a substantial increase in sudden death risk in young patients with HCM, although a relation between the frequency, duration, and rate of NSVT episodes could not be demonstrated.

Observer Agreement in Interpretation

The complexity of not only the human body but also the human mind has created measurements that, when applied to medical diagnosis, lead to observations with large variability (e.g., ST-segment displacement). The inherently subjective nature of these medical observations requires questioning of the results of most diagnostic methods—not only in regard to accuracy or validity but also agreement (among different interpreters for a given test). Attempts at describing or assessing agreement have been complex and variable, as evidenced in the literature by the numerous terms used: agreement, variability, consistency, within-observer correlation coefficients of agreement, and many others. Agreement has two subgroupings: intraobserver, referring to agreement of the individual observer with himself or herself on two separate occasions; and interobserver, referring to agreement among two or more individuals.

Blackburn[144] had 14 observers (from seven separate institutions) interpret 38 individual exercise ECG tests as normal, abnormal, or borderline. Five readers repeated the readings. In only 9 of the 38 exercise ECGs (24%) was there complete agreement among the 14 readers, and only 22 ECGs (58%) were read in agreement. This low value may be due to the fact that Blackburn's study did not allow a dichotomous decision because there was the third interpretation of borderline. In terms of intraobserver agreement there was a wide range from 58% to 92% and an average still less than ours for a dichotomous decision. Blackburn attributed this wide variation in both interobserver and intraobserver agreement to (1) the absence of defined criteria, (2) technical problems such as noise, and (3) differences in opinion as to ST-segment upsloping. Strict criteria such as the Minnesota code and computer analysis have been recommended as a means to increase agreement in electrocardiography.

Reproducibility of Treadmill Test Responses

Sullivan and colleagues[145] studied 14 male patients with exercise test–induced angina and ST-segment depression with treadmill testing on three consecutive days to evaluate the reproducibility of certain treadmill variables. Computerized ST-segment analysis and expired gas analysis, including anaerobic threshold, were evaluated for reproducibility using an intraclass correlation coefficient (ICC) analysis. The ICC is a generalization of the Pearson product-moment correlation that is not affected by the addition or multiplication of a given number of observations and provides a better indication of reproducibility than does the coefficient of variation. Oxygen uptake had a higher reliability coefficient ($r = .88$) and a smaller 90% confidence interval when compared with treadmill time ($r = .70$), consistent with a better correlation. The double product and heart rate were highly reproducible ($r = .90$ and $r = .94$, respectively). In addition, the 90% confidence interval for both double product and heart rate was small. The ST60 displacement in lead X and the lead of greatest displacement were highly reproducible ($r = .83$).

Measured oxygen uptake displayed better reproducibility than treadmill time at peak exercise, the onset of angina, and the gas exchange anaerobic threshold (ATGE). The double product, heart rate, and ST-segment displacement in lead X were found to be reproducible at peak exercise, the onset of angina, and the ATGE. Gas exchange analysis provided accurate physiologic determinants of exercise capacity in patients with angina pectoris. Noninvasive estimates of myocardial oxygen demand and

TABLE 4-10   Mean ± Standard Deviation of Exercise Test Variables at Maximal Angina-Limited Exercise

Variable	Mean and Standard Deviation				Intraclass Correlation Coefficient	
	Day 1	Day 2	Day 3	ANOVA $p < 0.05$*	r	90% Confidence Interval
Time (sec)	503 ± 72	516 ± 85	526 ± 66	0.35	0.70	0.48-0.86
VO_2	1.56 ± 0.29	1.55 ± 0.33	1.56 ± 0.29	0.99	0.88	0.76-0.95
Double product × 10³	18.9	19.6	18.9			
Heart rate (beats/min)	111 ±19	112 ±20	110 ±17	0.66	0.94	0.88-0.97
ST_{60} X (mV)	−0.14 ±0.11	−0.14 ±0.10	−0.14 ±0.10	0.99	0.83	0.63-0.92
ST_{60}GD (mV)	−0.19 ±0.08	−0.17 ±0.11	−0.20 ±0.09	0.17	0.82	0.60-0.92

Based on data from Sullivan M et al: The reproducibility of hemodynamic, electrocardiographic, and gas exchange data during treadmill exercise in patients with stable angina pectoris, Chest 86:375-382, 1984.
*$p > 0.05$ would indicate a significant change over three testing periods.
ANOVA, analysis-of-variance model to determine time trends; GD, lead of greatest ST-segment depression; ST_{60}, ST-segment depession at 60 msec after QRS end; VO_2, volume of oxygen; X, lead X (V5).

ischemia were reproducibly determined. These findings are summarized in Table 4-10.

Summary

The interpretation of the exercise test requires understanding exercise physiology and pathophysiology as well as expertise in electrocardiography. Certification is extremely important now that this technology is rapidly spreading beyond the subspecialty of cardiology. Training and experience are required as they are in other diagnostic procedures. For these reasons, the American College of Physicians and American College of Cardiology and the American Heart Association have published guidelines on clinical competence for physicians performing exercise testing (www.cardiologyonline.com/guidelines.htm, www.cardiology.org).[146-148]

All of the results of the exercise test must be considered. Attempts should be made to make the interpretation reliable by using good methods and following the aforementioned suggestions. When properly interpreted, the exercise test is one of the most important diagnostic and clinically helpful tests in medicine. Observer agreement is best when using dichotomous interpretations, and worst (most variable) when using more complex descriptions such as are involved in specifying location or overlapping areas. Computer analysis of the exercise ECG and measurement of gas exchange variables can be highly reproducible. However, as long as human judgment with all its complexities remains the basis for the final interpretation, there will always be some variation, and the human element will always be needed in medical diagnosis.

ST-segment depression is a representation of global subendocardial ischemia, with a direction determined largely by the placement of the heart in the chest. ST-segment depression does not localize coronary artery lesions. ST-segment depression in the inferior leads (II, aVF) is most often due to the atrial repolarization wave, which begins in the PR segment and can extend to the beginning of the ST segment. Severe transmural ischemia, resulting in wall motion abnormalities, causes a shift of the vector in the direction of the wall motion abnormality. However, preexisting areas of wall motion abnormality (i.e., scar), usually indicated by a Q wave, also cause such a shift, resulting in ST elevation without ischemia being present. When the resting ECG shows Q waves of an old MI, ST elevation is due to ischemia or wall motion abnormalities or both, whereas accompanying ST depression can be due to a second area of ischemia or reciprocal changes. When the resting ECG is normal, however, ST elevation is due to severe ischemia (spasm or a critical lesion), though accompanying ST depression is reciprocal. Such ST elevation is uncommon, is highly arrhythmogenic, and localizes. Exercise-induced ST depression loses its diagnostic power in patients with left bundle branch block, WPW, electronic pacemakers, ICDs with inverted T waves, and more than 1 mm of resting ST depression.

Exercise-induced R-wave and S-wave amplitude changes do not correlate with changes in left ventricular volume, ejection fraction, or ischemia. The consensus of many studies is that such changes do not have diagnostic value. ST-segment depression limited to the recovery period does not generally represent a "false positive" response. Inclusion of analysis during this time period increases the diagnostic yield of the exercise test. Other criteria, including downsloping ST changes in recovery and prolongation of depression, can improve test performance.

The evidence base for an exaggerated concern with silent ischemia is scant. Patients with silent ischemia (painless ST depression) usually have milder forms of coronary disease and a better prognosis. The evidence base for silent ischemia being more prevalent in diabetics is not as convincing as one would think given its widespread clinical acceptance. Many physicians believe that treadmill testing should be used for routine screening of diabetics.

As with resting ventricular arrhythmias, exercise-induced ventricular arrhythmias have an independent association with death in most patients with coronary disease and in asymptomatic individuals. The risk may be more delayed (> 6 years) than that associated with ST depression. Nonsustained ventricular tachycardia is uncommon during routine clinical treadmill testing and is usually well tolerated. In patients with a history of syncope, sudden death, physical examination with a large heart, murmurs, ECG showing prolonged QT, preexcitation, Q waves, and heart failure, ETIVAs are more worrisome. When healthy individuals exhibit PVCs during testing, do not react as if you were in a coronary care unit. The two available studies support the conclusion that ETISVAs are relatively rare compared with ventricular arrhythmias and appear to be benign except for their association with the development of atrial fibrillation in the future.

References

1. Einthoven W: Weiteres uber das elektrokardiogramm, *Arch fd ges Physiol* 122:517, 1908.
2. Simonson E: Electrocardiographic stress tolerance tests, *Prog Cardiovasc Dis* 13:269-292, 1970.
3. Blomqvist G: The Frank lead exercise electrocardiogram, *Acta Med Scand* 178:1-98, 1965.
4. Rautaharju PM et al: Waveform patterns in Frank-lead rest and exercise electrocardiograms of healthy elderly men, *Circulation* 48:541-548, 1973.
5. Simoons ML, Hugenholtz PG: Gradual changes of ECG waveform during and after exercise in normal subjects, *Circulation* 52:570-577, 1975.
6. Wolthuis RA et al: Normal electrocardiographic waveform characteristics during treadmill exercise testing, *Circulation* 60:1028-1035, 1979.
7. Gerson MC, Morris SN, McHenry PL: Relation of exercise induced physiologic ST-segment depression to R-wave amplitude in normal subjects, *Am J Cardiol* 46:778-782, 1980.
8. Kodama K et al: Transient U wave inversion during treadmill exercise testing in patients with left anterior descending coronary artery disease, *Angiology* 51(7):581-589, 2000.
9. Hayat NH, Salman H, Daimee MA, Thomas CS: Abolition of exercise induced positive U-wave after coronary angioplasty: clinical implication, *Int J Cardiol* 73(3):267-272, 2000.
10. Miwa K et al: Exercise-induced negative U waves in precordial leads as a marker of viable myocardium in patients with recent anterior myocardial infarction, *Int J Cardiol* 73(2):149-156, 2000.
11. Miwa K, Nakagawa K, Hirai T, Inoue H: Exercise-induced U-wave alterations as a marker of well-developed and well-functioning collateral vessels in patients with effort angina, *J Am Coll Cardiol* 35(3):757-763, 2000.
12. Fortuin NJ, Friesinger GC: Exercise-induced ST-segment elevation: clinical, electrocardiographic and arteriographic studies in twelve patients, *Am J Med* 49:459, 1970.
13. Hegge FN, Tuna N, Burchell HB: Coronary arteriographic findings in patients with axis shifts or ST-segment elevations on exercise testing, *Am Heart J* 86:603, 1973.
14. Chahine RA, Raizner AE, Ishimori T: The clinical significance of exercise-induced ST-segment elevation, *Circulation* 54:209, 1976.
15. Manvi KN, Ellestad MH: Elevated ST-segments with exercise in ventricular aneurysm, *J Electrocardiol* 5:317-323, 1972.
16. Sriwattanakomen S et al: ST-segment elevation during exercise: electrocardiographic and arteriographic correlation in 38 patients, *Am J Cardiol* 45:762-768, 1980.
17. Longhurst JC, Kraus WL: Exercise-induced ST elevation in patients without myocardial infarction, *Circulation* 60:616, 1979.
18. Waters DD, Chaitman BR, Bourassa MG, Tubau JF: Clinical and angiographic correlates of exercise-induced ST-segment elevation. Increased detection with multiple ECG leads, *Circulation* 61:286, 1980.

19. Bruce RA et al: Seattle Heart Watch initial clinical, circulatory and electrocardiographic response to maximal exercise, *Am J Cardiol* 33:459, 1974.

20. Bruce RA, Fisher LD: Unusual prognostic significance of exercise-induced ST elevation in coronary patients, *J Electrocardiol* 84-88, 1987.

21. De Feyter PJ et al: Clinical significance of exercise-induced ST-segment elevation, *Br Heart J* 46:84-92, 1981.

22. Bruce RA et al: ST-segment elevation with exercise: a marker for poor ventricular function and poor prognosis. Coronary Artery Surgery Study (CASS) confirmation of Seattle Heart Watch results, *Circulation* 4:897-905, 1988.

23. Braat SH, Kingma H, Brugada P, Wellens HJJ: Value of lead V4R in exercise testing to predict proximal stenosis of the right coronary artery, *J Am Coll Cardiol* 5:1308-1311, 1985.

24. Simoons M, Withagen A: The spatial association of ST shifts with nuclear perfusion. *Nuc Cardiol* 17:154-156, 1978.

25. Dunn RF et al: Exercise-induced ST-segment elevation in leads V1 or AVL. A predictor of anterior myocardial ischemia and left anterior descending coronary artery disease, *Circulation* 63:1357, 1981.

26. Mark DB et al: Localizing coronary artery obstructions with the exercise treadmill test, *Ann Intern Med* 106:53-55, 1987.

27. Hegge FN, Tuna N, Burchell HB: Coronary arteriographic findings in patients with axis shifts or S-T-segment elevations on exercise-stress testing, *Am Heart J* 5:603-615, 1973.

28. Gerwitz H et al: Role of myocardial ischemia in the genesis of exercise-induced ST-segment elevation in previous anterior myocardial infarction, *Am J Cardiol* 51:1293, 1983.

29. Caplin JL, Banim SO: Chest pain and electrocardiographic ST-segment elevation occurring in the recovery phase after exercise in a patient with normal coronary arteries, *Clin Cardiol* 8:228, 1985.

30. Hill JA, Conti CR, Feldman RL, Pepine CJ: Coronary artery spasm and its relationship to exercise in patients without severe coronary obstructive disease, *Clin Cardiol* 11:489-494, 1988.

31. Fox KM, Jonathan A, England D, Selwyn AP: Significance of exercise-induced ST-segment elevation in patients with previous myocardial infarction, *Am J Cardiol (Abstr)* 49:933, 1982.

32. Nobel RJ et al: Normalization of abnormal T-waves in ischemia, *Arch Intern Med* 136:391, 1976.

33. Sweet RL, Sheffield LT: Myocardial infarction after exercise-induced electrocardiographic changes in a patient with variant angina pectoris, *Am J Cardiol* 33:813, 1974.

34. McHenry PL, Morris SN: Exercise electrocardiography—current state of the art. In Schlant RC, Hurst JW, eds: *Advances in electrocardiography*, vol 2, New York, 1976, Grune & Stratton.

35. Maseri A et al: "Variant" angina: one aspect of a continuous spectrum of vasospastic myocardial ischemia, *Am J Cardiol* 42:1019-1025, 1978.

36. Detrano R et al: Factors affecting sensitivity and specificity of a diagnostic test: the exercise thallium scintigram, *Am J Med* 84:699-710, 1988.

37. Gutman RA, Bruce R: Delay of ST-depression after maximal exercise by walking for 2 minutes, *Circulation* 42:229, 1970.

38. Gibbons L, Cooper K: The safety of maximal exercise testing, *Circulation* 80:846, 1989.

39. Lachterman B, Lehmann KG, Abrahamson D, Froelicher VF: "Recovery only" ST-segment depression and the predictive accuracy of the exercise test, *Ann Intern Med* 112(1):11-16, 1990.

40. Karnegis JN, Matts J, Tuna N, Amplatz K, POSCH Group: Comparison of exercise-positive with recovery-positive treadmill graded exercise tests, *Am J Cardiol* 60:544-547, 1987.

41. Savage MP et al: Usefulness of ST-segment depression as a sign of coronary artery disease when confined to the post exercise recovery period, *Am J Cardiol* 60:1405-1406, 1987.

42. Froelicher VF et al: Value of exercise testing for screening asymptomatic men for latent coronary artery disease, *Prog Cardiovasc Dis* 18:265-276, 1976.

43. Ellestad M: *Stress testing: principles and practice,* ed 3, Philadelphia, 1986, FA Davis.

44. Rywik TM et al: Independent prognostic significance of ischemic ST-segment response limited to recovery from treadmill exercise in asymptomatic subjects, *Circulation* 97(21):2117-2122, 1998.

45. Lanza GA et al: Diagnostic and prognostic value of ST-segment depression limited to the recovery phase of exercise stress test, *Heart* 90(12):1417-1421, 2004.

46. Berman JA, Wynne J, Mellis G, Cohn PF: Improving diagnostic accuracy of the exercise test by combining R-wave changes with duration of ST-segment depression in a simplified index, *Am Heart J* 105:60-66, 1983.

47. Froelicher VF, Myers J, Follansbee WP, Labovitz AJ: *Exercise and the heart,* St Louis, 1993, Mosby, pp 48-69.

48. Hollenberg M et al: Influence of R-wave amplitude on exercise-induced ST-depression: need for a "gain factor" correction when interpreting stress electrocardiograms, *Am J Cardiol* 56:13-17, 1985.

49. Hakki A et al: R-wave amplitude: a new determinant of failure of patients with coronary heart disease to manifest ST-segment depression during exercise, *J Am Coll Cardiol* 3:1155-1160, 1984.

50. Jaffe MD: Effect of oestrogens on postexercise electrocardiogram, *Br Heart J* 38(12):1299-1303.

51. James FW: Exercise ECG test in children. In Chung EK, ed: *Exercise electrocardiography: a practical approach,* ed 2, Baltimore, 1983, Williams & Wilkins.

52. Sundqvist K, Atterhog JH, Jogestrand T: Effect of digoxin on the electrocardiogram at rest and during exercise in healthy subjects, *Am J Cardiol* 57:661-665, 1986.

53. Sundqvist K, Jogestrand T, Nowak J: The effect of digoxin on the electrocardiogram of healthy middle-aged and elderly patients at rest and during exercise—a comparison with the ECG reaction induced by myocardial ischemia, *J Electrocardiol* 35(3):213-217, 2002.

54. Tonkon MJ et al: Effects of digitalis on the exercise electrocardiogram in normal adult subjects, *Chest* 72:714-718, 1977.
55. Sketch MH et al: Digoxin-induced positive exercise tests: their clinical and prognostic significance, *Am J Cardiol* 48:655-659, 1981.
56. LeWinter M, Crawford M, O'Rourke R, Karliner J: The effects of oral propranolol, digoxin and combined therapy on the resting and exercise ECG, *Am Heart J* 93:202-209, 1977.
57. Whinnery JE, Froelicher VF, Stuart AJ: The electrocardiographic response to maximal treadmill exercise in asymptomatic men with left bundle branch block, *Am Heart J* 94:316, 1977.
58. Ibrahim NS, Selvester RS, Hagar JM, Ellestad MH: Detecting exercise-induced ischemia in left bundle branch block using the electrocardiogram, *Am J Cardiol* 82(6):832-835, 1998.
59. Vasey CG, O'Donnell J, Morris SN, McHenry P: Exercise-induced left bundle branch block and its relation to coronary artery disease, *Am J Cardiol* 56:892-895, 1985.
60. Grady TA et al: Prognostic significance of exercise-induced left bundle-branch block, *JAMA* 279(2):153-156, 1998.
61. Whinnery JE, Froelicher VF, Stuart AJ: The electrocardiographic response to maximal treadmill exercise in asymptomatic men with right branch bundle block, *Chest* 71:335, 1977.
62. Wolff L, Parkinson J, White P: Bundle branch block with short PR interval in healthy young people prone to paroxysmal tachycardia, *Am Heart J* 5:685-704, 1930.
63. Gazes PC: False positive exercise test in the presence of the Wolff-Parkinson-White syndrome, *Am J Cardiol* 78:13-15, 1969.
64. Poyatos ME et al: Exercise testing and thallium-201 myocardial perfusion scintigraphy in the clinical evaluation of patients with Wolff Parkinson White syndrome, *J Electrocardiol* 19:319-326, 1986.
65. Pappone C et al: Usefulness of invasive electrophysiologic testing to stratify the risk of arrhythmic events in asymptomatic patients with Wolff-Parkinson-White pattern, *J Am Coll Cardiol* 41:239-244, 2003.
66. Riff DP, Carleton RA: Effect of exercise on the atrial recovery wave, *Am Heart J* 82:759-763, 1971.
67. Sapin PM et al: Identification of false positive exercise tests with use of electrocardiographic criteria: a possible role for atrial repolarization waves, *J Am Coll Cardiol* 18:127-135, 1991.
68. Myrianthefs MM et al: False positive ST-segment depression during exercise in subjects with short PR segment and angiographically normal coronaries: correlation with exercise-induced ST-depression in subjects with normal PR and normal coronaries, *J Electrocardiol* 31(3):203-208, 1998.
69. McHenry PL, Cogan OJ, Elliott WC, Knoebel SB: False positive ECG response to exercise secondary to hyperventilation: cineangiographic correlation, *Am Heart J* 79(5):683-687, 1970.
70. McHenry PL et al: Evaluation of abnormal exercise electrocardiogram in apparently healthy subjects: labile repolarization (ST-T) abnormalities as a cause of false positive responses, *Am J Cardiol* 47(5):1152-1160, 1981.

71. Barnard R et al: Ischemic response to sudden strenuous exercise in healthy men, *Circulation* 48:936, 1973.

72. Foster C, Dymond DS, Carpenter J, Schmidt DH: Effect of warm-up on left ventricular response to sudden strenuous exercise, *J Appl Physiol* 53:380-383, 1982.

73. Abouantoun S et al: Can areas of myocardial ischemia be localized by the exercise electrocardiogram? A correlative study with thallium-201 scintigraphy, *Am Heart J* 108:933-941, 1984.

74. Fuchs RM et al: Electrocardiographic localization of coronary artery narrowings: studies during myocardial ischemia and infarction in patients with one-vessel disease, *Circulation* 66:1168-1175, 1982.

75. Weiner DA et al: The predictive value of anginal chest pain as an indicator of coronary disease during exercise testing, *Am Heart J* 96: 458-462, 1978.

76. Cole JP, Ellestad MH: Significance of chest pain during treadmill exercise; correlation with coronary events, *Am J Cardiol* 41:227-232, 1978.

77. Bodegard J et al: Possible angina detected by the WHO angina questionnaire in apparently healthy men with a normal exercise ECG: coronary heart disease or not? A 26 year follow up study, *Heart* 90(6):627-632, 2004.

78. Nesto RW et al: Angina and exertional myocardial ischemia in diabetic and nondiabetic patients: assessment by exercise thallium scintigraphy, *Ann Intern Med* 108(2):170-175, 1988.

79. Naka M et al: Silent myocardial ischemia in patients with non–insulin-dependent diabetes mellitus as judged by treadmill exercise testing and coronary angiography, *Am Heart J* 123(1):46-53, 1992.

80. Hikita H et al: Usefulness of plasma beta-endorphin level, pain threshold and autonomic function in assessing silent myocardial ischemia in patients with and without diabetes mellitus, *Am J Cardiol* 72(2):140-143, 1993.

81. Marchant B et al: Silent myocardial ischemia: role of subclinical neuropathy in patients with and without diabetes, *J Am Coll Cardiol* 22(5):1433-1437, 1993.

82. L'Huillier I et al: Predictive value of myocardial tomoscintigraphy in asymptomatic diabetic patients after percutaneous coronary intervention, *Int J Cardiol* 90(2-3):165-173, 2003.

83. Wackers FJ et al: Detection of silent myocardial ischemia in asymptomatic diabetic subjects: the DIAD study, *Diabetes Care* 27(8):1954-1961, 2004.

84. May O, Arildsen H, Damsgaard EM, Mickley H: Prevalence and prediction of silent ischaemia in diabetes mellitus: a population-based study, *Cardiovasc Res* 34(1):241-247, 1997.

85. Caracciolo EA et al: Diabetics with coronary disease have a prevalence of asymptomatic ischemia during exercise treadmill testing and ambulatory ischemia monitoring similar to that of nondiabetic patients. An ACIP database study, *Circulation* 93(12):2097-2105, 1996.

86. Falcone C et al: Silent myocardial ischemia in diabetic and nondiabetic patients with coronary artery disease, *Int J Cardiol* 90(2-3):219-227, 2003.

87. Lee DP, Fearon WF, Froelicher VF: Clinical utility of the exercise ECG in patients with diabetes and chest pain, *Chest* 119(5):1576-1581, 2001.

88. Fearon W, Voodi L, Atwood J, Froelicher V: The prognostic significance of silent ischemia detected by treadmill testing, *Am Heart J* 136:759-761, 1998.

89. Candinas RA, Podrid PJ: Evaluation of cardiac arrhythmias by exercise testing, *Herz* 15(1):21-27, 1990.

90. Kafka W, Petri H, Rudolph W: Exercise testing in the assessment of ventricular arrhythmias, *Herz* 7(3):140-149, 1982.

91. Hoffmann A, Wenk M, Follath F: Exercise-induced ventricular tachycardia as a manifestation of flecainide toxicity, *Int J Cardiol* 11(3):353-355, 1986.

92. Anastasiou-Nana MI et al: Occurrence of exercise-induced and spontaneous wide complex tachycardia during therapy with flecainide for complex ventricular arrhythmias: a probable proarrhythmic effect, *Am Heart J* 113(5):1071-1077, 1987.

93. Gosselink AT, Crijns HJ, Wiesfeld AC, Lie KI: Exercise-induced ventricular tachycardia: a rare manifestation of digitalis, *Clin Cardiol* 16(3):270-272, 1993.

94. Nazari J et al: Exercise induced fatal sinusoidal ventricular tachycardia secondary to moricizine, *Pacing Clin Electrophysiol* 15(10 pt 1):1421-1424, 1992.

95. Udall JA, Ellestad MH: Predictive implications of ventricular premature contractions associated with treadmill stress testing, *Circulation* 56:985-989, 1977.

96. Califf RM et al: Prognostic value of ventricular arrhythmias associated with treadmill testing in patients studied with cardiac catheterization for suspected ischemic heart disease, *J Am Coll Cardiol* 2:1060-1067, 1983.

97. Marieb MA et al: Clinical relevance of exercise-induced ventricular arrhythmias in suspected coronary artery disease, *Am J Cardiol* 66:172-178, 1990.

98. Schweikert RA et al: Association of exercise-induced ventricular ectopic activity with thallium myocardial perfusion and angiographic coronary artery disease in stable, low-risk populations, *Am J Cardiol* 83:530-534, 1999.

99. Sami M et al: Significance of exercise-induced ventricular arrhythmia in stable coronary artery disease: a coronary artery surgery study project, *Am J Cardiol* 54:1182-1188, 1984.

100. Casella G et al: Exercise-induced ventricular arrhythmias in patients with healed myocardial infarction, *Int J Cardiol* 40:229-235, 1993.

101. Jouven X et al: Long-term outcome in asymptomatic men with exercise-induced premature ventricular depolarizations, *N Engl J Med* 343:826-833, 2000.

102. Busby MJ, Shefrin EA, Fleg JL: Prevalence and long-term significance of exercise-induced frequent or repetitive ventricular ectopic beats in apparently healthy volunteers, *J Am Coll Cardiol* 14:1659-1665, 1989.

103. Froelicher VF et al: Epidemiologic study of asymptomatic men screened by maximal treadmill testing for latent coronary artery disease, *Am J Cardiol* 34:770-776, 1974.

104. Billman GE, Schwartz PJ, Gagnol JP, Stone HL: The cardiac response to submaximal exercise in dogs susceptible to sudden cardiac death, *J Appl Physiol* 59:890-897, 1985.

105. Friedwald VE, Spence DW: Sudden death associated with exercise: the risk-benefit issue, *Am J Cardiol* 66:183-188, 1990.

106. Verrier RL, Lown B: Behavorial stress and cardiac arrhythmias, *Annu Rev Physiol* 46:155-176, 1984.

107. Gettes LS: Electrolyte abnormalities underlying lethal and ventricular arrhythmias, *Circulation* 85(1 suppl):I70-I76, 1992.

108. Schwartz PJ, Billman GE, Stone HL: Autonomic mechanisms in VF due to acute myocardial ischemia during exercise in dogs with healed myocardial infarction: an experimental model for sudden cardiac death, *Circulation* 69:790-800, 1984.

109. Ranger S et al: Amplification of flecainide-induced ventricular conduction slowing by exercise. A potentially significant clinical consequence of use-dependent sodium channel blockade, *Circulation* 79(5):1000-1006, 1989.

110. Tuininga YS et al: Electrocardiographic patterns relative to initiating mechanisms of exercise-induced ventricular tachycardia, *Am Heart J* 126(2):359-367, 1993.

111. Kaufman ES et al: Electrocardiographic prediction of abnormal genotype in congenital long QT syndrome: experience in 101 related family members, *J Cardiovasc Electrophysiol* 12(4):455-461, 2001.

112. Laitinen PJ et al: Genes, exercise and sudden death: molecular basis of familial catecholaminergic polymorphic ventricular tachycardia, *Ann Med* 36(suppl 1):81-86, 2004.

113. Fleg JL, Lakatta EG: Prevalence and prognosis of exercise-induced nonsustained ventricular tachycardia in apparently healthy volunteers, *Am J Cardiol* 54(7):762-764, 1984.

114. Weiner DA, Levine SR, Klein MD, Ryan TJ: Ventricular arrhythmias during exercise testing: mechanism, response to coronary bypass surgery, and prognostic significance, *Am J Cardiol* 53:1553-1557, 1984.

115. McHenry PL, Morris SN, Kavalier M, Jordan JW: Comparative study of exercise-induced ventricular arrhythmias in normal subjects and patients with documented coronary artery disease, *Am J Cardiol* 37:609-616, 1976.

116. DeBusk RF, Davidson DM, Houston N, Fitzgerald J: Serial ambulatory electrocardiography and treadmill exercise testing after uncomplicated myocardial infarction, *Am J Cardiol* 45: 547-554, 1980.

117. Detry JR et al: Maximal exercise testing in patients with spontaneous angina pectoris associated with transient ST-segment elevation: risks and electrocardiographic findings, *Br Heart J* 37:897-905, 1975.

118. Bikkina M, Larson M, Levy D: Prognostic implications of asymptomatic ventricular arrhythmias: the Framingham Heart Study, *Ann Intern Med* 117:990-996, 1992.

119. Saini V, Graboys TB, Towne V, Lown B: Reproducibility of exercise-induced ventricular arrhythmia in patients undergoing evaluation for malignant ventricular arrhythmia, *Am J Cardiol* 63(11):697-701, 1989.

120. Faris JV, McHenry PL, Jordan JW, Morris SN: Prevalence and reproducibility of exercise-induced ventricular arrhythmias during maximal exercise testing in normal men, *Am J Cardiol* 37(4):617-622, 1976.

121. Condini M, Sommerfeldt L, Eybel C, Messer J: Clinical significance and characteristics of exercise-induced ventricular tachycardia, *Cathet Cardiovasc Diagn* 7:227-234, 1981.

122. Milanes J et al: Exercise tests and ventricular tachycardia, *West J Med* 145:473-476, 1986.

123. Fujiwara M et al: Clinical characteristics of ventricular tachycardia and ventricular fibrillation in exercise stress testing, *J Cardiol* 36(6):397-404, 2000.

124. Bunch TJ et al: The prognostic significance of exercise-induced atrial arrhythmias, *J Am Coll Cardiol* 43(7):1236-1240, 2004.

125. Maurer MS, Shefrin EA, Fleg JL: Prevalence and prognostic significance of exercise-induced supraventricular tachycardia in apparently healthy volunteers, *Am J Cardiol* 75(12):788-792, 1995.

126. Busby MJ, Shefrin EA, Fleg JL: Prevalence and long-term significance of exercise-induced frequent or repetitive ventricular ectopic beats in apparently healthy volunteers, *J Am Coll Cardiol* 14:1659-1665, 1989.

127. Froelicher VF et al: An epidemiological study of asymptomatic men screened with exercise testing for latent coronary heart disease, *Am J Cardiol* 34:770, 1974.

128. Froelicher VF et al: The value of exercise testing for screening asymptomatic men for latent CAD, *Prog Cardiovasc Dis* 18:265-276, 1976.

129. Morshedi-Meibodi A et al: Clinical correlates and prognostic significance of exercise-induced ventricular premature beats in the community: the Framingham Heart Study, *Circulation* 109(20): 2417-2422, 2004.

130. Frolkis JP, Pothier CE, Blackstone EH, Lauer MS: Frequent ventricular ectopy after exercise as a predictor of death, *N Engl J Med* 348(9): 781-790, 2003.

131. Sami M et al: Significance of exercise-induced ventricular arrhythmia in stable coronary artery disease: a coronary artery surgery study project, *Am J Cardiol* 54:1182, 1984.

132. Weiner DA, Levine SR, Klein MD, Ryan TJ: Ventricular arrhythmias during exercise testing: mechanism, response to coronary bypass surgery and prognostic significance, *Am J Cardiol* 53:1553, 1984.

133. Nair CK et al: Prognostic significance of exercise-induced complex ventricular arrhythmias in coronary artery disease with normal and abnormal left ventricular ejection fraction, *Am J Cardiol* 54:1136-1138, 1984.

134. Marieb MA et al: Clinical relevance of exercise-induced ventricular arrhythmias in suspected coronary artery disease, *Am J Cardiol* 66: 172-178, 1990.

135. Califf RM et al: Prognostic value of ventricular arrhythmias associated with treadmill exercise testing in patients studied with cardiac catheterization for suspected ischemic heart disease, *J Am Coll Cardiol* 2:1060-1067, 1983.

136. Partington S et al: Prevalence and prognostic value of exercise-induced ventricular arrhythmias, *Am Heart J* 145(1):139-146, 2003.

137. Beckerman J et al: Exercise-induced ventricular arrhythmias and cardiovascular death, *Ann Noninvasive Electrocardiol* 10(1):47-52, 2005.

138. Elhendy A et al: Functional and prognostic significance of exercise-induced ventricular arrhythmias in patients with suspected coronary artery disease, *Am J Cardiol* 90(2):95-100, 2002.

139. Yang JC, Wesley RC, Froelicher VF: Ventricular tachycardia during routine treadmill testing. Risk and prognosis, *Arch Intern Med* 151: 349-353, 1991.

140. Detry JR et al: Maximal exercise testing in patients with spontaneous angina pectoris associated with transient ST-segment elevation: risks and electrocardiographic findings, *Br Heart J* 37:897-905, 1975.

141. Tamakoshi K et al: Prevalence and clinical background of exercise-induced ventricular tachycardia during exercise testing, *J Cardiol* 39(4):205-212, 2002.

142. Detry JM, Abouantoun S, Wyns W: Incidence and prognostic implications of severe ventricular arrhythmias during maximal exercise testing, *Cardiology* 68(suppl 2):35-43, 1981.

143. Monserrat L et al: Non-sustained ventricular tachycardia in hypertrophic cardiomyopathy: an independent marker of sudden death risk in young patients, *J Am Coll Cardiol* 42(5):873-879, 2003.

144. Blackburn H, Technical Group on Exercise ECG: The exercise electrocardiogram: differences in interpretation, *Am J Cardiol* 24:871-880, 1968.

145. Sullivan M et al: The reproducibility of hemodynamic, electrocardiographic, and gas exchange data during treadmill exercise in patients with stable angina pectoris, *Chest* 86:375-382, 1984.

146. Schlant RC, Friesinger GC, Leonard JL: Clinical competence in exercise testing, *Circulation* 5:1884-1888, 1990.

147. COCATS guidelines: guidelines for training in adult cardiovascular medicine, Core Cardiology Training Symposium: June 27-28, 1994: American College of Cardiology [see comments], *J Am Coll Cardiol* 25:1-34, 1995.

148. Schlant RC, Friesinger GC, Leonard JJ: Clinical competence in exercise testing: a statement for physicians from the ACP/ACC/AHA Task Force on Clinical Privileges in Cardiology, *J Am Coll Cardiol* 16:1061-1065, 1990.

5   Diagnostic Applications of Exercise Testing

Introduction

Exercise can be considered a true test of the heart because it is the most common everyday stress that humans undertake. The exercise test is the most practical and useful procedure in the clinical evaluation of cardiovascular status. This chapter focuses on the most common use of the exercise test: to diagnose coronary artery disease (CAD) in patients with symptoms of ischemic CAD. The most common clinical presentation of CAD requiring diagnosis is angina pectoris, and the latest guidelines for evaluation of such patients still call for the standard exercise electrocardiogram (ECG) test as the first test.[1]

> **Key Point:** The standard exercise ECG test, bolstered by the application of scores, is the first test indicated for the diagnosis of CAD in the patient with chest pain or other possible ischemic symptoms unless the baseline ECG exhibits abnormalities that make ST analysis questionable.

Diagnostic Test Performance Definitions

Sensitivity and *specificity* are the terms used to define how reliably a test distinguishes diseased from nondiseased individuals. They are parameters of the accuracy of a diagnostic test. *Sensitivity* is the percentage of times that a test gives an abnormal (positive) result when those with the disease are tested. *Specificity* is the percentage of times that a test gives a normal (negative) result when those without the disease are tested. This is quite different from the colloquial use of the word *specific*.

The mnemonics SnNout and SpPin can be used to remember the performance of a test with high values of either sensitivity or specificity. When a test has a very high **Sen**sitivity, a **N**egative test rules **out** the diagnosis

TABLE 5-1   Definitions and Calculations of the Terms Used to Quantify the Discriminatory Characteristics of a Test

Sensitivity = (TP/TP + FN) × 100   Specificity = (TN/FP + TN) × 100

where
TP = those with abnormal test and disease (true positives)
TN = those with a normal test and no disease (true negatives)
FP = those with an abnormal test but no disease (false positives)
FN = those with a normal test but disease (false negatives)

$$TP + TN + FP + FN = \text{total population}$$

+ Likelihood ratio = ratio that a positive response is likely to have disease versus a negative response:

$$\frac{\text{sensitivity}}{1 - \text{specificity}}$$

− Likelihood ratio = ratio that a negative response is not likely to have disease versus a positive response:

$$\frac{1 - \text{sensitivity}}{\text{specificity}}$$

$$P(CAD) = \text{probability of CAD} \; = \; \frac{TP + FP}{\text{total population}}$$

$$P(\text{no CAD}) = 1 - P(\text{no CAD}) \; = \; \frac{TN + FP}{\text{total population}}$$

PV+ = percentage of those with an abnormal (positive) test result who have disease
PV− = percentage of those with a negative test that do not have disease
Predictive accuracy = percentage of correct classifications, both positive and negative
ROC = range of characteristics curve; plot of sensitivity versus specificity for the range of measurement cutpoints

$$\text{Predictive value of an abnormal test (PV+)} \; = \; \frac{TP}{TP + FP} \times 100$$

or

$$\text{Sensitivity} \times \frac{P(CAD)}{\text{Sensitivity} \times P(CAD)} + (1 + \text{Specificity})[1 - P(CAD)]$$

$$\text{Predictive accuracy} \; = \; \frac{TP + TN}{TP + TN + FP + FN} \times 100$$

or

$$[\text{Sensitivity} \times P(CAD)] + [\text{Specificity} \times [1 - P(CAD)]]$$

(SnNout); when a test has a very high **Sp**ecificity, a **P**ositive test rules **in** the diagnosis (SpPin).

The method of calculating the terms describing test performance is shown in Table 5-1.

There are established rules that should be considered when considering studies that have attempted to demonstrate the diagnostic characteristics of a test.[2-4] The two key rules are limitation of workup bias and avoidance of limited challenge. These rules can be followed by including all consecutive patients referred for diagnosis in the target population studying the test. If these rules have not been followed, the proposed sensitivity and specificity (as well as the range of characteristics curve and the area under the curve) can be exaggerated, and the test will not have the proposed characteristics when used clinically.

> **Key Point:** The diagnostic characteristics proposed for a new test or measurement must be assessed by determining if the rules for such studies were followed; otherwise the value of the new test or measurement in clinical practice is uncertain.

Cutpoint or Discriminant Value

A basic step in applying any testing procedure for the separation of normal individuals from patients with disease is to determine a value measured by the test (a threshold test result, or *cutpoint*) that best separates the two groups. A problem is that there is usually a considerable overlap of measurement values of a test in the groups with and without disease. Two bell-shaped normal distribution curves, one for the test variable in a population of normal individuals and the other for this variable in a population with disease, are illustrated in Figure 5-1. Along the vertical axis is the number of patients and along the horizontal axis could be the value for such measurements as Q-wave size, exercise-induced ST-segment depression, or creatine phosphokinase. Note that there is considerable overlap between the two curves. The optimal test would be able to achieve the most marked separation

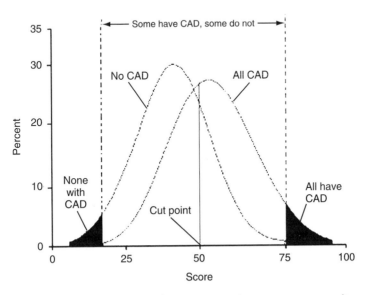

FIGURE 5-1 *Distribution of those with and without angiographic coronary artery disease according to values for a simple exercise test diagnostic score. Two bell-shaped normal distribution curves are illustrated, one for the test variable in a population of normal individuals and the other for this variable in a population with coronary artery disease.*

of these two bell-shaped curves, minimizing the overlap. Unfortunately, most of the tests currently used for the diagnosis of CAD, including the exercise test, have a considerable overlap of the range of measurements for the normal population and for those with heart disease. Therefore problems arise when a certain test measurement value (e.g., cutpoint) is used to separate these two groups (e.g., 0.1 mV of ST-segment depression or a probability level). The value can be set far to the right (e.g., 0.2 mV of ST-segment depression or a higher probability level) to identify nearly all the normal individuals as being free of disease. This gives the test a high specificity, but then a substantial number of those with the disease are called *normal*. The value can be chosen far to the left (i.e., 0.5 mm of ST-segment depression) to identify nearly all those with disease as being abnormal. This gives the test a high sensitivity, but then many normal individuals are identified as being abnormal.

There can be reasons for wanting to adjust a test to have a relatively higher sensitivity or relatively higher specificity. However, sensitivity and specificity are inversely related; that is, when sensitivity is the highest, specificity is the lowest, and vice versa. Any test has a range of inversely related sensitivities and specificities that can be chosen by specifying a certain discriminant or cutpoint value of the test measurement.

Further complicating the choice of a discriminant value is that many diagnostic procedures do not have values established that best separate normal individuals from those with disease. Even the Q wave on the standard resting ECG and exercise-induced ST-segment depression have uncertainty regarding what is the best discriminant value (or cutpoint) and what the sensitivity and specificity of the currently used criteria are. Arbitrary cutpoints have been selected to assist clinicians in distinguishing those with and without disease.

Key Point: Sensitivity and specificity are inversely related, and their relative values are determined by the cutpoint chosen for the criteria for normal or abnormal.

Receiver Operator or Range of Characteristic Curves

Plots of sensitivity versus specificity for a range of test measurement cutpoints provide an efficient way to compare test performance. Range of characteristics (ROC) curves are particularly helpful when optimal cutpoints for discriminating those with disease from those without disease need to be established to obtain particular sensitivities or specificities. A straight diagonal line indicates that the measurement or test has no discriminating power for the disease being tested. The greater the area of the curve below the diagonal line (i.e., area under the curve [AUC]), the greater its discriminating power. ROC curves make it possible to determine and then choose the appropriate cutpoints for the desired sensitivity or specificity and demonstrate the respective specificity and sensitivity. An example of an ROC curve is given in Figure 5-2. Cutpoints for a test measurement can be chosen from the curves that are associated with particular sensitivities and specificities. Population differences can shift the calibration for probability estimates or for the amount of ST-segment depression,

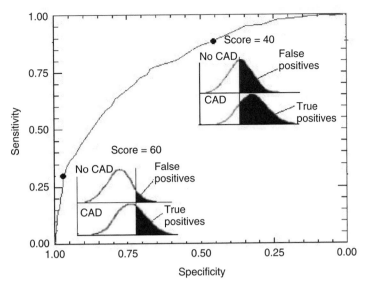

FIGURE 5-2   *Illustration of an ROC curve and how it can help choose cutpoints for different applications of a test or score.*

often without changing the ROC area. For instance, 1 mm of ST-segment depression can be associated with a sensitivity/specificity of 67%/72% in one population and 50%/90%, respectively, in another population because of differences in selection bias, but the ROC area of 0.70 can be maintained in both populations.

> **Key Point:** The diagnostic characteristics of a test can be illustrated by an ROC curve. A straight line with an area of 0.5 implies no discrimination. The greater the AUC, the greater the discriminatory value of the test or measurement. Falsely high AUC can be obtained if limited challenge applies to the study population. The ROC can be used to choose cutpoints with higher or lower relative sensitivities or specificities.

Predictive Accuracy

Predictive accuracy is the percentage of correct or true classifications out of all patients tested. It is the percentage of patients correctly classified as having or not having the disease (see Table 5-1). Mathematically, it is the sum of true positives and true negatives divided by the total population. Predictive accuracy depends on the prevalence of disease in the population tested. It simply is the percentage of times the test measurement correctly classifies those tested as having or not having disease.

The predictive accuracy of exercise-induced ST-segment depression can be demonstrated by analyzing the results obtained when exercise testing and coronary angiography have both been used to evaluate patients. From these studies, which usually represent an intermediate probability of disease (i.e., 50% prevalence), the exercise test cutpoints for horizontal or downsloping ST-segment depression have approximately a 70% predictive accuracy for angiographically significant CAD (an obstruction that causes ischemia with increased heart rate). In other words, the standard exercise ECG can classify those tested correctly as having or not having disease 70% of the time. As presented later, scores can significantly improve on predictive accuracy.

> **Key Point:** Predictive accuracy depends on the prevalence of the disease being diagnosed, whereas the AUC ROC is largely independent of disease prevalence.

Predictive Value

An additional term that helps define the diagnostic value of a test is the *predictive value* of a positive result. Table 5-1 also shows how this term is calculated. The predictive value of an abnormal test (positive predictive value) is the percentage of those persons with an abnormal test who have disease. Predictive value cannot be estimated directly from a test's demonstrated specificity or sensitivity. Predictive value depends on the prevalence of disease in the population tested. This is the test performance parameter most apparent to the physician, who can easily note how often someone with an abnormal test has disease.

Table 5-2 illustrates how a test with 50% sensitivity and 90% specificity performs in a population with a 5% prevalence of disease. Since 5% of 10,000 men have disease, 500 have disease. In the middle column are the numbers of men with abnormal tests and in the far right column are the

TABLE 5-2 Calculation of the Predictive Value of an Abnormal Test (Positive Predictive Value) Using a Test with a Sensitivity of 50% and a Specificity of 90% in Two Populations of 10,000 Patients: One with a CAD Prevalence of 5% and the Other with a 50% prevalence

CAD Prevalence	Subjects	Test Characteristics	Number with Abnormal Test Result	Number with Normal Test Result	Predictive Value of a Positive Result
5%	500 with CAD 9500 without CAD	50% sensitive 90% specific	250 (TP) 950 (FP)	250 (FN) 8550 (TN)	250/250+950 = 21%
50%	5000 with CAD 5000 without CAD	50% sensitive 90% specific	2500 (TP) 500 (FP)	2500 (FN) 4500 (TN)	2500/3000 = 83%

	Predictive Value of an Abnormal Test		Risk Ratio	
Disease prevalence sensitivity/specificity	5%	50%	5%	50%
70/90%	27%	88%	27 ×	3 ×
90/70%	14%	75%	14 ×	5 ×
90/90%	32%	90%	64 ×	9 ×
66/84%	18%	80%	9 ×	3 ×

CAD, Coronary artery disease; FN, those with a normal test but disease (false negatives); FP, those with an abnormal test but no disease (false positives); TN, those with a normal test and no disease (true negatives); TP, those with abnormal test and disease (true positives). This table demonstrates the important influence that prevalence has on the positive predictive value.

number with normal tests. Because the test is 50% sensitive, 250 of those with disease have abnormal tests and are true positives. The remaining 250 have normal tests and are false negatives. Because the test is 90% specific, 90% of the 9500 without disease are true negatives, whereas the remainder are false positives. To calculate the predictive value, the number of true positives is divided by the number of those with an abnormal test (true positives plus false positives). The predictive value of an abnormal response is directly related to the prevalence of the disease in the population tested. There are more false-positive responses when exercise testing is used in a population with a low prevalence than when it is used in a population with a high prevalence of disease. This fact explains the greater percentage of false positives found when using the test as a screening procedure. Screening applies the test in an asymptomatic group (with a low prevalence of CAD) as opposed to when using it as a diagnostic procedure in patients with symptoms most likely caused by CAD (higher prevalence of CAD).

As shown in Table 5-2, in a test with characteristics similar to those of the exercise ECG, the predictive value of 1 mm of ST depression increases from 21% when there is a 5% prevalence of disease to 83% when there is a 50% prevalence of disease. Thus four times as many with an abnormal test will have coronary disease when the patient population increases from a 5% prevalence of CAD to 50% prevalence.

> **Key Point:** Predictive value is the test performance parameter most apparent to the clinician administering a test, but it can also be misleading in terms of the value of the test for actual decision making.

Diagnostic Endpoints

Symptoms, History, or Findings Possibly Caused by Coronary Artery Disease

The flow diagram shown in Figure 5-3 illustrates the clinical logic for the diagnosis of CAD. Though the exercise test can be used to evaluate other disease processes, all of the available publications regarding diagnosis have addressed the issue of coronary disease. In fact, though a logical thought process can lead to performing exercise tests in other situations for diagnosis, studies have only evaluated test performance in patients with chest pain.

Diagnosis of Coronary Artery Disease

To evaluate a test for a disease, one must demonstrate how well the test distinguishes between those individuals with and those without the disease. Evaluation of exercise testing as a diagnostic test for CAD depends on the population tested, which must be divided into those with and those without CAD by independent techniques. Coronary angiography and clinical follow-up for coronary events are two methods of separating a population into those with and those without coronary disease. Surrogates for CAD such as other

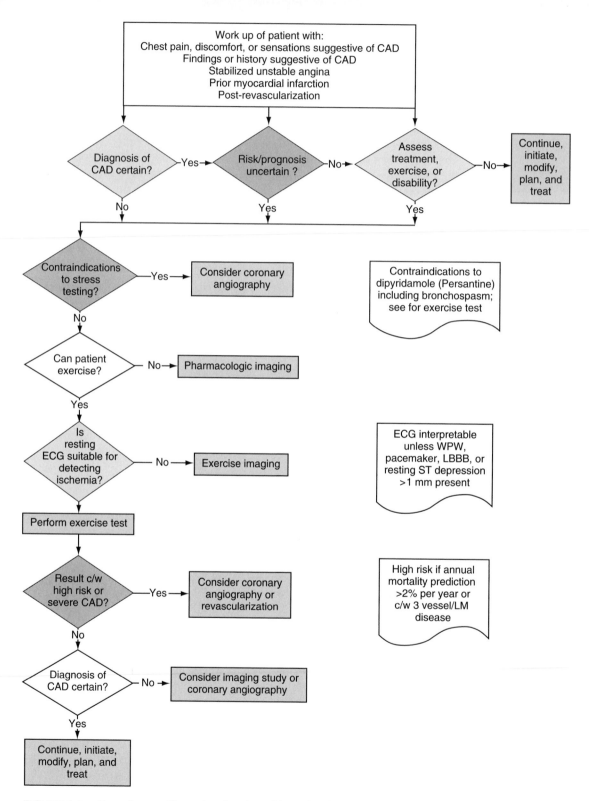

FIGURE 5-3 *Flow diagram illustrating the clinical logic for the diagnosis of CAD. (From the ACC/AHA exercise test guidelines.)*

test results or therapeutic interventions are not valid ways to discriminate those with and without disease for the purpose of evaluating a diagnostic procedure. One also must be clear regarding whether the test is diagnosing ischemia or CAD. Whereas the contrary is rarely true, CAD can be present and not cause ischemia. In fact, myocardial infarctions (MIs) or unstable angina can occur in patients with subcritical lesions because of spasm or thrombus. These lesions rarely cause death or major myocardial damage, but they are responsible for a portion of the morbidity of coronary disease. The mechanism is thought to be plaque rupture or fracturing, which releases thrombogenic material to the arterial surface. Neither the exercise test nor any other noninvasive tests available at this time can identify patients with subclinical atherosclerotic lesions; the tests should be able to recognize myocardial ischemia, however, due to flow-limiting lesions.

> **Key Point:** The diagnostic characteristics of the exercise test have only been studied in the subset of patients with chest pain; other ischemic manifestations such as dyspnea on exertion or fatigue have not been evaluated. Although coronary angiography has limitations, its findings are the target for the available interventions; therefore coronary obstructions remain the most clinically appropriate gold standard for exercise test performance.

Electrocardiogram Criteria

The standard criterion for an abnormal ECG response to exercise is horizontal or downward-sloping ST-segment depression of 0.1 mV or more for 80 msec. It appears to be due to generalized subendocardial ischemia. A "steal" phenomenon is likely from ischemic areas because of the effect of extensive collateralization in the subendocardium. ST-segment depression does not localize the area of ischemia (as does ST elevation), nor does it help indicate which coronary artery is occluded. The normal ST-segment vector response to tachycardia and to exercise is a shift rightward and upward. The degree of this shift appears to have a fair amount of biologic variation. Most normal individuals will have early repolarization at rest, which will shift to the isoelectric PR-segment line in the inferior, lateral, and anterior leads with exercise. This shift can be further influenced by ischemia and myocardial scars. When the later portions of the ST segment are affected, flattening or downward depression can be recorded. Both local effects and the direction of the spatial changes during repolarization cause the ST segment to have a different appearance at the many surface sites that can be monitored. The more leads with these apparent ischemic shifts, the more severe the disease.

The probability and severity of CAD are directly related to the amount of J-junction depression and are inversely related to the slope of the ST segment. Downsloping ST-segment depression is more serious than is horizontal depression, and both are more serious than upsloping depression. However, patients with upsloping ST-segment depression, especially when the slope is less than 1 mV/sec, probably are at increased risk. If a slowly ascending slope is used as a criterion for abnormal, the specificity of exercise testing is decreased (more false positives), although the test may become more sensitive. One electrode can show upsloping ST-segment depression while an adjacent electrode shows horizontal or downsloping depression. If an apparently borderline ST segment with an inadequate slope is recorded in a single precordial lead in a patient highly suspected of having CAD, multiple precordial leads should be scanned before the exercise test is called normal. An upsloping depressed ST segment may be the precursor to abnormal ST-segment depression in the recovery period or at higher heart rates during greater workloads.

> **Key Point:** ST-segment depression is the most common ECG manifestation of ischemia. It does not localize the site of ischemia, but the amount, number of leads,[5] and duration generally do reflect the amount of ischemia. Most abnormal ST-segment depression occurs in V4–5–6.[6-10] The probability of disease and its severity also are proportional to the slope of the ST segment, with downsloping depression being the most ominous. If ST depression occurs only in the inferior leads, it is usually due to atrial repolarization,[11] and a false positive must be considered.[12]

ST-Segment Interpretation Issues

Upsloping ST-Segment Depression
Patients with upsloping ST-segment depression, especially when the slope is less than 1 mV/sec, probably have an increased probability of coronary disease. If a slowly ascending slope is used as a criterion for abnormal, the specificity of exercise testing is decreased (more false positives), although the test becomes more sensitive.

Exercise-Induced ST Elevation
Early repolarization is a common resting pattern of ST elevation that occurs in normal individuals. Exercise-induced ST-segment elevation is always considered from the baseline ST level. ST elevation is relatively common after a Q-wave infarction, but ST elevation in leads without Q waves occurs in only 1 of every 1000 patients seen in a typical exercise laboratory.[13-19] ST elevation on a normal ECG (other than in aVR or V1) represents transmural ischemia (caused by spasm or a critical lesion), and in contrast to ST-segment depression, is very arrhythmogenic and localizes the ischemia. When it occurs in V2–4, the left anterior descending is involved; in the lateral leads, the left circumflex and diagonals are involved; and in II, III, and aVF, the right coronary artery is involved. This phenomenon appears to be 100% specific but is not very sensitive. When the resting ECG shows Q waves of an old MI, ST elevation is due to wall motion abnormalities and a large area of infarction, whereas accompanying ST depression can be due to a second area of ischemia or reciprocal changes.

R-Wave Changes
A multitude of factors affect the R-wave amplitude response to exercise,[20] and the response does not have diagnostic significance.[21,22] R-wave amplitude

typically increases from rest to submaximal exercise, perhaps to a heart rate of 130 beats per minute, and then decreases to a minimum at maximal exercise.[23] We have been unable to improve the diagnostic value of exercise-induced ST-segment depression by adjusting the amount of ST-segment depression by the R-wave height.

ST-Segment Depression in Recovery

ST-segment depression can occur during exercise or in recovery, and both are important to evaluate. It has been proposed that changes limited to the recovery period are more likely to represent false-positive responses[24] or are due to coronary artery spasm.[25] To facilitate imaging as soon as possible during recovery, studies including postexercise nuclear and echocardiographic imaging sometimes do not include an ECG evaluation after exercise.[26] Though a cool-down walk is known to obscure recovery ST shifts,[27] a cool-down walk has been implemented for safety concerns.[28]

These issues have now been resolved by a study from our laboratory (Lachterman and colleagues[29]) and others.[30-33] Abnormal ST-segment depression occurring only in recovery provides clinically useful information and is not more likely to represent a false-positive response. When considered with changes in exercise, changes in recovery increase the sensitivity of the exercise test without a decline in predictive value. A cool-down walk should be avoided after exercise testing, and exercise test scores and nuclear testing should consider recovery ST measurements. Avoidance of a cool-down walk has not resulted in an increased complication rate. The importance of recovery measurements made by computer was consistent with previous experience from visual analysis. That is, recovery changes are not generally false positives as previously thought, and they have excellent diagnostic value. Also, the ROC values for other ST measurements in recovery tended to be greater than comparable measurements during maximal exercise. The recovery time is probably so important because the conflicting impact of increasing heart rate during exercise "pulling" up the ST segment (resulting in a trend toward a positive slope) is no longer present. It is important to have the patient lie down immediately after exercise and not perform a cool-down walk for the recovery measurement to function as it did in our studies.

Data have also been presented supporting a correlation between prolonged ST-segment depression during recovery and more severe CAD.[34,35]

Influence of Other Factors on Test Performance

Medications

Drugs and resting ECG abnormalities can affect the results of exercise testing.

Digoxin

Digoxin has been shown to produce abnormal ST depression in response to exercise in 25% to 40% of apparently healthy individuals.[36-39] The prevalence of abnormal responses is directly related to age, and there is some evidence that digoxin can uncover subclinical coronary disease.[40] From a meta-analysis, the diagnostic characteristics of the exercise ECG are not affected sufficiently to negate the exercise test as the first test in the patient receiving digoxin with possible coronary disease. Although patients must be off the medication for at least 2 weeks for its effect to wash out, it is not necessary to do so before diagnostic testing.[39] The reason for which digoxin is administered can also affect test interpretation. However, the most common response of testing is a negative response, and this still has an important impact because sensitivity is not altered by digoxin.

Beta Blockers
For routine exercise testing in the clinical setting, it appears to be unnecessary for physicians to accept the risk of stopping beta blockers before testing when a patient is showing possible symptoms of ischemia. Stopping them in ischemic patients can precipitate an acute coronary syndrome (ACS) or cause blood pressure to be uncontrolled. Exercise test results are often considered "inadequate" or "nondiagnostic" in patients taking beta blockers and in patients who do not achieve 85% of their age-predicted maximal heart rate.[41] *The only way to maintain sensitivity with the standard exercise test in patients on beta blockers who fail to reach target heart rate is to use a treadmill score or 0.5 mm of ST depression as the criterion for abnormal.* Sensitivity and predictive accuracy of standard ST criteria significantly decrease in male patients taking beta blockers and do not reach target heart rate. In those who fail to reach target heart rate and are not beta blocked, sensitivity and predictive accuracy are maintained.

Other Medications
Various medications can affect test performance by altering the hemodynamic response of blood pressure, including antihypertensives and vasodilators. Acute administration of nitrates can attenuate the angina and ST depression associated with myocardial ischemia. Flecainide has been associated with exercise-induced ventricular tachycardia.[42,43] Anecdotal reports of the effects of other medications are unsubstantiated.

Effect of Baseline ECG Abnormalities

Left Bundle Branch Block
Exercise-induced ST-segment depression usually occurs with left bundle branch block (LBBB) and has no association with ischemia.[44] Even up to 1 cm can occur in healthy normal subjects.[45,46]

Exercise-Induced Left Bundle Branch Block
Exercise-induced LBBB independently was associated with a threefold higher risk of death and major cardiac events; however, this study did not reproduce the finding from the Krannert Institute, which suggested that CAD was more likely if the LBBB occurred below a heart rate of 125 beats per minute.[47] A review of the English- and French-language literature regarding intermittent

exercise-induced LBBB revealed that the mortality rate in the group with structural heart disease was 2.7% per year, whereas the mortality rate was 0.2% per year when no structural heart disease was identified, and that noninvasive testing had limited ability to detect or exclude CAD.[48]

Right Bundle Branch Block

Exercise-induced ST-segment depression usually occurs with right bundle branch block in the anterior chest leads (V1–3) and has no association with ischemia.[49] However, when ST-segment depression occurs in the left chest leads (V5–6) or the inferior leads (II, aVF), it has test characteristics similar to those seen when a normal resting ECG is present.

Resting ST-Segment Depression

Resting ST-segment depression has been identified as a marker for adverse cardiac events in patients with and without known CAD.[50-55] Per the guidelines, the test characteristics appear to be so degraded by 1 mm or more of resting ST depression that imaging should be added to the test. However, resting ST depression does not impair the prognostic characteristics of the test when other responses are considered in scores.

Key Point: Resting ST-segment depression is a marker for a higher prevalence and severity of CAD and is associated with a poor prognosis; standard exercise testing continues to be diagnostically useful in patients with less than 1 mm of resting ST depression. The published data appear to contain few patients with major resting ST depression (>1 mm). Exercise testing is unlikely to provide important diagnostic information in such patients, and exercise-imaging modalities are preferred in this subset of patients.

Clinical Factors

Gender

There has been controversy regarding the use of the standard exercise ECG test in women. In fact, some experts have recommended that only imaging techniques be used for testing women because of the impression that the standard exercise ECG did not perform as well for them as it does for men. The recent American College of Cardiology/American Heart Association (ACC/AHA) guidelines reviewed this subject in detail and came to another conclusion. The recent guidelines have stated that exercise testing for the diagnosis of significant coronary disease in adult men and women, with symptoms or other clinical findings suggestive of CAD, is a Class I indication (i.e., definitely indicated). The statement reads that adult male or female patients with an intermediate pretest probability of coronary disease (the intermediate probability based on gender, age, and chest pain symptoms) is a definite indication for the standard exercise test. Women in the intermediate classification are from 30 to 59 years old with typical or definite angina pectoris, from 30 to 69 years old with atypical or probable angina pectoris, and 60 to 68 years old with nonanginal chest pain (Table 5-3).

TABLE 5-3   Pretest Probability of Coronary Disease by Symptoms, Gender, and Age

Age	Gender	Typical/Definite Angina Pectoris	Atypical/Probable Angina Pectoris	Nonanginal Chest Pain	Asymptomatic
30-39 yr	Male	Intermediate	Intermediate	Low (<10%)	Very low (<5%)
	Female	Intermediate	Very low (<5%)	Very low	Very low
40-49 yr	Male	High	Intermediate	Intermediate	Low
	Female	Intermediate	Low	Very low	Very low
50-59 yr	Male	High (>90%)	Intermediate	Intermediate	Low
	Female	Intermediate	Intermediate	Low	Very low
60-69 yr	Male	High	Intermediate	Intermediate	Low
	Female	High	Intermediate	Intermediate	Low

High, <90%; intermediate, 10%-90%; low, <10%; very low, <5%.
No data exist for patients younger than 30 years or older than 69 years, but it can be assumed that coronary artery disease prevalence increases with age.

Numerous studies have now shown that equations or scores based on multivariable statistical analysis enable prediction of prognosis and improve the diagnostic characteristics of the exercise test. Equations that consider hemodynamic and clinical variables enable a better diagnosis of CAD in both men and women. Studies have shown that if estrogen status is considered, the diagnostic characteristics can be much improved in women. In general this means that women who are premenstrual or are receiving estrogen can obtain the same result from these equations if the exercise ST response is not considered. The Duke Treadmill Score has been validated in both genders as well.

> **Key Point:** Concern about false-positive ST responses in women may be addressed by careful assessment of pretest probability and selective use of stress imaging before proceeding to angiography. Scores from studies of exercise testing in women have exhibited test characteristics comparable with those of men when pretest probability is considered. Currently, insufficient data exist to justify a routine stress imaging test as the initial test in coronary disease in women.

Diabetics and Elderly

The standard exercise test appears to have similar test characteristics in patients with diabetes[56] and in the elderly.[57]

Meta-Analysis of Exercise Testing Studies

Focusing on the clinical and test methodologic issues, we investigated the variability of the reported diagnostic accuracy of the exercise ECG by applying meta-analysis.[58] One hundred forty-seven consecutively published reports, involving 24,074 patients who underwent both coronary angiography and exercise testing, were summarized. Details regarding population characteristics and methods, including publication year, number of ECG leads, exercise protocol, preexercise hyperventilation, definition of an abnormal ST response, exclusion of certain subgroups, and blinding of test interpretation, were quantified. Criteria for abnormal ST depression varied or at times were vague, but in general, 1 mm of horizontal or downsloping ST depression was used. Wide variability in sensitivity and specificity was found (the mean sensitivity was 68% with a range of 23% to 100% and a standard deviation of 16%; the mean specificity was 77% with a range of 17% to 100% and a standard deviation of 17%). The median predictive accuracy (percentage of total true calls) was approximately 73%.

Stepwise linear regression explained less than 35% of the variance in sensitivities and specificities reported in the 147 publications. This wide variability in the reported accuracy of the exercise ECG is not explained by the information available in the published reports. The wide variability in test performance makes it important that clinicians apply rigorous control of the methods they use for testing and analysis.

Results of Meta-Analysis in the Studies with MI Patients Removed

To more accurately portray the performance of the exercise test, the results in only 41 of the original 147 studies were considered. This is important because patients with MI can be assumed to have CAD and thus the diagnosis has been made. These 41 studies removed patients with a prior MI from this meta-analysis, fulfilling one of the criteria for evaluating a diagnostic test, and provided all of the numbers for calculating test performance. These 41 studies, including nearly 10,000 patients, demonstrated *a lower mean sensitivity of 68% and a lower mean specificity of 74%; this means that there also is a lower predictive accuracy of 71%*. Notice that the predictive accuracy has the least variation. In several studies where workup bias has been lessened, fulfilling the other major criteria, *the sensitivity of the test is approximately 50% and the specificity is 90%, with the predictive accuracy remaining about 70%*.[59]

> **Key Point:** This demonstrates that the key feature of the standard exercise ECG test for clinical utility is its high specificity and that the low sensitivity of the ST response must be enhanced by the use of scores.

The studies evaluating the exercise test were done as part of clinical practice. The degree of workup bias depends on how the physicians make clinical decisions at the institutions where the studies were performed. For instance, if the exercise test is used as a "gatekeeper," patients with an abnormal ST response and low exercise capacities will be selected for the cardiac catheterization laboratory, and others will be excluded. At another institution, where the exercise test is not as important in the decision-making process or where the study designers specifically tried to reduce workup bias (i.e., had patients with symptoms undergo both studies regardless of their results), there would be less workup bias. Thus graphing the percentage of abnormal exercise tests in a study against sensitivity and specificity is a valid way of evaluating the relationship of test characteristics relative to workup bias. Because this relationship was first detected in the studies of women, it was important to determine if this relationship also existed for men. We recalculated the data from the meta-analysis, so that we could plot the sensitivity and specificity versus the percentage of abnormal exercise tests. The same relationship existed in the 41 studies that largely consisted of men. Figure 5-4 is a box plot from these data. The data from the women is based on the 15 studies that only tested women. The studies that are listed for men are from the studies that largely were based on men, although they have a varying percentage of women in them, usually 25% or less. As you can see from the box plots, there is no significant difference between the sensitivity or specificity in the studies with men or women. However, notice that there is a slightly lower percentage of abnormal exercise test responses in the women's studies, which means that the specificity should be higher and the sensitivity lower in the women's studies, but they are not. This suggests that specificity is a little bit lower in women, but not enough to negate the exercise test as the first diagnostic test in women.

The workup bias is that not all patients seen with chest pain and undergoing exercise tests also get a cardiac catheterization because of good clinical practice. Excluded by workup bias are those with high exercise capacity and normal ST responses. Patients with low exercise capacity and abnormal ST responses are selected for further study. Though this is not 100% in any of the studies, tendencies for this to occur vary from study to study, and that is why different test performance characteristics have been obtained with the exercise test. In the studies that have removed workup bias by protocol, these differences are very clearly seen. As you can see in Table 5-4, approximately 12,000 patients are included in the 58 studies with varying

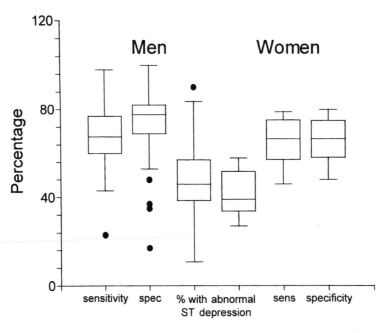

FIGURE 5-4   Box plots of the results of the angiographic correlative studies in men and women. From the box plots, there is no significant difference between the sensitivity or specificity in the studies with men or women.

TABLE 5-4   Effect of Workup Bias on the Standard Exercise ECG Test

Studies	No. of Patients	Sensitivity	Specificity
With workup bias: 58	12,000	67%	72%
Without workup bias: 2	2,000	45%	90%

degrees of workup bias. The mean sensitivity is 67% and mean specificity is 72%. The two studies that removed workup bias by protocol included 2000 patients and have considerably different test characteristics.

Multivariable Techniques to Diagnose Angiographic Coronary Disease

Since Ellestad and colleagues[60] demonstrated that the accuracy of the test could be improved by combining other clinical and exercise parameters along with the ST responses, many clinical investigators have published studies proposing multivariable equations to enhance the accuracy of the standard exercise test. Studies using modern statistical techniques have demonstrated that combinations of clinical and exercise test variables could more accurately predict the probability of angiographic CAD than the standard ST-depression criteria.

Multivariable analysis is a statistical technique that seeks to separate subjects into different groups on the basis of measured variables.[61] Clinical investigators have commonly used two types of analysis: discriminate function and logistic regression analysis. Logistic regression has been preferred because it models the relationship to a sigmoid curve (which often is the mathematical relationship between a risk variable and an outcome) and its output is between 0 and 1 (i.e., from 0% to 100% probability of the predicted outcome). The appropriate values are inserted into the following logistic regression formula to calculate an estimate of the probability for angiographic coronary disease:

$$\text{Probability (0 to 1) of disease} = 1/(1+e^{-(a+bx+cy...)})$$

where a = intercept, b and c are coefficients, and x and y are variable values. Thus the output of a discriminate function prediction equation is a unitless numerical score, whereas a logistic regression equation provides an actual probability.

Over a 15-year period from 1980 through 1995, 30 articles were published that used multivariable statistical analysis for the diagnosis of the presence of any or of severe angiographic CAD.[62] Because some did both, 24 studies predicted the presence of angiographic CAD and 13 studies predicted disease extent or severe angiographic CAD.

In 16 of the 24 studies predicting the presence of angiographic disease, patients with prior MI were excluded, as they should be, and in 5 studies they were improperly included. In the remaining 3 studies, exclusions were unclear.

In 16 studies that excluded patients with prior MI, MI it was defined by history in 6 studies, by ECG findings in 1 study, and by either criterion in 5 studies. In the remaining 5 studies the criteria for MI exclusion were unclear. Ten of the 24 studies clearly excluded patients with previous coronary artery bypass surgery or prior percutaneous coronary intervention (PCI); in the remainder, this was unclear. The definition of *significant coronary angiographic stenosis* ranged from 50% to 80%, and in one study a coronary angiographic score was used instead. The prevalence of angiographic disease ranged from 30% to 78%. The percentages of patients with one-vessel, two-vessel, and three-vessel disease were provided in only 13 of the 24 studies.

Comparison of Clinical and Exercise Test Variables

Table 5-5 lists and counts the predictors of disease presence in 24 studies that considered exercise test and clinical variables to predict presence of any angiographic disease. Thirty equations were created, but not all of the models were given all of the variables for consideration. The denominator is the number of equations that considered the variable, and the numerators are the numbers of equations that chose the specific variable to be significant.

The discriminating power of the variables listed previously that appear in more than 50% of the equations can be assumed as occurring more than

TABLE 5-5   Clinical and Exercise Test Variables Considered in Studies Using Multivariable Statistical Techniques to Predict the Presence of Angiographically Determined CAD

Clinical Variables	Number of Positive Studies/ Number of Equations*	Significant Predictor*
Gender	20/20	100%
Chest pain	17/18	94%
Age	19/27	70%
Elevated cholesterol	8/13	62%
Diabetes mellitus	6/14	43%
Smoking history	4/12	33%
Abnormal resting ECG	4/17	24%
Hypertension	1/8	13%
Family history of CAD	0/7	0%

Exercise Test Variables	Number of Positive Studies/ Number of Equations*	Significant Predictor*
ST-segment slope	14/22	64%
ST-segment depression	17/28	61%
Maximal heart rate	16/28	57%
Exercise capacity	11/24	46%
Exercise-induced angina	11/26	42%
Double product	2/13	15%
Maximal systolic BP	1/12	8%

BP, Blood pressure; *CAD,* coronary artery disease, *ECG,* electrocardiogram.
*The denominator is the number of published equations that considered the variable as a candidate for consideration, and the numerator is the number of studies that found the variable to be an independently significant predictor.

by chance. However, the predictive power of other variables remains undecided. The differences in the variables chosen for predicting presence and severity of coronary disease are discussed in Chapter 7.

Summary of the Multivariate Diagnostic Prediction Studies

These studies consistently demonstrate that the multivariable equations outperform simple ST-segment diagnostic criteria. These equations generally provide an ROC area of about 0.80. That they will function accurately in a clinic or office practice is uncertain because workup bias will never be totally removed. This selection process results in patients with abnormal ST responses or chest pain being more likely to be chosen, whereas patients with high exercise capacities would be excluded from such studies, resulting in a relatively higher prevalence of disease than seen in a clinic population. Thus the coefficients for exercise capacity and ST-segment depression are probably not totally appropriate. In addition, although the discriminating power of the equations may persist when they are applied to another population, the calibration can be off.[63] For instance, the equation may predict a 50% chance of coronary disease given a set of variables in one population when a 70% chance is more appropriate in another population with the same variables.

Exercise Test Scores

The ACC/AHA guidelines suggest the use of scores to enhance the predictive ability of exercise tests. A variety of statistical tools are available to create diagnostic and prognostic scores, and the use of exercise testing scores has been well studied; the applicability and reliability of scores is key to their optimal use.[64]

Statistical Techniques to Develop Scores

When developing a score or prediction rule, variables should be considered that are believed to predict the occurrence of an outcome and then those found to have discriminating power should be applied.[65] The standard approach for creating an exercise test score is to use a combination of clinical information and exercise test results to form an algorithm for estimating the probability of disease.

Pretest Scores

The exercise ECG test is the recommended test for diagnosing CAD in patients with an intermediate probability for it. In the ACC/AHA exercise test guidelines, the Diamond-Forrester tabular method is used to determine pretest probability with consideration of age, gender, and chest pain characteristics. The intermediate pretest probability category was assigned a Class I indication, whereas the low and high pretest probability categories were assigned Class IIb indications for exercise testing. The Morise score for

Variable		Choose response	Sum
Age Men Women			
<40	<50	3	
40-54	50-64	6	
≥55	≥65	9	
Women only		Negative = +3	
Angina History		Typical = 5	
Diamond Method		Atypical = 3	
		Non-anginal = 1	
Diabetes?		2	
Hyperlipidemia?		1	
Hypertension?		1	
Smoking? (Any)		1	
Family Hx CAD? 1°		1	
Obesity? BMI>27		1	
		Total Score:	

Pretest

Choose only one per group

≤8=low probability

9-15= intermediate probability

≥16=high probability

Am J Med 1997;102:350
Am Heart J 1999;138:740

FIGURE 5-5   *Calculation of the simple pretest clinical score for angiographic coronary disease. Choose only one per group. Morise, A. P. Comparison of the Diamond-Forrester method and a new score to estimate the pretest probability of coronary disease before exercise testing, Am Heart J 138:740–745, 1999.*

categorizing patients as to pretest probability of angiographic disease (Figure 5-5) appears to be superior to the tabular method.[66]

Management Strategy Using Scores

Exercise test scores can also assist in managing patients with possible CAD by placing them into three categories of risk rather than just dichotomizing them as positive or negative. Low-risk patients can be treated safely with medical management of coronary risk factors and watchful waiting before further testing. High-risk patients should be considered candidates for more aggressive management that may include cardiac catheterization. In patients with an intermediate-probability treadmill score, imaging tests are of value for further risk stratification.

"Simplified" Score Derivation

Simplified scores derived from multivariable equations have been developed to determine the probability of disease and prognosis. All variables are coded with the same number of intervals so that the coefficients will be proportional. For instance, if 5 is the chosen interval, dichotomous variables are 0 if not present and 5 if present. Continuous variables such as age and maximal heart rate are coded in five groups associated with increasing prevalence of disease. The relative importance of the selected variables is obvious, and the health care provider merely compiles the variables in the score, multiplies by the appropriate number, and then adds up the products. Calculation of the "simple" exercise test score can be done using Figure 5-6 for men and Figure 5-7 for women.[67,68]

Scores Compared with Physicians' Estimates

If physicians can estimate the probability of CAD and prognosis as well as the scores, there is no reason to add this complexity to test interpretation. Two early studies compared a prediction equation with clinicians' estimates. A computer algorithm for estimating probabilities of any significant coronary obstruction and triple-vessel/left main obstructions was derived, validated, and compared with the assessments of clinician cardiologists.[69] The algorithm performed at least as well as the clinicians when the latter knew the identity of the patients whose angiograms they had decided to perform. Hlatky and colleagues[70] attempted to validate two available methods of probability calculation by comparing their diagnostic accuracy with that of cardiologists. Ninety-one cardiologists evaluated the clinical summaries of eight randomly selected patients. Average diagnostic accuracy was best for the computer program.

With these two studies as background, we used our database to compare exercise test scores and ST measurements with a physician's estimation of the probability of the presence and severity of angiographic disease and the risk

Variable	Circle response	Sum	
Maximal Heart Rate	Less than 100 bpm = 30		**Men**
	100 to 129 bpm = 24		
	130 to 159 bpm = 18		
	160 to 189 bpm = 12		
	190 to 220 bpm = 6		
Exercise ST Depression	1-2mm = 15		<40 =
	> 2mm = 25		Low
Age	>55 yrs = 20		Probability
	40 to 55 yrs = 12		
Angina History	Definite/Typical = 5		40-60 =
	Probable/atypical = 3		Intermediate
	Non-cardiac pain = 1		Probability
Hypercholesterolemia?	Yes = 5		
Diabetes?	Yes = 5		>60 =
Exercise Test Induced Angina?	Occurred = 3		High
	Reason for stopping = 5		Probability
	Total Score:		

FIGURE 5-6   *Calculation of the "simple" exercise test score for men for predicting the presence of angiographic coronary disease. Choose only one per group.*

Variable	Circle response	Sum	
Maximal Heart Rate	Less than 100 bpm = 20		**Women**
	100 to 129 bpm = 16		
	130 to 159 bpm = 12		
	160 to 189 bpm = 8		
	190 to 220 bpm = 4		
Exercise ST Depression	1-2mm = 6		<37 =
	> 2mm =10		Low
Age	>65 yrs = 25		Probability
	50 to 65 yrs = 15		
Angina History	Definite/Typical = 10		37-57 =
	Probable/atypical = 6		Intermediate
	Non-cardiac pain = 2		Probability
Hypercholesterolemia?	Yes = 10		
Diabetes?	Yes = 10		>57 =
Exercise Test Induced Angina?	Occurred = 9		High
	Reason for stopping =15		Probability
Estrogen Status	Positive=-5, Negative=5		
	Total Score:		

FIGURE 5-7 *Calculation of the "simple" exercise test score for women for predicting the presence of angiographic coronary disease. Choose only one per group.*

of death.[71,72] When probability estimates for presence and severity of angiographic disease were compared, in general, the treadmill scores were superior to physicians' and ST analysis at predicting severe angiographic disease. When prognosis was estimated, treadmill prognostic scores did as well as expert cardiologists and better than most other physician groups (internists, family practice).

Duke Treadmill Score

The Duke Treadmill Score (DTS) is a composite index that was designed to provide survival estimates based on results from the exercise test. To calculate the score, subtract five times the amount of ST-segment depression and four times the chest pain score (2 points if chest pain was the reason the test was stopped, 1 if angina occurred) from peak METs achieved. To test its potential usefulness for providing diagnostic estimates, Duke researchers used a logistic regression model to predict significant ($\geq75\%$ stenosis) and severe (three-vessel or left main) CAD.[73] After adjustment for baseline clinical risk, the DTS was effectively diagnostic for significant and severe CAD. For low-risk patients (score: ≤5), 60% had no coronary stenosis and 16% had single-vessel stenosis. By comparison, 74% of high-risk patients (score: 11) had three-vessel or left main coronary disease. Five-year mortality rates were 3%, 10%, and 35% for low-, moderate-, and high-risk DTS groups. The area under the ROC curves for predicting significant CAD was 0.70 for ST deviation alone, 0.76 for the score alone, and 0.91 for the score plus clinical history prediction.

> **Key Point:** The DTS provides accurate diagnostic and prognostic information for the evaluation of symptomatic patients evaluated for clinically suspected CAD. The DTS should be included as part of the test summary report.

ACC/AHA Guidelines for the Diagnostic Use of the Standard Exercise Test

The task force to establish guidelines for the use of exercise testing has met and produced guidelines in 1986, 1997, and 2002. The 1997 publication had some dramatic changes from the first, including the recommendation that the standard exercise test be the first diagnostic procedure in women and in most patients with resting ECG abnormalities rather than performing imaging studies. The 2002 update added two items to **Class I** indications. The following is a synopsis of these evidence-based guidelines:

Class I (definitely appropriate)—Conditions for which there is evidence or general agreement that the standard exercise test is useful and helpful for the diagnosis of CAD

1. Adult male or female patients (including those with complete right bundle branch block or with less than 1 mm of resting ST depression) with an intermediate *pretest probability* (see Table 5-3) of CAD based on gender, age, and symptoms (specific exceptions are noted under Classes II and III)
2. Patients with suspected or known CAD, previously evaluated, now with significant change in clinical status
3. ACS patients 8 to 12 hours after presentation who have been free of active ischemic or congestive heart failure (CHF) symptoms (level of evidence: B)
4. Intermediate-risk ACS patients 2 to 3 days after presentation who have been free of active ischemic or CHF symptoms (level of evidence: B)

Class IIa (probably appropriate)—Conditions for which there is conflicting evidence or a divergence of opinion that the standard exercise test is useful and helpful for diagnosis but the weight of evidence for usefulness or efficacy is in favor of the exercise test

1. Intermediate-risk unstable angina patients who have initial cardiac markers that are normal, repeat ECG that is unchanged, and cardiac markers that are normal at up to 12 hours and no other evidence of ischemia (level of evidence: B)
2. Patients with vasospastic angina . . . *(removed in 2002)*

Class IIb (may be appropriate)—Conditions for which there is conflicting evidence or a divergence of opinion that the standard exercise test is useful and helpful for the diagnosis of CAD but the usefulness/efficacy is less well established

1. Patients taking digoxin with less than 1 mm of baseline ST depression *(removed in 2002)*
2. Patients with the following ECG abnormalities: Wolff-Parkinson-White syndrome (WPW), electronic pacing, 1 mm or less ST-segment depression, complete LBBB, or any intraventricular conduction defect (IVCD) >120 msec
3. Patients with stable clinical course who undergo periodic monitoring to guide therapy
4. Patients with a low pretest probability of CAD by age, symptoms, and gender

Class III (not appropriate)—Conditions for which there is evidence or general agreement that the standard exercise test is not useful and helpful for the diagnosis of CAD and in some cases may be harmful

1. To use the ST-segment response in the diagnosis of CAD in patients who demonstrate the following baseline ECG abnormalities *(removed in 2002 though acknowledged to be inappropriate)*: preexcitation (WPW) syndrome; electronically paced ventricular rhythm; more than 1 mm of resting ST-segment depression; complete LBBB; patients with comorbidities likely to limit life expectancy and candidacy for interventions
2. High-risk ACS patients (level of evidence: C)

Pretest probability was determined from the Diamond-Forrester estimates tabulated in the guidelines per Table 5-3.

Immediate Management of Acute Coronary Syndrome Patients

The exercise test has been recommended as part of the diagnostic workup of selected patients with ACS. The 2002 guidelines list the following recommendations:

Class I

1. The history, physical examination, 12-lead ECG, and initial cardiac marker tests should be integrated to assign patients with chest pain into one of four categories: a noncardiac diagnosis, chronic stable angina, possible ACS, and definite ACS. (Level of evidence: C)
2. Patients with definite or possible ACS, but whose initial 12-lead ECG and cardiac marker levels are normal, should be observed in a facility with cardiac monitoring (e.g., chest pain unit), and a repeat ECG and cardiac

marker measurement should be obtained 6 to 12 hours after the onset of symptoms. (Level of evidence: B)

3. **In patients in whom ischemic heart disease is present or suspected, if the follow-up 12-lead ECG and cardiac marker measurements are normal, a stress test (exercise or pharmacologic) to provoke ischemia may be performed in the emergency department, in a chest pain unit, or on an outpatient basis shortly after discharge. Low-risk patients with a negative stress test can be managed as outpatients. (Level of evidence: C)**

4. Patients with definite ACS and ongoing pain, positive cardiac markers, new ST-segment deviations, new deep T-wave inversions, hemodynamic abnormalities, or a positive stress test should be admitted to the hospital for further management. (Level of evidence: C)

5. Patients with possible ACS and negative cardiac markers who are unable to exercise or who have an abnormal resting ECG should undergo a pharmacologic stress test. (Level of evidence: B)

6. Patients with definite ACS and ST-segment elevation should be evaluated for immediate reperfusion therapy. (Level of evidence: A)

By integrating information from the history, physical examination, 12-lead ECG, and initial cardiac marker tests, clinicians can assign patients into one of four categories: noncardiac diagnosis, chronic stable angina, possible ACS, and definite ACS.

Chronic stable angina may also be diagnosed in this setting, and patients with this diagnosis should be managed according to the ACC/AHA guidelines for the management of patients with chronic stable angina.[74]

Studies published since the guidelines were printed include the excellent review from Amsterdam and colleagues[75] and other reports that have described the use of immediate exercise testing to evaluate a large, heterogeneous group of low-risk patients with chest pain.[76-79]

Summary

Newer diagnostic modalities should be compared with the standard exercise test because it is a mature, established technology. The equipment and personnel for performing it are readily available. Exercise testing equipment is relatively inexpensive so that replacement or updating is not a major limitation. The test can be performed in the doctor's office and does not require injections or exposure to radiation. It can be an extension of the medical history and physical examination, providing more than simply diagnostic information. Furthermore, it can determine the degree of disability and impairment to quality of life, as well as be the first step in rehabilitation and altering a major risk factor (physical inactivity).

Some of the newer add-ons or substitutes for the exercise test have the advantage of being able to localize ischemia, as well as diagnose coronary disease when the baseline ECG negates ST analysis (>1 mm of ST-segment depression, LBBB, WPW). Also, nonexercise stress techniques permit diagnostic assessment of patients unable to exercise. Although the newer technologies appear to have better diagnostic characteristics, this is not always the case, particularly when more than the ST segments from the exercise test are used in scores.

The ACC/AHA guidelines for the diagnostic use of the standard exercise test have stated that it is appropriate for testing of adult male or female patients (including those with complete right bundle branch block or with <1 mm of resting ST-segment depression) with an intermediate pretest probability of CAD based on gender, age, and symptoms.

The purpose of methodologic standards for diagnostic tests is to improve patient care, reduce health care costs, improve the quality of diagnostic test information, and eliminate useless tests or testing methodologies. The two most important to consider when evaluating such studies are limited challenge and workup bias. Limited challenge usually results in exaggerated values for sensitivity, specificity, predictive accuracy, and ROC curve area. Workup bias results in shifting cutpoint performance further along the ROC curve and when removed shows that the exercise test has a high specificity in office practice. The mnemonics SnNout and SpPin help one to remember the performance of a test with high values of either sensitivity or specificity. When a test has a very high **Sen**sitivity, a **N**egative test rules **out** the diagnosis (SnNout); when a test has a very high **Sp**ecificity, a **P**ositive test rules **in** the diagnosis (SpPin). The ACP Journal Club has published an excellent roadmap for systematic reviews of diagnostic test evaluations.[80]

In studies that took into account the number of coronary arteries involved, all found increasing sensitivity of the test as more vessels were involved. The most false negatives have been found among patients with single-vessel disease, particularly if the diseased vessel was not the left anterior descending artery. No matter what techniques are used, there is a reciprocal relationship between sensitivity and specificity. The more specific a test is (i.e., the more able it is to determine who is disease free), the less sensitive it is, and vice versa. The values for adjusting the criterion can alter sensitivity and specificity for the cutpoint used for abnormal. For instance, when the criterion for an abnormal exercise-induced ST-segment response is altered to 0.2 mV depression, making it more specific for CAD, the sensitivity of the test will be reduced by half.

With patients subgrouped according to beta-blocker administration as initiated by their referring physician, no differences in test performance were found in a consecutive group of males being evaluated for possible CAD. However, the only way to maintain sensitivity with the standard exercise test in the beta-blocker group who failed to reach target heart rate was to use a treadmill score or 0.5 mm of ST-segment depression as the criterion for abnormal. Thus, in our most recent study of the effects of beta blockade and heart rate response, we found the sensitivity and predictive accuracy of standard ST criteria for exercise-induced ST-segment depression to be significantly decreased in male patients taking beta blockers who did not reach an adequate heart rate. In those who failed to reach target heart rate and were not beta blocked, sensitivity and predictive accuracy were maintained. Though perhaps useful for particular patients, for routine exercise testing it appears unnecessary for physicians to accept the risk of stopping beta blockers before testing when a patient is exhibiting possible symptoms of ischemia.

Concern about false-positive ST responses when testing women may be addressed by careful assessment of pretest probability and selective use of a stress imaging test before proceeding to angiography. The optimal strategy for circumventing false-positive test results for the diagnosis of coronary disease in women requires the use of scores, and there are insufficient data to justify routine stress imaging tests as the initial test for women.

Studies considering non-ECG data consistently demonstrate that the multivariable equations outperform simple ST diagnostic criteria. These equations generally provide a predictive accuracy of 80% (ROC area of 0.80). To obtain the best diagnostic characteristics with the exercise test, clinical and non-ECG test responses should be considered. We have validated simple scores for both men and women at other institutions and have compared them with physicians' estimates. They should be applied during every test along with the DTS because they are easy to use and significantly improve the prediction of angiographic CAD.

Exercise-induced ST-segment depression in inferior limb leads is a poor marker for CAD in and of itself.[81] Precordial lead V5 alone consistently outperforms the inferior leads and the combination of leads V5 and II, because lead II was shown to have a high false-positive rate. In patients without prior MI and normal resting ECGs, ST-segment depression in precordial lead V5, along with V4 and V6, is a reliable marker for CAD, and the monitoring of inferior limb leads adds little additional diagnostic information (although elevation inferiorly should not be ignored). In patients with a normal resting ECG, exercise-induced ST-segment depression confined to the inferior leads is of limited value for the identification of coronary disease.

Although the concept of acute coronary syndromes (ACSs) has altered the clinical milieu, the Consiglio Nazionale delle Ricerche (CNR) Cardiology Research group in Italy reviewed the literature to determine if evidence still supports the use of the exercise ECG as the first-choice stress testing modality for ACS.[82] The research group concluded that a large body of evidence supports the use of the exercise ECG as a cost-effective tool for prognostic purposes and for quality-of-life assessment following ACS. This is consistent with the ACC/AHA guidelines.

The guidelines state that patients who are pain free, have either a normal or nondiagnostic ECG or one that is unchanged from previous tracings, and have a normal set of initial cardiac enzymes are candidates for further evaluation to screen for nonischemic chest discomfort versus a low-risk ACS. If the patient is low risk and does not experience any further ischemic discomfort, and a follow-up 12-lead ECG and cardiac marker measurements after 6 to 8 hours of observation are normal, the patient may be considered for an early exercise test to provoke ischemia. This test can be performed before discharge and should be supervised by an experienced physician. Alternatively, the patient may be discharged and return for the test as an outpatient within 3 days.

References

1. Snow V et al: Evaluation of primary care patients with chronic stable angina: guidelines from the American College of Physicians, *Ann Intern Med* 141:57-64, 2004.
2. Philbrick JT, Horwitz RI, Feinstein AR: Methodologic problems of exercise testing for coronary artery disease: groups, analysis and bias, *Am J Cardiol* 46:807, 1980.
3. Reid M, Lachs M, Feinstein A: Use of methodological standards in diagnostic test research, *JAMA* 274:645-651, 1995.
4. Guyatt GH: Readers' guide for articles evaluating diagnostic tests: what ACP Journal Club does for you and what you must do yourself, *ACP Journal Club* 115:A-16, 1991.
5. Weiner DA, McCabe CH, Ryan TJ: Prognostic assessment of patients with coronary artery disease by exercise testing, *Am Heart J* 105:749-755, 1983.
6. Blackburn H, Katigbak R: What electrocardiographic leads to take after exercise? *Am Heart J* 67:184-188, 1964.
7. Miller TD, Desser KB, Lawson M: How many electrocardiographic leads are required for exercise treadmill tests? *J Electrocardiol* 20:131-137, 1987.
8. Simoons ML, Block P: Toward the optimal lead system and optimal criteria for exercise electrocardiography, *Am J Cardiol* 47:1366-1374, 1981.
9. Viik J et al: Correct utilization of exercise electrocardiographic leads in differentiation of men with coronary artery disease from patients with a low likelihood of coronary artery disease using peak exercise ST-segment depression, *Am J Cardiol* 81:964-969, 1998.
10. Mark DB et al: Localizing coronary artery obstructions with the exercise treadmill test, *Ann Intern Med* 106:53-55, 1987.
11. Riff DP, Carleton RA: Effect of exercise on the atrial recovery wave, *Am Heart J* 81:759-763, 1971.
12. Miranda CP et al: Usefulness of exercise-induced ST-segment depression in the inferior leads during exercise testing as a marker for coronary artery disease, *Am J Cardiol* 69:303-308, 1992.
13. Fortuin NJ, Friesinger GC: Exercise-induced ST-segment elevation: clinical, electrocardiographic and arteriographic studies in twelve patients, *Am J Med* 49:459, 1970.
14. Hegge FN, Tuna N, Burchell HB: Coronary arteriographic findings in patients with axis shifts or ST-segment elevations on exercise testing, *Am Heart J* 86:603, 1973.
15. Chahine RA, Raizner AE, Ishimori T: The clinical significance of exercise-induced ST-segment elevation, *Circulation* 54:209, 1976.
16. Longhurst JC, Kraus WL: Exercise-induced ST elevation in patients without myocardial infarction, *Circulation* 60:616, 1979.
17. Mark DB et al: Localizing coronary artery obstructions with the exercise treadmill test, *Ann Intern Med* 106:53-55, 1987.
18. Bruce RA, Fisher LD: Unusual prognostic significance of exercise-induced ST elevation in coronary patients, *J Electrocardiol* 74:84-88, 1987.
19. De Feyter PJ et al: Clinical significance of exercise-induced ST-segment elevation, *Br Heart J* 46:84-92, 1981.

20. Kentala E, Luurela O: Response of R wave amplitude to posture changes and to exercise, *Ann Clin Res* 7:258-263, 1975.
21. Bonoris PE et al: Evaluation of R wave amplitude changes versus ST-segment depression in stress testing, *Circulation* 57:904-910, 1978.
22. Eenige van MJ, De Feyter PJ, Jong JP, Roos JP: Diagnostic incapacity of exercise-induced QRS wave amplitude changes to detect coronary artery disease and left ventricular dysfunction, *Eur Heart J* 3:9-16, 1982.
23. Myers J, Ahnve S, Froelicher V, Sullivan M: Spatial R wave amplitude during exercise: relation with left ventricular ischemia and function, *J Am Coll Cardiol* 6:603-608, 1985.
24. McHenry PL, Morris SN: Exercise electrocardiography—current state of the art. In Schlant RC, Hurst JW, eds: *Advances in electrocardiography,* vol 2, New York, 1976, Grune & Stratton.
25. Maseri A et al: "Variant" angina: one aspect of a continuous spectrum of vasospastic myocardial ischemia, *Am J Cardiol* 42:1019-1025, 1978.
26. Detrano R et al: Factors affecting sensitivity and specificity of a diagnostic test: the exercise thallium scintigram, *Am J Med* 84:699-710, 1988.
27. Gutman RA, Bruce R: Delay of ST-depression after maximal exercise by walking for 2 minutes, *Circulation* 42:229, 1970.
28. Gibbons L, Cooper K: The safety of maximal exercise testing, *Circulation* 80:846, 1989.
29. Lachterman B, Lehmann KG, Abrahamson D, Froelicher VF: "Recovery only" ST-segment depression and the predictive accuracy of the exercise test, *Ann Intern Med* 112:11-16, 1990.
30. Karnegis JN et al: Comparison of exercise-positive with recovery-positive treadmill graded exercise tests, *Am J Cardiol* 60:544-547, 1987.
31. Savage MP et al: Usefulness of ST-segment depression as a sign of coronary artery disease when confined to the post exercise recovery period, *Am J Cardiol* 60:1405-1406, 1987.
32. Rywik TM et al: Independent prognostic significance of ischemic ST-segment response limited to recovery from treadmill exercise in asymptomatic subjects, *Circulation* 97:2117-2122, 1998.
33. Lanza GA et al: Diagnostic and prognostic value of ST-segment depression limited to the recovery phase of exercise stress test, *Heart* 90:1417-1421, 2004.
34. Goldschlager N, Selzer A, Cohn K: Treadmill stress tests as indicators of presence and severity of coronary artery disease, *Ann Intern Med* 85:277-286, 1976.
35. Callaham PR, Thomas L, Ellestad MH: Prolonged ST-segment depression following exercise predicts significant proximal left coronary artery stenosis, *Circulation* 76(suppl IV):IV-253, 1987 (abstract).
36. LeWinter M, Crawford M, O'Rourke R, Karliner J: The effects of oral propanolol, digoxin and combined therapy on the resting and exercise ECG, *Am Heart J* 93:202-209, 1977.
37. Tonkon MJ et al: Effects of digitalis on the exercise electrocardiogram in normal adult subjects, *Chest* 72:714-718, 1977.
38. Sketch MH et al: Digoxin-induced positive exercise tests: their clinical and prognostic significance, *Am J Cardiol* 48:655-659, 1981.

39. Sundqvist K, Atterhog JH, Jogestrand T: Effect of digoxin on the electrocardiogram at rest and during exercise in healthy subjects, *Am J Cardiol* 57:661-665, 1986.

40. Meyers DG, Bendon KA, Hankins JH, Stratbucker RA: The effect of baseline electrocardiographic abnormalities on the diagnostic accuracy of exercise-induced ST-segment changes, *Am Heart J* 119:272-276, 1990.

41. Gauri AJ et al: Effects of chronotropic incompetence and beta-blocker use on the exercise treadmill test in men, *Am Heart J* 142:136-141, 2001.

42. Cantwell JD, Murray PM, Thomas RJ: Current management of severe exercise-related cardiac events, *Chest* 93:1264-1269, 1988.

43. Anastasiou-Nana MI et al: Occurrence of exercise-induced and spontaneous wide complex tachycardia during therapy with flecainide for complex ventricular arrhythmias: a probable proarrhythmic effect, *Am Heart J* 113:1071-1077, 1987.

44. Whinnery JE, Froelicher VF, Stuart AJ: The electrocardiographic response to maximal treadmill exercise in asymptomatic men with left bundle branch block, *Am Heart J* 94:316, 1977.

45. Ibrahim NS, Selvester RS, Hagar JM, Ellestad MH: Detecting exercise-induced ischemia in left bundle branch block using the electrocardiogram, *Am J Cardiol* 82:832-835, 1998.

46. Richter WS, Aurisch R, Munz DL: Septal myocardial perfusion in complete left bundle branch block: case report and review of the literature, *Nuklearmedizin* 37(4):146-150, 1998.

47. Grady TA et al: Prognostic significance of exercise-induced left bundle-branch block, *JAMA* 279:153-156, 1998.

48. Munt B, Huckell VF, Boone J: Exercise-induced left bundle branch block: a case report of false positive MIBI imaging and review of the literature, *Can J Cardiol* 13:517-521, 1997.

49. Whinnery JE, Froelicher VF, Stuart AJ: The electrocardiographic response to maximal treadmill exercise in asymptomatic men with right branch bundle block, *Chest* 71:335, 1977.

50. Blackburn H: Importance of the electrocardiogram in populations outside the hospital, *Can Med Assoc J* 108:1262-1265, 1973.

51. Cullen K, Stenhouse NS, Wearne KL, Compston GN: Electrocardiograms and 13 year cardiovascular mortality in Busselton study, *Br Heart J* 47:209-212, 1982.

52. Aronow WS: Correlation of ischemic ST-segment depression on the resting electrocardiogram with new cardiac event rates in 1,106 patients over 62 years of age, *Am J Cardiol* 64:232-233, 1989.

53. Califf RM et al: Importance of clinical measures of ischemia in the prognosis of patients with documented coronary artery disease, *J Am Coll Cardiol* 11:20-26, 1988.

54. Harris PJ et al: Survival in medically treated coronary artery disease, *Circulation* 60:1259-1269, 1979.

55. Miranda CP, Lehmann KG, Froelicher VF: Correlation between resting ST-segment depression, exercise testing, coronary angiography, and long-term prognosis, *Am Heart J* 122:1617-1626, 1991.

56. Lee DP, Fearon WF, Froelicher VF: Clinical utility of the exercise ECG in patients with diabetes and chest pain, *Chest* 119:1576-1581, 2001.
57. Lai S et al: Treadmill scores in elderly men, *J Am Coll Cardiol* 43:606-615, 2004.
58. Gianrossi R et al: Exercise-induced ST-depression in the diagnosis of coronary artery disease: a meta-analysis, *Circulation* 80:87-98, 1989.
59. Morise A, Diamond GA: Comparison of the sensitivity and specificity of exercise electrocardiography in biased and unbiased populations of men and women, *Am Heart J* 130:741-747, 1995.
60. Ellestad MH, Savitz S, Bergdall D, Teske J: The false positive stress test. Multivariate analysis of 215 subjects with hemodynamic, angiographic and clinical data, *Am J Cardiol* 40:681-687, 1977.
61. Concato J, Feinstein AR, Holford TR: The risk of determining risk with multivariate models, *Ann Intern Med* 118:201-210, 1993.
62. Yamada H, Do D, Morise A, Froelicher V: Review of studies utilizing multi-variable analysis of clinical and exercise test data to predict angiographic coronary artery disease, *Prog Cardiovasc Dis* 39:457-481, 1997.
63. Harrell FE Jr, Lee KL, Mark DB: Multivariable prognostic models: issues in developing models, evaluating assumptions and adequacy, and measuring and reducing errors, *Stat Med* 15:361-387, 1996.
64. Froelicher V, Shetler K, Ashley E: Better decisions through science: exercise testing scores, *Prog Cardiovasc Dis* 44:395-414, 2002.
65. Swets JA, Dawes RM, Monahan J: Better decisions through science, *Scientific American,* Oct 2000, pp 82-87.
66. Morise A: Comparison of the Diamond-Forrester method and a new score to estimate the pretest probability of coronary disease before exercise testing, *Am Heart J* 138:740-745, 1999.
67. Raxwal V, Shetler K, Do D, Froelicher V: A simple treadmill score, *Chest* 113:1933-1940, 2000.
68. Morise AP, Lauer MS, Froelicher VF: Development and validation of a simple exercise test score for use in women with symptoms of suspected coronary artery disease, *Am Heart J* 144:818-825, 2002.
69. Detrano R et al: Computer probability estimates of angiographic coronary artery disease: transportability and comparison with cardiologists' estimates, *Comput Biomed Res* 25:468-485, 1992.
70. Hlatky M, Bovinick E, Brundage B: Diagnostic accuracy of cardiologists compared with probability calculations using Bayes' rule, *Am J Cardiol* 49:192-197, 1982.
71. Lipinski M et al: Comparison of exercise test scores and physician estimation in determining disease probability, *Arch Intern Med* 161:2239-2244, 2001.
72. Lipinski M et al: Comparison of treadmill scores with physician estimates of diagnosis and prognosis in patients with coronary artery disease, *Am Heart J* 143:650-658, 2002.
73. Shaw LJ et al: Use of a prognostic treadmill score in identifying diagnostic coronary disease subgroups, *Circulation* 98:1622-1630, 1998.

74. Gibbons RJ et al: ACC/AHA 2002 guideline update for the management of patients with chronic stable angina: a report of the American College of Cardiology/American Heart Association Task Force on Practice Guidelines (Committee to Update the 1999 Guidelines for the Management of Patients with Chronic Stable Angina), *J Am Coll Cardiol* 41:159-168, 2003.
75. Amsterdam EA et al: Early exercise testing in the management of low risk patients in chest pain centers, *Prog Cardiovasc Dis* 46:438-452, 2004.
76. Prina LD et al: Outcome of patients with a final diagnosis of chest pain of undetermined origin admitted under the suspicion of acute coronary syndrome: a report from the Rochester Epidemiology Project, *Ann Emerg Med* 43:59-67, 2004.
77. Sanchis J et al: Predictors of short-term outcome in acute chest pain without ST-segment elevation, *Int J Cardiol* 92:193-199, 2003.
78. Aroney CN, Dunlevie HL, Bett JH: Use of an accelerated chest pain assessment protocol in patients at intermediate risk of adverse cardiac events, *Med J Aust* 178:370-374, 2003.
79. Amsterdam EA et al: Immediate exercise testing to evaluate low-risk patients presenting to the emergency department with chest pain, *J Am Coll Cardiol* 40:251-256, 2002.
80. Pai M, McCulloch M, Enanoria W, Colford JM Jr: Systematic reviews of diagnostic test evaluations: what's behind the scenes? *ACP J Club* 141:A11-A13, 2004.
81. Miranda CP et al: Usefulness of exercise-induced ST-segment depression in the inferior leads during exercise testing as a marker for coronary artery disease, *Am J Cardiol* 69:303-308, 1992.
82. Bigi R, Cortigiani L, Desideri A: Exercise electrocardiography after acute coronary syndromes: still the first testing modality? *Clin Cardiol* 26:390-395, 2003.

6 Prognostic Applications of Exercise Testing

Rationale

There are two principal reasons for estimating prognosis. The first is to provide accurate answers to patients' questions regarding the probable outcome of their illness. Though discussion of prognosis is inherently delicate, and probability statements can be misunderstood, most patients find this information useful in planning their affairs regarding work, recreational activities, personal estate, and finances. The second reason to determine prognosis is to identify those patients in whom interventions might improve outcome.

Although improved prognosis equates with increased quantity of life, quality-of-life issues must also be taken into account. In that regard, it is apparent that in certain clinical settings, catheter or surgical interventions provide better therapy than medication. However, when misapplied these interventions can have a negative impact on the quality of life (inconvenience, complications, and discomfort), as well as creating a financial burden to the individual and to society.

> **Key Point:** Although some patients ask how long they have to live and this question can never be answered with certainty, nearly all patients hope for a reasonable estimate of their chances for longevity from their health care provider.

Exercise Testing as Part of the Basic Patient Evaluation

Patients with known or suspected coronary disease are usually evaluated initially after a careful cardiac history and physical examination with an exercise test. The test can be performed safely and inexpensively and even accomplished in the physician's office. In addition to diagnostic information, the test gives practical and clinically valuable information regarding exercise capacity and response to therapy. The indications for angiography have dramatically changed since the 1980s. Now, with drug-eluting stents, the risk of reocclusion has been reduced to single digits. The possibility of putting patients at higher risk by performing an intervention has drastically dropped. Fewer patients with coronary artery disease (CAD) are experiencing angina pectoris than ever before because of progress in interventional cardiology.

Only certain groups of patients with specific CAD patterns are conferred a survival benefit from bypass surgery.[1] Because of the lack of certainty and the need for a "road map" for coronary intervention, coronary angiography is considered the gold standard for evaluating patients for the presence of coronary disease and determining which patients might benefit from interventional therapy. Angiography defines static anatomy because it is performed at rest, but the insertion of flow wires into the coronary arteries can quantitate coronary blood flow.[2]

Key Point: Even if the exercise test is done for diagnostic reasons, the prognostic information obtained can be helpful.

Statistical Methods Used for Survival Analysis

To answer questions appropriately regarding patient decisions, follow-up studies must be performed and special statistical methods called *survival analysis* applied. Survival analysis consists of a group of univariate and multivariate mathematical techniques that consider person-time of exposure and calculations of "hazard" or risk. The key difference between hazard analysis and other statistical methods is censoring, or removal from exposure. Censoring is done at time of "lost to follow-up," removal from risk (i.e., coronary artery bypass surgery [CABS], percutaneous coronary intervention [PCI]), or termination of the study. The two most commonly used techniques are Kaplan-Meier survival curves for univariate analysis and the Cox proportional hazard model for multivariable analysis. Multivariable analysis is necessary because many of the variables interact. Univariately, variables can be associated with death and generate a risk ratio, but the association may be through other variables.

Endpoints and Censoring

The relative prognostic importance of the ischemic variables can be minimized by not censoring on interventions for ischemia (i.e., removal of intervened patients from observation when the intervention occurs in follow-up) because the intervention stops patients from dying. Consideration of all-cause mortality instead of cardiovascular (CV) mortality can have the same effect. This may explain why the ischemic variables included in the Duke score that clearly had diagnostic power do not predict all-cause mortality.[3] Although all-cause mortality has advantages over CV mortality as an endpoint for interventional studies,[4] the Duke score was generated using the endpoints of infarction and CV death.[5] Interventions such as bypass surgery or catheter procedures were censored in the Duke study (that is, subjects were removed from the survival analysis when interventions occurred). Such censoring should increase the association of ischemic variables with outcome by removing patients whose disease has been alleviated, and thereby would not be as likely to experience the outcome. Often researchers do not censor patients if they had a CV procedure during follow-up because they do not have that information. In a study in a Veterans Administration (VA) patient population with an annual all-cause mortality rate of 3%, our group found that 75% of deaths were CV deaths, and that 6% of patients were censored in follow-up because of bypass surgery.[6] If the proportions are similar in a more current population, it would not be unreasonable to expect a bias against the predictive power of these variables. The use of coronary interventions as endpoints falsely strengthens the association of ischemic variables with endpoints because the ischemic responses clinically result in the intervention being performed. Although some investigators have justified their use by requiring a time period to expire after the test before using the intervention/procedure as an endpoint, this still influences the associations. Another problem is that variables predicting infarction can be different than those predicting death, creating a situation where one variable's contrasting effects with respect to two endpoints can cancel each other out.

All-Cause versus Cardiovascular Mortality

Recent studies of prognosis have actually not been superior to the earlier studies that considered CV endpoints and removed patients from observation who had interventions. This is because death data are now relatively easy to obtain whereas previously investigators had to follow the patients and contact them or review their records. Thus, prognostic studies were uncommon because of the expense of follow-up, but more recently all-cause mortality has become available through the Social Security Death Index. In addition, CV mortality can be determined by death certificates, often available from state governments. Although death certificates have limitations, in general they classify those with accidental, gastrointestinal, pulmonary, and cancer deaths so that those remaining are most likely to have died of CV causes. This endpoint is more appropriate when studying a test for CV disease. Whereas all-cause mortality is a more important endpoint for intervention studies, CV mortality is more appropriate for evaluating a CV test (i.e., the exercise test). Identifying those at risk of death of any cause does not make it possible to identify those who might benefit from CV interventions, one of the major goals of prognostication.

Key Point: The statistical methods used in a given study need to be assessed before the results are put into clinical practice.

Prediction of High Risk or Poor Prognosis in Patients with Stable Coronary Heart Disease

The following types of prognostic studies based on endpoint classification using exercise testing in patients with stable coronary heart disease are discussed:

- Cardiovascular disease (CVD) endpoints
- Coronary angiographic findings
- Improved survival with CABS

In addition, specialized situations for predicting prognosis, including silent ischemia, diabetes, and the elderly, are considered separately.

Follow-up Studies Predicting Cardiovascular Disease Endpoints

Since the pioneering studies from the University of Alabama,[7,8] numerous investigators have used clinical, exercise test, and catheterization data to predict prognosis in patients with CAD. Hammermeister and colleagues[9] assessed 733 medically treated patients by going stepwise first through clinical markers and then the exercise test. Heart failure (HF) was the most important clinical variable, and maximal double product was the most important treadmill variable. Cox regression analysis showed ejection fraction, age, number of diseased vessels, and resting ventricular arrhythmia in that order to be most predictive. Gohlke and colleagues[10] followed 1034 patients with CAD and found exercise workload, angina during the exercise test, and maximal heart rate to independently predict risk of death. Exercise-induced ST depression was only independently predictive in the subgroup with three-vessel disease and normal ventricular function. Brunelli and colleagues[11] reported their findings in 1083 patients younger than 65 years old followed for a mean of 5 years. Exercise-induced ST depression was not considered independently but rather was combined with angina and exercise capacity in order to create a marker associated with CV death. Weiner and colleagues[12] analyzed 4083 patients from the Coronary Artery Surgery Study (CASS) registry of patients with no previous coronary surgery who were able to undergo a treadmill test within 1 month of their catheterization. When all 30 variables were analyzed jointly, HF was the most potent clinical predictor of survival when the clinical and exercise test variables were analyzed. Such findings have led us today to consider HF patients separately when doing prognostic evaluation studies.

The Duke Prognostic Study
Mark and colleagues[13] studied 2842 consecutive patients who underwent cardiac catheterization and exercise testing and whose data were entered into the Duke computerized medical information system. Seventy percent of the study patients were men, and the median age was 49 years. Two thirds had stable angina and one third had progressive anginal symptoms. A history of myocardial infarction (MI) was present in 29%, and 22% had

pathologic Q waves. At catheterization, the mean ejection fraction was 60%, and 27% had three-vessel or left main CAD. The median follow-up for the study population was 5 years and the follow-up was 98% complete. A treadmill angina index was assigned a value of 0 if angina was absent, 1 if typical angina occurred during exercise, and 2 if angina was the reason the patient stopped exercising. Before the test, 54% of the patients had taken beta blockers and 11% had taken digoxin. ST measurements considered were the sum of the largest net ST depression and elevation, the sum of the ST displacements in all 12 leads, the number of leads showing ST displacement of 0.1 mV or more, and the product of the number of leads showing ST displacement and the largest single ST displacement in any lead. To make the score apply to other treadmill protocols, it is necessary to convert minutes in the Bruce protocol to METs with the following equation:

$$METs = 1.3 \text{ (minutes)} - 2.2$$

or

$$\text{Minutes in the Bruce protocol} = METs + 2.2 \div 1.3$$

Six steps were used to derive the prognostic treadmill score. First, the patient population was randomly split into two groups: a training sample of 1422 patients and a validation sample of 1420 patients. Second, the Cox proportional hazards regression model was used in the training sample to assess the strength of association between the primary study endpoint (death of CV cause) and treadmill responses. Treadmill responses were then ranked using the likelihood ratio derived from the Cox model. Third, the most important treadmill response was entered into a Cox regression model and the remaining responses were then entered in order until the model represented the independent prognostic information available from the exercise test. Fourth, the regression coefficients from this regression model were used to form a linear treadmill score. Fifth, the new score was tested to determine if patients with different levels of scores had a survival pattern similar to that seen in the training sample. Finally, the score was recalculated based on variables derived from the test results in all patients. In the 24% of the patients who had coronary artery surgery, the follow-up was measured to the time of surgery and then they were removed from observation. The largest net ST deviation recorded during exercise in any one of the 12 leads proved to be the single most important variable for predicting prognosis. After adjusting for maximum net ST deviation using the Cox model, only two other variables contained additional prognostic information: the treadmill angina index and METs. The results did not change substantially when patients taking beta blockers or digoxin were excluded. The results also remained unchanged when patients treated surgically were excluded from the study. A score was calculated as follows:

$$\text{Exercise time} - (5 \times \text{maximum ST depression}) - (4 \times \text{angina index})$$

where exercise time is measured in minutes and ST deviation in millimeters. Patients at high risk with a score of −11 or lower had a 5-year survival rate of 72%. Patients at moderate risk with a score of −10 to +4 had a 5-year survival

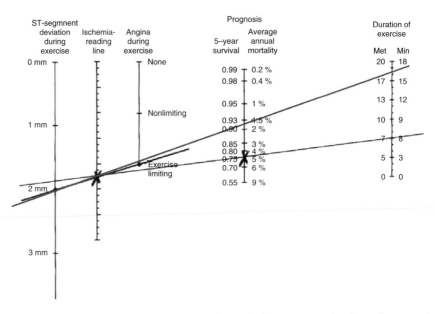

FIGURE 6-1 *Nomogram that can be used to calculate CV mortality from the DTS. This sample patient is a 55-year-old government employee with atypical chest pain. He had 2 mm of horizontal ST depression. The test was stopped at 7 METs because of angina. The red line shows the importance of METs because elevated values drastically improve prognosis. Beware any nomogram with equally spaced lines because the spacing is critical to the relationships with the prediction variables. Another caveat is that the ischemic elements do not appear to be predictive in the elderly. This nomogram has been validated in women and patients with resting ST depression.*

rate of 91%, and patients at low risk with a score of +5 or greater had a 5-year survival rate of 97%. When total cardiac events were considered, the high-risk group had a 5-year survival rate of 65%, the moderate-risk group had a 5-year survival rate of 86%, and the low-risk group had a 5-year survival rate of 93%. The treadmill score contained prognostically important information even after the information provided by clinical and catheterization data was considered. This score has been implemented in a nomogram (Figure 6-1).

> **Key Point:** The Duke Treadmill Score (DTS) has been judged by many experts to be one of the most important advances in exercise testing in the past 20 years. It has been incorporated into all the major guidelines and should be calculated as part of every exercise test.

Other Prognostic Studies

The VA randomized trial of CABS reported a 7-year follow-up of 245 patients randomized to medical management who had a baseline treadmill test.[14] Univariately and using Cox analysis, ST depression (> 2 mm), exercise-induced premature ventricular contractions (PVCs), and final heart rate greater than 140 beats per minute were significant predictors of mortality. These results are important to consider because PVCs have not had independent predictive power in all studies, high heart rates have been protective rather than associated with risk, and a poor exercise capacity was not predictive. These results might be explained by their failure to censor on interventions.

From Buenos Aires, Lerman and colleagues[15] reported on 190 patients with exercise test and coronary angiograms who were followed for 6 years. Their patients had a high annual mortality rate and a low rate of interventions, yet exercise-induced ST depression failed to predict prognosis. Maximal systolic blood pressure (SBP) less than 130 mm Hg was the strongest predictor of death.

Wyns and colleagues[16] evaluated the independent prognostic information provided by exercise testing by calculating the survival rates with the life table method in 372 men referred for coronary angiography. A previous MI was noted in 146, and 248 had typical angina. During a mean follow-up of 2 years, 32 patients died and 27 patients had nonfatal events. Typical angina pectoris and/or an old MI and an abnormal exercise test (angina and/or ST-segment shifts occurred) had significant prognostic value. Cox regression analysis was performed, and age and maximal workload were the only variables predictive for survival or cardiac events. Exercise capacity provided prognostic information that was not available either from the history or from cardiac catheterization.

A second study from Saint-Luc Hospital in Brussels included 470 consecutive males without a prior MI but with complaints of chest pain who underwent a maximal exercise perfusion test and coronary angiography.[17] During follow-up (up to 8 years), 32 patients died of CV causes and 30 had a nonfatal MI. Of historical variables, only age was chosen as significant multivariately, and angina and pretest likelihood were also chosen univariately. An exercise test score based on maximal heart rate, ST60 at maximal exercise, angina during the test, maximal workload, and ST slope was chosen in multivariate analysis.

At our VA Medical Center, 588 male patients who underwent exercise testing and cardiac catheterization were followed to determine whether CV mortality rate could be predicted by clinical and exercise test data.[18] Over a mean follow-up period of 4 years, there were 39 CV deaths and 45 nonfatal MIs. The Cox proportional hazard model demonstrated the following characteristics to have a significant independent hazard ratio: history of heart failure (relative risk = 4X), ST depression on the resting electrocardiogram (ECG) (relative risk = 3X), and a drop of SBP below rest during exercise (relative risk = 5X). Exercise-induced ST depression was not associated with either death or nonfatal MI. From cardiac catheterization, only the ejection fraction added independent information to the model. A simple score based on one item of clinical information (history of HF), a resting ECG finding (ST depression), and exertional hypotension stratified our patients from 75% with a low risk (annual cardiac mortality rate of 1%), to 17% with a moderate risk (annual mortality rate of 7%), and 1% with a high risk (annual cardiac mortality rate of 12%; hazard ratio of 20).

Summarizing These Follow-up Prognostic Studies

Nine studies (Table 6-1) have used clinical, exercise test, and catheterization data to predict prognosis in patients with CAD. Some investigators combined variables, and others did not consider key variables or excluded patients with certain clinical features (e.g., HF). Nevertheless, two of the nine found a history of HF, two found exercise SBP, and one found resting ST depression to be associated with death, as we did. In contrast to the Long Beach Veterans Affairs Medical Center (VAMC) study, however, three found exercise-induced ST depression and six of the nine found poor exercise capacity to be predictive of death. Unfortunately, the Duke study did not have maximal SBP collected for comparison. The choice of variables in the Cox hazard models from these studies is tabulated in Table 6-2. Age is not chosen by most of the studies because of the narrow age range for patients submitted for cardiac catheterization. This is the first time exertional hypotension was chosen by a Cox model rather than just observed univariately.

Effect of Workup Bias on the Follow-up Prognostic Studies

All of the aforementioned studies selected patients by requiring that they underwent both exercise testing and coronary angiography. This would mean that they consisted of a higher risk group with a higher prevalence of serious CAD, because patients who were not catheterized would be selected for milder disease and symptoms. To evaluate the effect of this selection process, the Duke group repeated their analysis in an outpatient population that did not undergo cardiac catheterization.[19] The same variables were chosen in their Cox model and the same equation was derived. Similarly, we analyzed 2546 male patients who underwent noninvasive evaluation. Over a mean follow-up period of 2.8 years, there were 119 CV deaths and 44 nonfatal MIs. Significant independent hazard ratios were associated with history of HF or taking digoxin (or both), exercise-induced ST depression, peak METs, and peak SBP during exercise. A simple score based on these four factors stratified patients from low risk (annual cardiac mortality rate < 1%) to high risk (annual cardiac mortality rate of 7%).

The first Duke study used inpatients, all of whom had a catheterization, whereas the later report only included outpatients evaluated before the decision for cardiac catheterization. Their score, based on treadmill time, exercise-induced ST depression, and angina score during the test, performed as well for prognostication as it did in the first paper. Therefore workup bias did not affect their prognostication model. We have attempted the same type of validation in a VA population. In contrast to the Duke group, we included exercise SBP and clinical data in our model. Though history of HF/digoxin was the most powerful variable in both of our VA studies, surprisingly, different exercise test variables were chosen. The model from our first VA study in patients selected for catheterization only chose exertional hypotension, whereas the model from this second VA study (only noninvasive clinical

TABLE 6-1 Population Descriptors Including Clinical Variables and Results from Exercise Testing and Coronary Angiography in the Follow-up Studies of Multivariate Prediction of Cardiac Events

Descriptors	LB VAMC (No Catheter)	LB VAMC	VA CABS	CASS	DUKE
Clinical					
Years entered	1984–1990	1984–1990	1970–1974	1974–1979	1969–1981
Population size	2546	588	245	4083	2842
Age	59	59 (mean)	51 (mean)	50	49 (median)
Males (%)	100	100%	100%	80%	70%
Congestive heart failure	5%	8%	9%	8%	4%
Myocardial infarction	23%	45%	54%	40%	29%
Q waves (at least one)	21%	37%	38%	22%	22%
Digoxin	8%	8%	NA	14%	11%
Beta blockers	22%	35%	14%	40%	54%
Typical angina	21%	52%	100%	50%	47%
Exercise Test					
% with 1 mm ST-segment depression	22%	58%	72%	44%	35%
% angina	4%	35%	66%	80%	50%
Maximal heart rate (beats/min)	137	124	125	138	134
Maximal systolic blood pressure (mm Hg)	175	159	156	171	160
METs	8.4	6.6	5.7	NA	7
Premature ventricular contractions	5%	12%	19%	12%	6%
Cardiac Catheterization Findings					
Three-vessel disease (%)	NA	14%	55%	23%	22%
Left main artery disease (%)	NA	7%	13%	7%	5%
No significant lesion (%)	NA	26%	0%	34%	40%
Ejection fraction	NA	60 (mean)		57%	60 (median)
Significant lesion criteria	NA	70%	50%	70%	75%
Follow-up					
Years	5	5	7	5	5
Coronary artery bypass surgery	2%	20%	24%	36%	24%
Annual cardiovascular mortality rate	1.5%	2.7%	NA	1%	1.6%
Annual total mortality rate	2.8%	3.5%	4%	1.6%	1.8%
Independent Predictors of Mortality by Priority					
	CHF/digoxin	CHF	E-I PVCs	CHF	E-I ST dep
	METs	SBP drop	MHR >140	Treadmill stage	Angina index
	Max SBP	Resting ST dep	E-I ST dep >2mm	E-I ST dep	Treadmill time
	E-I ST dep				

AP, Angina pectoris; *CABS,* coronary artery bypass surgery; *CASS,* Coronary Artery Surgery Study; *CHF,* congestive heart failure; *dep,* depression; *E-I,* exercise-induced; *LB,* Long Beach; *METs,* metabolic equivalents; *MHR,* maximal heart rate; *MI,* myocardial infarction; *PVCs,* premature ventricular contractions; *SBP,* systolic blood pressure; *VA,* Veterans Affairs; *VAMC,* Veterans Affairs Medical Center.

TABLE 6-1 Population Descriptors including Clinical Variables and Results from Exercise Testing and Coronary Angiography in the Follow-up Studies of Multivariate Prediction of Cardiac Events—Cont'd

Italian	Belgian	Belgian (No MI)	German	Seattle	Buenos Aires
1976–1979	1972–1977	1978–1985	1975–1978	1971–1974	1972–1982
1083	372	470	1238	733	180
49 (mean)	48	52	50 (mean)	52 (mean)	51 (mean)
90%	100%	100%	90%	80%	96%
Excluded	1%		Excluded	13%	Excluded
42%	39%	Excluded	>50%	40%	64%
37%	39%	Excluded	50%	45%	
	0%	Excluded	8%	18%	
	0%				
95%	67%	75%	95%	86%	71%
42%	27%	54%	56%		65%
60%	49%	44%	61%		60%
130	148	140	118	145	128
171	NA	186	182	160	151
5.4	9	8	5	6.5	5.2
15%	2%	NA		18%	21%
5%	34%	26%	33%	12%	44%
5%	8%	8%	0%		8
26%	18%	22%	0%	39%	0%
60	NA	65	60	60	
75%	50%	50%	50%	70%	75%
5.5	5	5	5	3.5	6
15%	28%	29%			9%
1.5%	1.8%	2%		2.6%	4.6%
2%	2.4%		2.4%	3.1%	
Q-wave	Age	Age	Exercise capacity	CHF	Max SBP <130
Prior MI	Exercise capacity	Max exercise score (–2 to +2)	Angina	Max double product	ST elevation
Effort ischemia		(MHR, ST60, AP, watts, ST slope)	MHR	Max SBP	<4 METs
Exercise capacity				Angina Resting ST dep	Inappropriate dyspnea

TABLE 6-2 Meta-analysis of Prognosis in Patients with Stable Coronary Artery Disease Requiring Exercise Test and Coronary Angiography

Poor exercise capacity	6 of 9 studies
Congestive heart failure	3 of 9
ST-segment depression	
Resting	2 of 9
Exercise	3 of 9
Exercise systolic blood pressure	3 of 9

evaluation) found exercise-induced ST depression, exercise SBP, and exercise capacity to have predictive power.

The workup bias inherent in choosing patients for cardiac catheterization in our first study resulted in a sicker, older, and more disabled group with a higher annual cardiac mortality rate (2.6% vs. 1.5%). This second study included a population with a near-normal age-adjusted exercise capacity whereas the first study population had an average age-adjusted exercise capacity 75% of normal.

Key Point: Workup bias can explain some of the differences in the studies, but the DTS and the VA treadmill score have been validated in circumstances where workup bias was minimized. HF patients and the elderly should be considered separately.

Long-Beach VA Follow-up Study

In a manner similar to the Duke study that developed the DTS, we developed a score in the VA.[20] In a population of 2546 veterans, using stepwise selection, the Cox model was allowed to build on each variable group to arrive at the final model, which chose history of HF/digoxin, change in SBP score, METs, and exercise-induced ST depression. The coefficients from the Cox model weighted the variables as follows: $5 \times$ (HF/digoxin [yes = 1, no = 0]) + (exercise-induced ST depression in millimeters) + (change in SBP score) − (METs). Three groups were formed using the score: <−2 (low risk), −2 to +2 (moderate risk), and >2 (high risk). The Kaplan-Meier survival curves are illustrated in Figure 6-2. This score enabled identification of a low-risk group (80% of the population) with an annual mortality rate of less than 1% over the first 3 years after their exercise test. In addition, a moderate-risk group (14% of the population), with a 4% annual mortality rate over the 3 years after their exercise test, and a high-risk group (6% of the population), with a 7% annual mortality rate over the 3 years after their exercise test, were identified.

In addition, the DTS was calculated for each of our veteran patients. The treadmill angina index was modified because we did not have angina coded as the reason for stopping; it was coded as 0 for not present, and 1 as occurring during the test. We also used METs instead of minutes of exercise. In Figure 6-3 are the range of characteristics (ROC) curves for the Duke score and the VA score predicting CV deaths in the total group ($n = 3134$). The area under the VA score curve (0.76) was significantly greater than the area under the Duke score curve (0.68). These scores are summarized in Table 6-3.

Score Comparison

Unfortunately, one of the only studies to also compare these two scores was in post-MI patients, and the follow-up was only for 6 months. The Gruppo Italiano per lo Studio della Sopravvivenza nell'Infarto Miocardico (GISSI) investigators compared the performance of the DTS and the VAMC score in predicting 6-month death in GISSI-2 study survivors of acute MI treated with thrombolytic agents to a simple predictive scoring system developed from the same database.[21] Patients in the GISSI-2 study ($n = 6251$) performed a symptom-limited exercise test 1 month after MI. They calculated for each

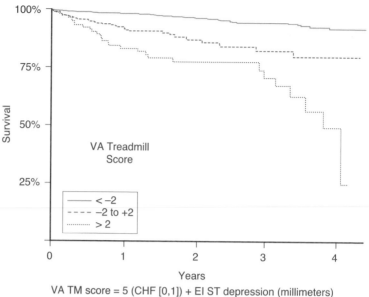

VA TM score = 5 (CHF [0,1]) + EI ST depression (millimeters) + change SBP score (0–5) – METs

FIGURE 6-2   The Kaplan-Meier survival curves from the VA follow-up study. Three groups were formed using the score: < –2 (low risk), –2 to +2 (moderate risk), and >2 (high risk). The score enabled identification of a low-risk group (80% of the population) with an annual mortality rate of less than 1% over the first 3 years after their exercise test. In addition, a moderate-risk group (14% of the population) with a 4% annual mortality rate and a high-risk group (6% of the population) with a 7% annual mortality rate over the 3 years after their exercise test were identified.

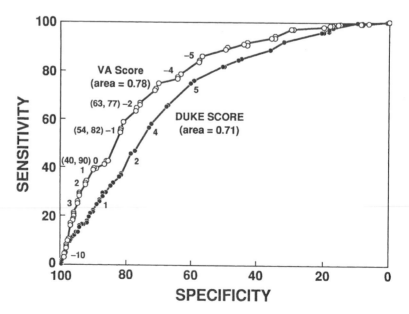

FIGURE 6-3   The ROC curves for the Duke score and the VA score predicting CV deaths in the total group (n = 3134).

TABLE 6-3   The Two Prognostic Scores from Properly Designed and Analyzed Follow-up Studies

Duke score = METs − 5 × (mm E-I ST depression) − 4 × (TM AP index)
VA score = 5 × (CHF/digoxin) + mm E-I ST depression + change in SBP score − METs

Treadmill angina pectoris (TM AP) score: 0 if no angina; 1 if angina occurred during test; 2 if angina was the reason for stopping.
Change in systolic blood pressure (SBP) score: from 0 for rise greater than 40 mm Hg to 5 for drop below rest.

patient the DTS, the VAMC score, and the new GISSI score. All three scores were able to stratify risk (from a low risk of < 1%, to a moderate risk of 2%, to a high risk of 5%). The investigators concluded that exercise test prognostic scores could stratify risk in survivors of MI who received thrombolytic drugs.

However, Morise and Jalisi[22] compared our new simple scores for predicting angiographic CAD with the DTS for predicting all-cause mortality. They used 4640 patients without known coronary disease whose mortality rate was 3% with 3 years of follow-up. All three scores stratified patients into low-, intermediate-, and high-risk groups. No differences were seen when patients were evaluated as subgroups according to gender, diabetes, beta blockers, or inpatient status. Low-risk patients defined by the DTS had consistently higher mortality rates and absolute number of deaths compared with low-risk patients using other scores. In addition, the DTS had less incremental stratifying value than the new exercise scores. The authors concluded that simple pretest and exercise scores risk-stratified patients with suspected coronary disease in accordance with published guidelines and better than the DTS. These results extended to diabetics, inpatients, women, and patients on beta blockers. It would be beneficial to see these same analyses performed predicting infarct-free survival with censoring for cardiac interventions.

Prognosis Prediction for "All-Comers" to the Exercise Laboratory

Previous prognostic scores were developed in specific subsets of patients, so we analyzed all patients referred for evaluation at our exercise laboratory between 1987 and 2000.[23] There were 6213 males (mean age 59 ± 11 years) who had standard exercise ECG treadmill tests over the study period with a mean 6-year follow-up. There were no complications of testing in this clinically referred population, 78% of whom were referred for chest pain, risk factors, or signs or symptoms of CAD. Overlapping thirds had typical angina or history of MI, 579 had prior CABG, and 522 had a history of HF. Twenty percent died for an average annual mortality rate of 2.6%. The following variables in rank order were chosen: peak METs less than 5, older than 65 years old, history of HF, and history of MI. A score based on simply adding these variables classified patients into low-, medium-, and high-risk groups. The high-risk group (score of 3 or more) had a hazard ratio of 5 and a 5-year mortality rate of 31% (Figure 6-4). When CV mortality rate was

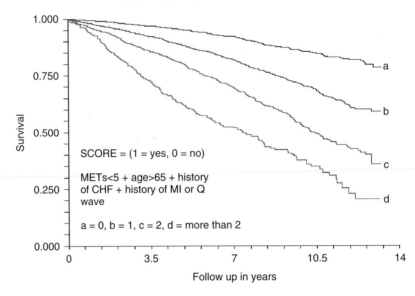

FIGURE 6-4 *Kaplan-Meier survival curves for the "all-comers" prognostic score using all-cause mortality as the endpoint.*

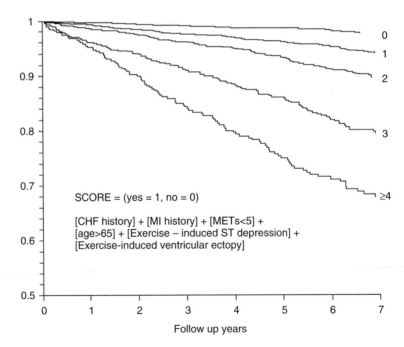

FIGURE 6-5 *Kaplan-Meier survival curves for the "all-comers" prognostic score using CV mortality as the endpoint. Two additional treadmill responses appeared as independently significant: exercise-induced ST depression and arrhythmias.*

available, we repeated these analyses. Two additional treadmill responses appeared as independently significant: exercise-induced ST depression and arrhythmias (Figure 6-5).

Predicting Prognosis in Women

Clinical presentation, performance in diagnostic tests, and prevalence of CAD are different between men and women with chest pain. Duke University researchers analyzed data from 976 women referred for evaluation of chest pain who underwent exercise treadmill testing and cardiac catheterization.[24] Women and men differed significantly in the DTS, disease prevalence (32% vs. 72% significant CAD), and 2-year mortality rate (1.9% for women compared with 4.9% for the men). Mortality rate increased for higher-risk DTS groups in both genders. The 2-year mortality rate for women was 1%, 2.2%, and 3.6%, respectively, for low-, moderate, and high-risk groups. The 2-year mortality rate for men was 1.7%, 5.8%, and 16.6%, respectively, for low-, moderate-, and high-risk groups. Because of the differences in disease prevalence, women had better survival at all values of the DTS. Although women had better survival than men, the DTS actually performed better in women than in men for excluding disease, with fewer low-risk women having mild or severe disease.

As part of the Women's Ischemia Syndrome Evaluation (WISE) study, Morise and colleagues[25] evaluated 563 women undergoing coronary angiography for suspected myocardial ischemia. The prevalence of angiographic CAD was 26%. Overall, 189 women underwent treadmill testing. Prognostic endpoints included death, MI, stroke, and revascularization. The simple scores and the DTS score stratified women into three probability groups according to the prevalence of coronary disease:

- Pretest: low 20/164 (12%), intermediate 53/245 (22%), high 75/154 (49%)
- Exercise test: low 11/83 (13%), intermediate 22/74 (30%), high 17/32 (53%)

However, the DTS did not stratify as well. When pretest and exercise scores were considered together, the best stratification with the exercise test score was in the intermediate pretest group. The DTS did not stratify this group at all. Pretest and exercise test scores also stratified women according to prognostic endpoints. Exercise test scores are most useful in women with an intermediate pretest score, consistent with American College of Cardiology/American Heart Association (ACC/AHA) guidelines.

Predicting Prognosis in Patients with Resting ST Depression

Kwok and colleagues[26] demonstrated that the DTS can effectively risk-stratify patients with ST-T abnormalities on the resting ECG. When patients with ST-T abnormalities were classified into risk groups according to DTS, there were significant overall differences among the risk groups for all outcome endpoints. The 7-year event-free survival rates were 94%, 88%, and 69% for the low-, intermediate-, and high-risk groups, respectively. More patients with ST-T changes were classified as high risk (5% vs. 2%) and their 7-year survival was lower than that of the control population high-risk patients (76% vs. 93%).

The Elderly

The decline in function that accompanies aging is a consequence of age-related decrements in CV, pulmonary, and musculoskeletal structure. Ultimately, these result in impaired physical function in the elderly.[27] The DTS was validated in patients in the age range when CAD first appears, but data are limited in the elderly. To determine the prognostic value the treadmill test in the elderly, researchers from the Mayo Clinic and the Olmsted Medical Group compared the prognostic value of the test in patients younger than 65 and older than 65 years of age.[28] Elderly ($n = 514$) and younger ($n = 2593$) patients who underwent treadmill testing between 1987 and 1989 were identified retrospectively and followed for 6 years. Compared with younger patients, elderly patients had more comorbid conditions, had a higher prevalence of abnormal ST depression (28% vs. 9%), and achieved a lower exercise capacity (6 METs vs. 11 METs). A poor exercise capacity and angina during the exercise test were associated with future cardiac events. Exercise-induced ST depression did not carry significant value in the elderly and was associated with future cardiac events only in younger patients. An increase of 1 MET in exercise capacity was associated with a 14% decrease in risk for a cardiac event in younger patients and with an 18% risk reduction among the elderly. After adjustment for clinical factors, there was a strong inverse association between exercise capacity and outcome. METs achieved was the only treadmill exercise test variable that provided prognostic information for both mortality rate and cardiac events. In the elderly, exercise capacity was also inversely associated with the likelihood of nursing home placement. Spin and colleagues[29] also demonstrated the strong association between METs achieved from exercise testing and all-cause mortality rate in the elderly.

Kwok and colleagues[30] found that the DTS could not predict death, MI, and cardiac interventions in patients 75 years or older. Lai and colleagues[31] considered both death and angiographic endpoints and found age-specific scores to be necessary in the elderly. What can explain why exercise test variables other than exercise capacity do not provide prognostic information in those over 75 years of age? Possibly it is due to the many competing causes of mortality in the elderly compared with younger subjects, who are more likely to die of one cause. It is also possible that the elderly are survivors who, for instance, have coronary disease but have extensive collaterals that protect them from death though not ischemia. Reduced exercise capacity in the elderly is partially explained by the high prevalence of coexisting medical problems, such as deconditioning, muscle weakness, orthopedic problems, neurologic problems, and peripheral vascular disease.

To further study this issue, we classified our patients into subsets based on age. Exercise capacity was chosen by Cox hazard model most consistently in the age-groups using either endpoint. Even when age was added to the DTS, prediction of death did not improve in those over 70 years of age because of the nonlinear relationship between ages, exercise test variables, and time to death. The most important age cutpoints for clinically important differences in exercise test predictors appeared to be 70 and 75 years of age. In patients 70 to 75 years of age, METs was the only variable predictive of all-cause

TABLE 6-4   Results of Cox Hazard Model with CV Mortality as the Endpoint for Age Groupings Illustrating How the Predictive Power of the Treadmill Responses Change with Age

	<45	45-55	55-65	65-75	>75	
Age						
N	619	987	1081	717	174	
CV death	8	35	72	77	22	
METs	−0.22	−0.18	−0.13	−0.13	NS	Regression coefficient
	0.81	0.83	0.87	0.87		Hazard
	0.67-0.97	0.75-0.93	0.81-0.94	0.80-0.95		95% CI
Exercise-induced ST depression	NS	0.61	NS	NS	NS	
		1.85				
		1.39-2.46				
Duke angina score	NS	NS	NS	NS	NS	
Maximal SBP	NS	0.014	NS	NS	NS	
		1.01				
		1-1.03				
Maximal heart rate	NS	NS	NS	NS	NS	1st in Cox
						2nd in Cox
						3rd in Cox
Resting ST depression	NS	NS	NS	0.81	NS	
				2.27		
				1.26-4.07		

CI, Confidence intervals. Modified from Yamazaki T, Myers J, Froelicher VF. Effect of age and end point on the prognostic value of the exercise test, *Chest* 125:1920–1928, 2004.

mortality and exercise-induced ST depression was the only predictor of CV death; in patients older than 75 years of age, none of the exercise test responses were predictive of either death outcome (Table 6-4). None of the treadmill variables were selected as a predictor of outcome in those 45 years old or younger. This is probably due to the small number of deaths and the lack of data regarding cardiac interventions during follow-up. Exercise-induced ST depression was significantly more prevalent in those who died, but it was independently associated with CV mortality only in those 45 to 55 years old. The failure of the DTS to have prognostic value in our population remains a mystery because in the same population it is one of the important predictors for the presence of angiographic disease.[32]

> **Key Point:** Age and the endpoint used in the Cox hazard analyses affect the variables chosen when creating prognostic scores. Age has a nonlinear relationship with the predictor variables and outcomes such that adding age to scores does not improve prediction in the elderly. The DTS probably does not predict outcome well in the elderly because other clinical predictors (comorbidities, psychosocial factors, and subclinical conditions) overpower the treadmill responses.

Diabetics and Those with Silent Ischemia

These two situations are discussed together because of the widespread belief that silent ischemia is more common in diabetics. An open mind should be kept in this regard, however, because the evidence basis for this belief is not conclusive.

Preliminary studies led to the hypothesis that "silent" myocardial ischemia had a worse prognosis than angina pectoris because patients with it do not have an intact "warning system." However, in studies of patients referred for diagnostic purposes or with stable coronary syndromes, silent myocardial ischemia detected by exercise testing has been associated with either a lesser or similar prognosis compared to patients with angina pectoris. Since exercise testing has advantages over ambulatory monitoring in regard to the leads monitored, chest pain description, and fidelity of the recording apparatus, confirmation of these findings would help resolve the controversy over the relative prognostic impact of silent myocardial ischemia. Exercise testing studies provide one means of evaluating the risk of silent ischemia. Unfortunately, these exercise test studies do not evaluate patients with true silent ischemia. The patients are being tested because of some symptoms, usually angina; however, the patient with silent ischemia does not have angina at the time of the test. Importantly, though, patients with only silent ischemia are rare. Therefore the following data from exercise test studies give us a good idea of how the usual patients seen in clinical practice with silent ischemia, at least on some occasions, are likely to do.[33,34] Silent ischemia on the treadmill is not a benign finding (average annual mortality rate 2.8%), but CAD patients with silent ischemia had a less aggressive anginal course, less CAD, and a better prognosis. Other, smaller angiographic studies agree with this finding.[35,36]

To further evaluate this issue, another analysis from the CASS registry was performed.[37] Patients with either silent or symptomatic ischemia during exercise testing had a similar risk of developing an acute MI or sudden death—except in those with three-vessel CAD, where the risk was greater in those with silent ischemia. We took the opportunity to determine whether differences in the prevalence of silent ischemia and its impact on prognosis could be explained by age or by MI and diabetes mellitus status.[38] Patients in the angina plus ST depression and silent ischemia groups had significantly higher overall 2-year mortality rate than patients without ST-segment depression. Overall mortality rate in the angina plus ST depression and silent ischemia patients was not significantly different. We recently repeated these analyses in our larger data set of veterans with a longer follow-up (Figure 6-6). Furthermore, it has been consistently found that patients with symptomatic ischemia have a higher prevalence of severe angiographic disease than patients with silent ischemia.[39-41]

> **Key Point:** Therapy should not be guided by the false hypothesis that patients with silent ischemia are at higher risk for death than those with angina and ST depression. A consistent finding has been that patients with symptomatic ischemia have a higher prevalence of severe angiographic disease than patients with silent ischemia.

Not all studies have shown a difference in the prevalence of silent myocardial ischemia between diabetics and the general population. In a landmark Danish study, the prevalence of ischemia was compared in a random sample of 120 users of insulin and 120 users of oral hypoglycemic agents age 40 to 75 years.[42] The observed prevalence of silent ischemia on treadmill or Holter testing in diabetics was 13.5% and was not different in

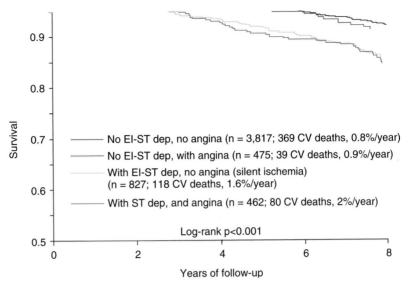

FIGURE 6-6 *Kaplan-Meier curves for the general population of 6000 male veterans divided and classified by angina and exercise-induced (EI) ST depression.*

matched controls. No association was found between silent ischemia and gender or diabetes type. Although hypertension was highly predictive of silent ischemia in the diabetic subjects, other variables did not have predictive value. This finding is hard to explain. Scandinavian populations have previously been noted to outlie in CVD prevalence,[43] and it is possible that a high level of baseline disease in the nondiabetic population masks the population differences seen in other studies.

Data from the Asymptomatic Cardiac Ischemia Pilot (ACIP) study revealed that asymptomatic ST-segment depression during Holter monitoring was 94% in diabetics and 88% in nondiabetics.[44] In addition, the time to onset of 1 mm of ST-segment depression and time to onset of angina were similar in both groups. Unlike the previous study, however, entry into the ACIP study required a cardiac event, so the disease was not consistently silent.

> **Key Point:** Silent myocardial ischemia has been found to be associated with the same, lower, and higher risk relative to nonsilent (i.e., painful) ischemia. It has been found to occur with the same and higher frequency in diabetics. What is clear, however, is that, whether silent or not, ischemia during treadmill testing in the general population predicts increased risk for death. However, in general these patients were tested because they had chest pain symptoms. That is, their ischemia was "silent" only with respect to the exercise test itself.

A New Prognostic Marker: Heart Rate Recovery
Recent studies have highlighted the prognostic value of heart rate recovery (HRR), or the drop in heart rate after an exercise test. Although earlier

physiologic studies suggested a rapid HRR response to exercise to be a marker of physical fitness, only recently has its prognostic value been reported. The rate of heart rate return to baseline after exercise is theorized to be due to high vagal tone associated with fitness and good health. Although the prognostic value of HRR has recently been highlighted, its relative value compared with other treadmill responses and its diagnostic value remain uncertain. Table 6-5 shows comparisons of the HRR studies across a number of important parameters. In the first study, Cole and colleagues[45] studied 2428 adults who had been referred for exercise nuclear perfusion scans. They found that using a drop of 12 beats per minute or less as the definition of an abnormal response and abnormal responders exhibited a relative risk of 4 for death. The group having a value less than 12 beats per minute had a mortality rate of 19%, and the group with a value higher than 12 beats per minute had a mortality rate of 5% over the 6-year period. The study employed the symptom-limited Bruce protocol with a 2-minute cool-down walk, and HRR was measured at 1 minute after peak exercise. Patients on beta blockers were included in the study, and no difference was seen in the ability of the test to discriminate between low- and high-risk patients in those patients on beta blockers. The investigators used all-cause mortality and performed survival analysis both with and without censoring of interventions (CABS and PCI), and found no difference in results.

The same investigators then studied a different patient population.[46] Asymptomatic patients enrolled in the Lipid Research Clinics Prevalence Study underwent exercise testing. The tests were stopped when 85% to 90% of peak heart rate was achieved, and there was no cool-down walk. HRR was a strong predictor of all-cause mortality; patients with an abnormal value had a mortality rate of 10% whereas patients with a normal value had a mortality rate of 4% over 12 years of follow-up.

To further elucidate the power of HRR in distinct populations, investigators from the Cleveland Clinic published a study using patients referred for standard treadmill testing.[47] Using the same methods as the original study, the investigators found similar results, although notably the cutoff value for an abnormal test was different. Patients with abnormal HRR had an 8% mortality rate at 5.2 years, whereas patients with normal HRR had only a 2% mortality rate. Neither this nor the previous study censored for CABS or PCI, and 8% of the patients had CABS while 75% were asymptomatic. The investigators also compared the prognostic ability of HRR with that of the DTS. Whereas the ischemic components of the DTS did not have prognostic power, peak METs did, because the DTS produced similar survival curves to HRR. In patients with an abnormal DTS and an abnormal HRR, survival was even further compromised.

We attempted to validate the use of HRR for prognosis in a male veteran population.[49] The mortality rate in our study was higher than that in previous studies. Using similar statistical analyses, we found that an HRR of less than 22 beats per minute at 2 minutes of recovery identified a high-risk group of patients. We also found that beta blockers had no significant impact on the prognostic value of HRR. Similar to Cole and colleagues,[45] we found that a low exercise capacity was the most powerful predictor of mortality.

TABLE 6-5 Major Published Prognostic Studies Relating to the Decrease of Heart Rate after Exercise

Study	Population	Sample Size (% Women)	Exclusion Criteria	Years of Follow-up	Test Protocol/ Recovery status	Minutes of Recovery/ Cutpoint	Mortality (All Causes)	Sensitivity/Specificity for Death
Cole[45] NEJM	Referral for exercise perfusion; 9% with known CAD	2428 (37)	CABS, angiography, CHF/digoxin use, LBBB	6	Bruce, with 2-minute cool-down, symptom-limited	1 min/12 beats/min	213 (9%)	(cutpoint = 12 beats/min) 56%/77% (cutpoint = 8 beats/min) 33%/90%
Cole[46] Annals	Participants in Lipid Research Clinics Prevalence Study, asymptomatic	5234 (39)	Beta blockers, other cardiac medications, h/o cardiovascular disease	12	Bruce, without cool-down 85% age-predicted heart rate	2 min/42 beats/min	325 (6.2%), 36% believed to be cardiovascular Follow-up 100%	54%/69%
Nishime[47] JAMA	Referral for ETT; 8% prior CABS, 75% screening asymptomatic, 9% prior MI	9454 (22)	CHF, LBBB, digoxin, valvular heart disease	5.2	Bruce, with 2-minute cool-down, symptom-limited	1 min/12 beats/min	312 (3%)	49%/81%
Watanabe[48] Circulation	Referral for ETT-echo	5785 (37)	CHF, valve disease, afib, pacer	3	N/A No cool-down	1 min/18 beats/min	190 (3.5%)	33%/87%
Shetler[49] JACC	Referral for standard ETT; 42% with prior MI	2193 (all men)	CABS, angiography, LBBB, pacer	6.8	Ramp without cool-down, symptom-limited	2 min/22 beats/min	413 (19%)	35%/83%

CABS, coronary artery bypass surgery; *CHF,* congestive heart failure; *ETT,* exercise treadmill test; *h/o,* history of; *LBBB,* left bundle branch block; *MI,* myocardial infarction.

When entered stepwise as continuous variables, however, HRR at 2 minutes of recovery was chosen ahead of age and exercise capacity.

A distinct advantage over previous studies is that we selected a group of patients who underwent coronary angiography. This made it possible to evaluate the diagnostic ability of HRR. Surprisingly, HRR was not selected among the standard variables to be included in a logistic model, and its ROC curve did not indicate any discriminatory value. Thus, although HRR has been validated as an important prognostic variable, it did not help in diagnosing coronary disease in this study. In general, these studies did not censor on events or consider event-free survival; therefore HRR may well just be a surrogate for physical fitness/activity level predicting outcome along with medical therapy.

The following later studies addressed the issues of the ability of HRR to predict CV disease/events rather than all-cause mortality and its performance in women and diabetics. Because no prior study considered the association of HRR after exercise with the incidence of coronary heart disease (CHD) and CV disease, 2967 Framingham study subjects (1400 men, mean age 43 years) free of CVD were analyzed.[50] During 15 years of follow-up, 214 subjects experienced a CHD event, 312 developed a CVD event, and 167 died. In multivariable models, continuous HRR indexes were not associated with the incidence of CHD or CVD events or with all-cause mortality. However, in models evaluating quintile-based cutpoints, the top quintile of HRR (greatest decline in heart rate) at 1 minute after exercise was associated with half the CHD and CVD of the bottom quintile, but not all-cause mortality.

A total of 2994 asymptomatic women without CVD, 30 to 80 years old, performed a near-maximal treadmill test as part of the Lipid Research Clinics Prevalence Study (1972–1976).[51] They were followed for 20 years with CV and all-cause mortality as the endpoints. There were 427 deaths (14%), 147 of which were due to CV causes. Low exercise capacity, low HRR, and not achieving target heart rate were independently associated with increased all-cause and CV mortality. There was no increased CV death risk for exercise-induced ST-segment depression, but there was an age-adjusted 20% increase in CV death for every MET decrease and a 36% increase in CV mortality rate per 10 beats per minute decrement in HRR. After adjusting for multiple other risk factors, women who were below the median for both exercise capacity and HRR had a 3.5-fold increased risk of CV death. Among women with low-risk Framingham scores, those with below median levels of both METs and HRR had significantly increased risk compared with women who had above median levels of these two exercise variables (45 and 4 CV deaths per 10,000 person-years, respectively, hazard ratio of 13).

In a study of male diabetics, 2333 men with diabetes were studied.[52] Hazard ratios for CV and all-cause death were adjusted for age, METs, resting heart rate, fasting blood glucose, body mass index, smoking, alcohol consumption, lipids, and history of CV disease. During 15 years of follow-up, there were 142 CV deaths and 287 total deaths. Compared with men in the highest quartile of HRR, the adjusted hazard ratio was 1.5 to 2 for CV death.

> **Key Point:** An abnormal HRR appears to have greater prognostic power for all-cause mortality than age and exercise capacity. It should be calculated as part of every exercise test. However, it appears to predict non-CV death better than CV death.

Predicting Severe Angiographic Disease

Exercise Test Responses

Many studies have tried to predict left main disease using exercise testing,[53-55] and different criteria have been used with varying results. Predictive value here refers to the percentage of those with the abnormal criteria who actually had left main disease. Naturally, most of the "false positives" actually had CAD, but less severe forms. Sensitivity here refers to the percentage of those with left main disease only that are detected. These criteria have been refined over time, and the last study by Weiner and colleagues[56] using the CASS data deserves further mention.

A markedly positive exercise test (Table 6-6) defined as 0.2 mV or more of downsloping ST-segment depression beginning at 4 METs or less, persisting for at least 6 minutes into recovery, and involving at least five ECG leads had the greatest sensitivity (74%) and predictive value (32%) for left main coronary disease. This abnormal pattern identified either left main or three-vessel disease with a sensitivity of 49%, a specificity of 92%, and a predictive value of 74%.

Blumenthal and colleagues[57] validated the ability of a strongly positive exercise test to predict left main coronary disease even in patients with minimal or no angina. The criteria for a markedly positive test included the following: (1) early ST-segment depression, (2) 0.2 mV or more of depression, (3) downsloping ST depression, (4) exercise-induced hypotension, (5) prolonged ST changes after the test, and (6) multiple areas of ST depression. Although Lee and colleagues[58] included many clinical and exercise test variables, only three variables were found to help predict left main disease: angina type, age, and the amount of exercise-induced ST-segment depression.

It appears that individual clinical or exercise test variables are unable to detect left main coronary disease because of their low sensitivity or predictive value. However, a combination of the amount, pattern, and duration of ST-segment response has been highly predictive and reasonably sensitive for left main or three-vessel coronary disease. The question still remains of how to identify those with abnormal resting ejection fractions, and those who will benefit the most with prolonged survival after CABS. Perhaps those with a normal resting ECG will not need surgery for increased longevity because of the associated high probability of normal ventricular function.

TABLE 6-6   Markedly Positive Treadmill Test Responses

More than 0.2 mV downsloping ST-segment depression
ST depression involving five or more leads
ST depression occurring at less than 5 METs
ST depression prolonged late into recovery

Meta-Analysis of Studies Predicting Angiographic Severity

To evaluate the variability in the reported accuracy of the exercise ECG for predicting severe coronary disease, Detrano and colleagues[59] applied meta-analysis to 60 consecutively published reports comparing exercise-induced ST depression with coronary angiographic findings. The 60 reports included 62 distinct study groups comprising 12,030 patients who underwent both tests. Both technical and methodologic factors were analyzed. Wide variability in sensitivity and specificity was found (mean sensitivity was 86% [range 40% to 100%] and mean specificity was 53% [range 17% to 100%]) for left main or three-vessel disease. All three variables found to be significantly and independently related to test performance were methodologic. Exclusion of patients with right bundle branch block and receiving digoxin improved the prediction of three-vessel or left main CAD, and comparison with a "better" exercise test decreased test performance.

Hartz and colleagues[60] compiled results from the literature on the use of the exercise test to identify patients with severe CAD. Pooled estimates of sensitivity and specificity were derived for the ability of the exercise test to identify three-vessel or left main CAD. Using a 1 mm criterion for ST depression averaged a sensitivity of 75% and a specificity of 66%, whereas using a 2 mm criterion averaged a sensitivity of 52% and a specificity of 86%. There was great variability among the studies examined in the estimated sensitivity and specificity for severe CAD that could not be explained by their analysis.

Key Point: ST analysis alone has limited sensitivity and specificity for severe forms of angiographic disease. Scores are necessary to improve test performance.

Multivariable Equations and Scores to Predict Severe Angiographic Disease

The most common statistical methods employed include Bayesian statistics, logistic regression, and discriminant function analysis. The Bayesian approach, which considers pretest clinical variables, is a logical method in clinical practice and helps one decide which tests are appropriate. However, it appears that logistic regression or discriminant function analysis permits a more robust prediction of disease.

There are statistical techniques to separate subjects into different groups on the basis of measured variables.[61] Two commonly used types of analysis are discriminant function and logistic regression analysis. Logistic regression has been preferred because it models the relationship to a sigmoid curve (which often is the mathematical relationship between a risk variable and an outcome) and its output is between 0 and 1 (i.e., from 0% to 100% probability of the predicted outcome). Thus the output of a discriminant function is a unitless numerical score whereas a logistic regression provides an actual probability, which, however, may vary from one population to another.

Logistic regression results in an equation that takes the following form:

$$\text{Probability} = 1/(1 + e^{-(a + bx + cy...)})$$

where a = intercept, b and c are coefficients, and x and y are variable values such as 0 or 1 for gender, diabetes, or chest pain and a continuous value for age or heart rate.

Since 1979, at least 12 studies have been performed combining the patient's medical history, symptoms of chest pain, hemodynamic data, exercise capacity, and exercise test responses to calculate the probability of severe angiographic CAD.[62-73] The results are summarized in Table 6-7. Nine of the 13 studies excluded patients with previous CABS or prior PCI, and in the remaining 4 studies, exclusions were unclear. The percentage of patients with one-vessel, two-vessel, and three-vessel disease was described in 10 of the 13 studies. The definition of *severe disease* or *disease extent* also differed. In 5 of the 13 studies, *disease extent* was defined as multivessel disease. In the remaining 8 studies, it was defined as three-vessel or left main disease, and in one study as only left main artery disease. In another study the impact of disease in the right coronary artery on left main disease was considered. The prevalence of severe disease ranged from 16% to 48% in the studies defining *disease extent* as multivessel disease and from 10% to 28% in the studies using the more strict criterion of three-vessel or left main disease.

Surprisingly, some of the variables chosen for predicting severe disease are different than those for predicting disease presence for diagnosis. Whereas gender and chest pain were chosen to be significant in more than half of the severity studies, age was less important, and resting ECG abnormalities and diabetes were the only other variables chosen in more than half the studies. In contrast, the most consistent clinical variables chosen for diagnosis were age, gender, chest pain type, and hypercholesterolemia. ST depression and slope were frequently chosen for severity, but exercise capacity and heart

TABLE 6-7 Summary of Results from 13 Studies Predicting Disease Severity

	Clinical Variables	Significant Predictor
Predictors of Disease Severity in 13 Studies (14 Equations)		
Gender	7/9	78%
Chest pain symptoms	8/11	73%
Diabetes mellitus	6/10	60%
Age	8/14	57%
Abnormal resting ECG	4/8	50%
Elevated cholesterol	4/10	40%
Family history of CAD	1/4	25%
Smoking history	2/8	25%
Hypertension	1/6	17%
Exercise Test Variables		
ST-segment depression	11/14	79%
ST-segment slope	6/8	75%
Double product	4/7	57%
Delta systolic BP	5/11	45%
Exercise capacity	4/13	31%
Exercise-induced angina	4/13	31%
Maximal heart rate	1/10	10%
Maximal systolic BP	0/4	0%

rate were less consistently chosen for diagnosis. Double product and delta SBP were chosen as independent predictors in more than half of the studies predicting severity.

Predicting Improved Survival with Coronary Artery Bypass Surgery

Which exercise test variables indicate those patients who would have an improved prognosis if they underwent CABS? The limitation of the available studies is that patients have not been randomized to surgery according to their exercise test results and the analyses are retrospective.

Bruce and colleagues[74] assessed noninvasive screening criteria for patients who had improved 4-year survival rate after CABS. Their data came from 2000 men with coronary heart disease enrolled in the Seattle Heart Watch who had a symptom-limited maximal treadmill test; these subjects received usual community care, which resulted in 16% of them having CABS in nonrandomized fashion. Patients with cardiomegaly, less than a 5 MET exercise capacity, and/or a maximal SBP of less than 130 would have a better outcome if treated with surgery. Presence of two or more of these parameters presents the highest risk and the greater differential for improved survival with bypass. The 4-year survival rate in this group would be 94% for those who had surgery versus 67% for those who received medical management (in those who had two or more of the parameters). In the European surgery trial,[75] patients who had an exercise test response of 1.5 mm of ST-segment depression had improved survival with surgery. This also extended to those with baseline ST-segment depression and those with claudication.

From the CASS study group,[76] in more than 5000 nonrandomized patients, though there were definite differences between the surgical and nonsurgical groups, survival could be accounted for by stratification in subsets. The surgical benefit regarding mortality was greatest in the 789 patients with 1 mm of ST-segment depression at less than 5 METs. Among the 398 patients with three-vessel disease with this exercise test response, the 7-year survival rate was 50% in those medically managed versus 81% in those who underwent CABS. *There was no difference in mortality rate in randomized patients able to exceed 10 METs.* In the VA surgery randomized trial,[77] there was a 79% survival rate with CABS versus 42% for medical management in patients with two or more of the following: 2 mm or more of ST depression, heart rate of 140 beats per minute or greater at 6 METs, and/or exercise-induced PVCs. The results from those four studies are summarized in Table 6-8.

Comparison of Prediction Equations with Cardiologists' Predictions

To study the accuracy with which long-term prognosis can be predicted in patients with CAD, prognostic predictions from a data-based multivariable statistical model were compared with predictions from senior cardiologists.[78] Test samples of 100 patients each were selected from a large series of medically treated patients with significant coronary disease. Using detailed

TABLE 6-8 Studies Evaluating Exercise Test Responses Associated with Improved Survival Rates with Coronary Artery Bypass Surgery

Study	Markers of Patients Who Will Have Improved Survival with Bypass Surgery
Seattle Heart Watch	Cardiomegaly, < 5 METs exercise capacity; maximal systolic blood pressure < 130 mm Hg
European Surgery Trial	ST-segment depression at rest; 1.5 mm ST-segment depression with exercise, or claudication
Coronary Artery Surgery Study (CASS)	1 mm of ST-segment depression at < 5 METs; no difference if 10 METs exceeded
Veterans Affairs Coronary Artery Bypass Surgery Study	Two or more of the following: • 2 mm of ST-segment depression • Heart rate < 140 beats/min at 6 METs • Exercise-induced premature ventricular contractions

case summaries, five senior cardiologists each predicted 1- and 3-year survival and infarct-free survival probabilities for 100 patients. Fifty patients appeared in multiple samples for assessing interphysician variability. Cox regression models, developed using patients not in the test samples, predicted corresponding outcome probabilities for each test patient. Overall, model predictions correlated better with actual patient outcomes than did the doctors' predictions. For 3-year survival, rank correlations were 0.61 (model) and 0.49 (doctors). For 3-year infarct-free survival predictions, correlations with outcome were 0.48 (model) and 0.29 (doctors). Comparisons by individual doctor revealed that Cox model 3-year survival predictions were better than those of four of five doctors (model predictions added significant prognostic information to the doctor's predictions, whereas the converse was not true). For infarct-free survival, the Cox model was superior to all five doctors. Where multiple doctors made predictions, the interphysician variability was substantial.

A computer algorithm for estimating probabilities of any significant coronary obstruction and three-vessel/left main obstructions was derived, validated, and compared with the assessments of cardiac clinician angiographers.[79] The algorithm performed at least as well as the clinicians when the latter knew the identity of the patients whose angiograms they had decided to perform. The clinicians were more accurate when they did not know the identity of the subjects but worked from tabulated objective data. Referral and value-induced bias may affect physician judgment in assessing disease probability. Application of computer aids or consultation with cardiologists not directly involved with patient management may assist in more rational assessments and decision making.

Using these two papers as a starting point, we used our database to compare exercise test scores and ST measurements with a physician's estimation of the probability of the presence and severity of angiographic disease and the risk of death.[80,81] A clinical exercise test was performed and an angiographic database was used to print patient summaries and treadmill reports. The clinical/treadmill test reports were sent to expert cardiologists and to two other groups, including randomly selected cardiologists and internists. They classified the patients summarized in the reports as having a high, low, or intermediate probability for the presence of any and also severe angiographic disease using a numerical probability from 0% to 100%. Twenty-six percent of the patients had severe angiographic disease, and the annual mortality rate for the population was 2%. Forty-five expert cardiologists returned estimates on 473 patients, 37 randomly chosen practicing cardiologists returned estimates on 202 patients, 29 randomly chosen practicing internists returned estimates on 162 patients, 13 academic cardiologists returned estimates on 145 patients, and 27 academic internists returned estimates on 272 patients. When probability estimates for presence and severity of angiographic disease were compared, in general, the treadmill scores were superior to physicians' estimates and ST analysis at predicting severe angiographic disease. Treadmill prognostic scores did as well as expert cardiologists and better than most other physician groups.

Key Point: Scores do as well as expert physicians and better than other physicians in predicting CAD, its severity, and prognosis.

ACC/AHA Guidelines for the Prognostic Use of the Standard Exercise Test

The task force to establish guidelines for the use of exercise testing has met and produced guidelines in 1986, 1997, and 2002. The following is a synopsis of these evidence-based guidelines regarding use of the exercise test for prognosis.

Indications for exercise testing to assess risk and prognosis in patients with symptoms or a prior history of CAD:

Class I (definitely appropriate)—Conditions for which there is evidence or general agreement that the standard exercise test is useful and helpful to assess risk and prognosis in patients with symptoms or a prior history of CAD

- Patients undergoing initial evaluation with suspected or known CAD (specific exceptions are noted in Class IIb)
- Patients with suspected or known CAD previously evaluated with significant change in clinical status

Class IIb (may be appropriate)—Conditions for which there is conflicting evidence or a divergence of opinion that the standard exercise test is useful and helpful to assess risk and prognosis in patients with symptoms or a prior history of CAD but the usefulness/efficacy is less well established

- Patients who demonstrate the following ECG abnormalities:
  - Preexcitation (Wolff-Parkinson-White) syndrome
  - Electronically paced ventricular rhythm

- More than 1 mm of resting ST depression
- Complete left bundle branch block
- Patients with a stable clinical course who undergo periodic monitoring to guide management

Class III (not appropriate)—Conditions for which there is evidence or general agreement that the standard exercise test is not useful and helpful to assess risk and prognosis in patients with symptoms or a prior history of CAD and in some cases may be harmful

- Patients with a severe comorbidity likely to limit life expectancy or candidacy for revascularization

Summary

The two principal reasons for estimating prognosis are to provide accurate answers to patients' questions regarding the probable outcome of their illness and to identify those patients in whom interventions might improve outcome. There is a lack of consistency in the available studies because patients die along a pathophysiologic spectrum ranging from those who die from HF with little myocardium remaining to those who die from an ischemic-related event with ample myocardium remaining. Clinical and exercise test variables most likely associated with HF deaths (HF markers) include a history or symptoms of HF, prior MI, Q waves, and other indicators of left ventricular dysfunction. Variables most likely associated with ischemic deaths (ischemic markers) are angina, and rest and exercise ST depression. Some variables can be associated with either type of CV death; these include exercise capacity, maximal heart rate, and maximal SBP. The latter variables may explain why they are reported most consistently in the available studies. A problem exists that ischemic deaths occur later in follow-up and are more likely to occur in those lost to follow-up, whereas HF deaths are more likely to occur early (within 2 years) and are more likely to be classified. Workup bias probably explains why exercise-induced ST depression fails to be a predictor in most of the angiographic studies. Ischemic markers are associated with a later and lesser risk, whereas HF or left ventricular dysfunction markers are associated with a sooner and greater risk of death.

Recent studies of prognosis have actually not been superior to the earlier studies that considered CV endpoints and removed patients from observation who had interventions. This is because death data are now relatively easy to obtain whereas previously investigators had to follow the patients and contact them or review their records. CV mortality can be determined by death certificates. Although death certificates have their limitations, in general they classify those with accidental, gastrointestinal, pulmonary, and cancer deaths so that those remaining are most likely to have died of CV causes. This endpoint is more appropriate when studying a test for CV disease. Whereas all-cause mortality is a more important endpoint for intervention studies, CV mortality is more appropriate for evaluating a CV test (i.e., the exercise test). Identifying those at risk of death of any cause does not make it possible to identify those who might benefit from CV interventions, one of the two goals of prognostication.

Rather than the differences perhaps it is better to stress the consistencies. Considering simple clinical variables can assess risk. A good exercise capacity, no evidence or history of HF or ventricular damage (Q waves, history of HF), and no ST depression, or only one of these clinical findings, are associated with a very low risk. These patients are low risk in exercise programs and need not be considered for interventions to prolong their life. High-risk patients can be identified by groupings of the clinical markers (i.e., two or more). Exertional hypotension is particularly ominous. Identification of high risk implies that such patients in exercise training programs should have lower goals and should be monitored. Such patients should also be considered for coronary interventions to improve their longevity. Furthermore, with each decrease in the MET value achieved there is a 10% to 20% increase in mortality rate, so simply considering exercise capacity has consistent importance in all patient groups.

The mathematical models for determining prognosis are usually more complex than those used for identifying severe angiographic disease. Diagnostic testing can use multivariate discriminant function analysis to determine the probability of severe angiographic disease being present or not. Prognostic testing must use survival analysis, which includes censoring for patients with uneven follow-up due to "lost to follow-up" or other cardiac events (i.e., CABS, PCI) and must account for time-person units of exposure. Survival curves must be developed, and the Cox proportional hazards model is often preferred. We have proposed the rules in Table 6-9 to assess prognostic studies. The newest important marker of risk, heart rate recovery, has yet to be adequately validated with the more appropriate endpoint of CV mortality.

From this perspective, it is obvious that there is much information supporting the use of exercise testing as the first noninvasive step after the history, physical examination, and resting ECG in the prognostic evaluation of CAD patients. It accomplishes both purposes of prognostic testing: to provide information regarding the patient's status and to help make recommendations for optimal management. The exercise test results help one to make reasonable decisions for selection of patients who should undergo coronary angiography. Because the exercise test can be performed in the doctor's office and provides valuable information for clinical management in regard to activity levels, response to therapy, and disability, the exercise test is the reasonable first choice for prognostic assessment. This assessment should always include calculation of the estimated annual mortality risk using the Duke Treadmill Score, though its ischemic elements have less power in the elderly.

TABLE 6-9 Proposed Criteria for Studies Assessing Prognostic Value of Clinical and Exercise Test Variables

1. *Study population:* Inclusion criteria such as catheterization should be specified. Prevalences of congestive heart failure, congestive heart failure-associated conditions (prior myocardial infarction, Q waves on resting ECG), and angina should be stated.
2. *Avoidance of workup bias:* Limited study populations such as patients referred for catheterization should be avoided, or validation studies in different populations or bootstrapping techniques should be used.
3. *Exercise testing procedures:* Protocols used and criteria for abnormal values should be well described.
4. *Clinical and exercise test variables:* Variables must be clearly defined and entered into the statistical analysis separately.
5. *Study endpoints:* Cardiovascular death and nonfatal myocardial infarction should be used.
6. *Avoidance of "overfitting the data":* The ratio of events to the number of variables studied should be at least 10 to ensure enough "hard" outcomes per given variable studied.
7. *Follow-up:* Length and completeness should be documented.
8. *Treatment of interventions:* Coronary artery bypass surgery and percutaneous transluminal coronary angioplasty should not be used as endpoints.
9. *Censoring:* Patients should be censored on interventions (coronary artery bypass surgery or percutaneous transluminal coronary angioplasty) and on "lost to follow-up."
10. *Relationship between censored events and studied variables:* It should be determined whether censoring is random or correlated with specific clinical and exercise test markers.
11. *Multivariate survival analysis techniques:* Cox proportional hazard model or discriminate analysis should be used.
12. *Concordance with the hierarchic nature of clinical data acquisition:* Variables should be entered into multivariate analysis in an order similar to clinical practice (i.e., clinical parameters followed by exercise test variables and then invasive test variables).
13. *Interactions between variables:* Associations between variables (e.g., digoxin use and congestive heart failure or ST elevation over Q waves) should be noted and treated appropriately.
14. *Avoidance of test-review bias:* Investigators should be blinded to patient characteristics and results of other diagnostic and prognostic tests.

References

1. Yusuf S et al: Effect of coronary artery bypass graft surgery on survival: overview of 10-year results from randomised trials by the Coronary Artery Bypass Graft Surgery Trialists Collaboration, *Lancet* 344(8922):563-570, 1994.
2. Marcus ML, Wilson FR, White CW: Methods of measurement of myocardial blood flow in patients: a critical review, *Circulation* 76:245-251, 1987.
3. Shaw LJ et al: Use of a prognostic treadmill score in identifying diagnostic coronary disease subgroups, *Circulation* 98(16):1622-1630, 1998.
4. Lauer MS, Blackstone E, Young J, Topol E: Cause of death in clinical research: time for a reassessment? *J Am Coll Cardiol* 34(3):618-620, 1999.
5. Mark DB et al: Prognostic value of a treadmill exercise score in outpatients with suspected coronary artery disease, *N Engl J Med* 325(12):849-853, 1991.
6. Froelicher VF et al: Prediction of artherosclerotic cardiovascular death in men using a prognostic score, *Am J Cardiol* 73(2):133-138, 1994.
7. Oberman A et al: Natural history of coronary artery disease, *Bull N Y Acad Med* 48:1109-1125, 1972.
8. Reeves TJ, Oberman A, Jones WB, Sheffield LT: Natural history of angina pectoris, *Am J Cardiol* 33:423-430, 1974.

9. Hammermeister KE, DeRouen TA, Dodge HT: Variables predictive of survival in patients with coronary disease. Selection by univariate and multivariate analyses from the clinical, electrocardiographic, exercise, arteriographic, and quantitative angiographic evaluation, *Circulation* 59:421-430, 1979.

10. Gohlke H, Samek L, Betz P, Roskamm H: Exercise testing provides additional prognostic information in angiographically defined subgroups of patients with coronary artery disease, *Circulation* 68:979-985, 1983.

11. Brunelli C, Cristofani R, L'Abbate A, for the ODI Study Group: Long-term survival in medically treated patients with ischemic heart disease and prognostic importance of clinical and electrocardiographic data (the Italian CNR Multicenter Prospective Study ODI), *Eur Heart J* 10:292-303, 1989.

12. Weiner DA et al: Prognostic importance of a clinical profile and exercise test in medically treated patients with coronary artery disease, *J Am Coll Cardiol* 3:772-779, 1984.

13. Mark DB et al: Exercise treadmill score for predicting prognosis in coronary artery disease, *Ann Intern Med* 106:793-800, 1987.

14. Peduzzi P, Hultgren H, Thomsen J, Angell W: Prognostic value of baseline exercise tests, *Prog Cardiovasc Dis* 28:285-292, 1986.

15. Lerman J, Svetlize H, Capris T, Perosio A: Follow-up of patients after exercise test and catheterization, *Medicina* (Buenos Aires) 46:201-211, 1986.

16. Wyns W et al: Progostic value of symptom limited exercise testing in men with a high prevalence of coronary artery disease, *Eur Heart J* 6:939-945, 1985.

17. Detry JM et al: Non-invasive data provide independent prognostic information in patients with chest pain without previous myocardial infarction: findings in male patients who have had cardiac catheterization, *Eur Heart J* 9:418-426, 1988.

18. Morris CK et al: Prediction of cardiovascular death by means of clinical and exercise test variables in patients selected for cardiac catheterization, *Am Heart J* 125(6):1717-1726, 1993.

19. Marks D et al: Prognostic value of a treadmill exercise score in outpatients with suspected coronary artery disease, *N Engl J Med* 325:849-853, 1991.

20. Morrow K, Morris CK, Froelicher VF, Hideg A: Prediction of cardiovascular death in men undergoing noninvasive evaluation for CAD, *Ann Intern Med* 118(9):689-695, 1993.

21. Villella M et al: Ergometric score systems after myocardial infarction: prognostic performance of the Duke Treadmill Score, Veterans Administration Medical Center Score, and of a novel score system, GISSI-2 Index, in a cohort of survivors of acute myocardial infarction, *Am Heart J* 145(3):475-483, 2003.

22. Morise AP, Jalisi F: Evaluation of pretest and exercise test scores to assess all-cause mortality in unselected patients presenting for exercise testing with symptoms of suspected coronary artery disease, *J Am Coll Cardiol* 42(5):842-850, 2003.

23. Prakash M et al: Clinical and exercise test predictors of all-cause mortality: results from >6,000 consecutive referred male patients, *Chest* 120(3):1003-1013, 2001.
24. Alexander K et al: Value of exercise treadmill testing in women, *J Am Coll Cardiol* 32(6):1657-1664, 1998.
25. Morise AP et al: Validation of the accuracy of pretest and exercise test scores in women with a low prevalence of coronary disease: the NHLBI-sponsored Women's Ischemia Syndrome Evaluation (WISE) study, *Am Heart J* 147(6):1085-1092, 2004.
26. Kwok JM et al: Prognostic value of a treadmill exercise score in symptomatic patients with nonspecific ST-T abnormalities on resting ECG, *JAMA* 282(11):1047-1053, 1999.
27. Brechue W, Pollock M: Exercise training for coronary artery disease in the elderly, *Clin Geriatr Med* 12(1):207-229, 1996.
28. Goraya T et al: Prognostic value of treadmill exercise testing in elderly persons, *Ann Intern Med* 132:862-870, 2000.
29. Spin JM et al: The prognostic value of exercise testing in elderly men, *Am J Med* 112(6):453-459, 2002.
30. Kwok JM et al: Prognostic value of the Duke Treadmill Score in the elderly, *J Am Coll Cardiol* 39:1475-1481, 2002.
31. Lai S et al: Treadmill scores in elderly men, *J Am Coll Cardiol* 43(4):606-615, 2004.
32. Raxwal V et al: Simple treadmill score to diagnose coronary disease, *Chest* 119(6):1933-1940, 2001.
33. Weiner DA et al: Significance of silent myocardial ischemia during exercise testing in patients with coronary artery disease, *Am J Cardiol* 59:725-729, 1987.
34. Mark DB et al: Painless exercise ST deviation on the treadmill: long-term prognosis, *J Am Coll Cardiol* 14:885-892, 1989.
35. Falcone C et al: Clinical significance of exercise-induced silent myocardial ischemia in patients with coronary artery disease, *J Am Coll Cardiol* 9(2):295-299, 1987.
36. Visser FC et al: Silent versus symptomatic myocardial ischemia during exercise testing: a comparison with coronary angiographic findings, *Int J Cardiol* 27(1):71-78, 1990.
37. Weiner DA et al: Risk of developing an acute myocardial infarction or sudden coronary death in patients with exercise-induced silent myocardial ischemia. A report from the Coronary Artery Surgery Study (CASS) registry, *Am J Cardiol* 62:1155-1158, 1988.
38. Callaham P et al: Exercise-induced silent ischemia, *J Am Coll Cardiol* 14:1175-1180, 1989.
39. Visser FC et al: Silent versus symptomatic myocardial ischemia during exercise testing: a comparison with coronary angiographic findings, *Int J Cardiol* 27:71-78, 1990.
40. Miranda C et al: Comparison of silent and symptomatic ischemia during exercise testing in men, *Ann Intern Med* 114:649-656, 1991.
41. Karnegis JN et al: Positive and negative exercise test results with and without exercise-induced angina in patients with one healed myocardial

infarction: analysis of baseline variables and long-term prognosis, *Am Heart J* 122:701-708, 1991.

42. May O, Arildsen H, Damsgaard EM, Mickley H: Prevalence and prediction of silent ischaemia in diabetes mellitus: a population-based study, *Cardiovasc Res* 34(1):241-247, 1997.

43. Keys A: Coronary heart disease in seven countries, *Circulation* 41-42: I1-I211, 1970.

44. Caracciolo EA et al: Diabetics with coronary disease have a prevalence of asymptomatic ischemia during exercise treadmill testing and ambulatory ischemia monitoring similar to that of nondiabetic patients. An ACIP database study, *Circulation* 93(12):2097-2105, 1996.

45. Cole CR et al: Heart-rate recovery immediately after exercise as a predictor of mortality, *N Engl J Med* 341(18):1351-1357, 1999.

46. Cole CR, Foody JM, Blackstone EH, Lauer MS: Heart rate recovery after submaximal exercise testing as a predictor of mortality in a cardiovascularly healthy cohort, *Ann Intern Med* 132(7):552-555, 2000.

47. Nishime EO et al: Heart rate recovery and treadmill exercise score as predictors of mortality in patients referred for exercise ECG, *JAMA* 284(11):1392-1398, 2000.

48. Watanabe J et al: Heart rate recovery immediately after treadmill exercise and left ventricular systolic dysfunction as predictors of mortality: the case of stress echocardiography, *Circulation* 104(16):1911-1916, 2001.

49. Shetler K et al: Heart rate recovery: validation and methodologic issues, *J Am Coll Cardiol* 38(7):1980-1987, 2001.

50. Morshedi-Meibodi A et al: Heart rate recovery after treadmill exercise testing and risk of cardiovascular disease events (the Framingham Heart Study), *Am J Cardiol* 90(8):848-852, 2002.

51. Mora S et al: Ability of exercise testing to predict cardiovascular and all-cause death in asymptomatic women: a 20-year follow-up of the lipid research clinics prevalence study, *JAMA* 290(12):1600-1607, 2003.

52. Cheng YJ et al: Heart rate recovery following maximal exercise testing as a predictor of cardiovascular disease and all-cause mortality in men with diabetes, *Diabetes Care* 26(7):2052-2057, 2003.

53. Cheitlin MD et al: Correlation of "critical" left coronary artery lesions with positive submaximal exercise tests in patients with chest pain, *Am Heart J* 89(3):305-310, 1975.

54. Goldschlager N, Selzer A, Cohn K: Treadmill stress tests as indicators of presence and severity of coronary artery disease, *Ann Intern Med* 85:277-286, 1976.

55. NcNeer JF et al: The role of the exercise test in the evaluation of patients for ischemic heart disease, *Circulation* 57:64-70, 1978.

56. Weiner DA, McCabe CH, Ryan TJ: Identification of patients with left main and three vessel coronary disease with clinical and exercise test variables, *Am J Cardiol* 46:21-27, 1980.

57. Blumenthal DS, Weiss JL, Mellits ED, Gerstenblith G: The predictive value of a strongly positive stress test in patients with minimal symptoms, *Am J Med* 70:1005-1010, 1981.
58. Lee TH, EF Cook, Goldman L: Prospective evaluation of a clinical and exercise-test model for the prediction of left main coronary artery disease, *Med Decis Making* 6:136-144, 1986.
59. Detrano R et al: Exercise-induced ST-segment depression in the diagnosis of multivessel coronary disease: a meta analysis, *J Am Coll Cardiol* 14:1501-1508, 1989.
60. Hartz A, Gammaitoni C, Young M: Quantitative analysis of the exercise tolerance test for determining the severity of coronary artery disease, *Int J Cardiol* 24:63-71, 1989.
61. Concato J, Feinstein AR, Holford TR: The risk of determining risk with multivariate models, *Ann Intern Med* 118:201-210, 1993.
62. Cohn K et al: Use of treadmill score to quantify ischemic response and predict extent of coronary disease, *Circulation* 59:286-296, 1979.
63. Fisher L et al: Diagnostic quantification of CASS (Coronary Artery Surgery Study) clinical and exercise test results in determining presence and extent of coronary artery disease, *Circulation* 63:987-1000, 1981.
64. McCarthy D, Sciacca R, Blood D, Cannon P: Discriminant function analysis using thallium 201 scintiscans and exercise stress test variables to predict the presence and extent of coronary artery disease, *Am J Cardiol* 49:1917-1926, 1982.
65. Lee T, Cook E, Goldman L: Prospective evaluation of a clinical and exercise test model for the prediction of left main coronary artery disease, *Med Decis Making* 6:136-144, 1986.
66. Hung J et al: A logistic regression analysis of multiple noninvasive tests for the prediction of the presence and extent of coronary artery disease in men, *Am Heart J* 110:460-469, 1985.
67. Christian T, Miller T, Bailey K, Gibbons R: Exercise tomographic thallium-201 imaging in patients with severe coronary artery disease and normal electrocardiograms, *Ann Intern Med* 121:825-832, 1994.
68. Morise A, Bobbio M, Detrano R, Duval R: Incremental evaluation of exercise capacity as an independent predictor of coronary artery disease presence and extent, *Am Heart J* 127:32-38, 1994.
69. Morise A, Diamond G, Detrano R, Bobbio M: Incremental value of exercise electrocardiography and thallium-201 testing in men and women for the presence and extent of coronary artery disease, *Am Heart J* 130:267-276, 1995.
70. Moussa I, Rodriguez M, Froning J, Froelicher VF: Prediction of severe coronary artery disease using computerized ECG measurements and discriminant function analysis, *J Electrocardiol* 25:49-58, 1992.
71. Detrano R et al: Algorithm to predict triple-vessel/left main coronary artery disease in patients without myocardial infarction, *Circulation* 83(3):89-96, 1991.
72. Christian TF, Miller TD, Bailley KR, Gibbons RJ: Noninvasive identification of severe coronary artery disease using exercise tomographic thallium-201 imaging, *Am J Cardiol* 70:14-20, 1992.

73. Hung J et al: Noninvasive diagnostic test choices for the evaluation of coronary artery disease in women: a multivariate comparison of cardiac fluoroscopy, exercise electrocardiography and exercise thallium myocardial perfusion scintigraphy, *J Am Coll Cardiol* 4:8-16, 1984.

74. Bruce RA, Hossack KF, DeRouen TA, Hofer V: Enhanced risk assessment for primary coronary heart disease events by maximal exercise testing: 10 years' experience of Seattle Heart Watch, *J Am Coll Cardiol* 2:565-573, 1983.

75. European Cooperative Group: Long-term results of prospective randomized study of coronary artery bypass surgery in stable angina pectoris, *Lancet* 2:1173-1180, 1982.

76. Weiner DA et al: The role of exercise testing in identifying patients with improved survival after coronary artery bypass surgery, *J Am Coll Cardiol* 8(4):741-748, 1986.

77. Hultgren HN, Peduzzi P, Detre K, Takaro T: The 5 year effect of bypass surgery on relief of angina and exercise performance, *Circulation* 72:V79-V83, 1985.

78. Lee KL et al: Predicting outcome in coronary disease. Statistical models versus expert clinicians, *Am J Med* 80(4):553-560, 1986.

79. Detrano R et al: Computer probability estimates of angiographic coronary artery disease: transportability and comparison with cardiologists' estimates, *Comput Biomed Res* 25(5):468-485, 1992.

80. Lipinski M et al: Comparison of exercise test scores and physician estimation in determining disease probability, *Arch Intern Med* 161(18):2239-2244, 2001.

81. Lipinski M et al: Comparison of treadmill scores with physician estimates of diagnosis and prognosis in patients with coronary artery disease, *Am Heart J* 143(4):650-658, 2002.

7   Exercise Testing of Patients with Left Ventricular Dysfunction

Pathophysiology

Myocardial damage or dysfunction is the pathophysiologic basis of heart muscle disease. Myocardial damage or dysfunction can be divided into systolic and diastolic dysfunction. Systolic function relates to the emptying characteristics of the left ventricle, and diastolic function relates to its filling properties. Systolic dysfunction caused by myocardial damage is most common in clinical practice and usually leads to left ventricular dilation. The ventricle dilates as a compensatory mechanism to take advantage of the Frank-Starling relationship (i.e., increased contractility with stretching of the sarcomeres), which can eventually worsen ventricular performance over time. Anything that causes ventricular damage or scarring (e.g., muscle loss) usually leads to systolic dysfunction.

Approximately 70% of patients with the syndrome of chronic heart failure (HF) have systolic dysfunction, and the rest have diastolic dysfunction. In patients with the latter, systolic function and ejection fraction (EF) can be normal but filling pressure is usually elevated because of a stiff, noncompliant ventricle.[1] Usually, diastolic dysfunction is secondary to hypertension, pathologic hypertrophy, infiltrative diseases of the myocardium, and, at times, ischemia. All patients with systolic dysfunction have some degree of diastolic dysfunction, and when systolic dysfunction is compensated, diastolic dysfunction often remains. Currently, the treatment for acute congestive heart failure (CHF) in both conditions is the same. This is fortunate because they can be difficult to distinguish clinically without echocardiography. However, it appears that treatment and prognosis with diastolic dysfunction are more related to the conditions underlying it and the treatment of these conditions,[2] whereas the treatment of systolic dysfunction has been clarified by numerous randomized trials. An issue requiring further clarification is whether ischemic systolic dysfunction can be improved by revascularization.

Several randomized trials are in progress comparing percutaneous coronary intervention and coronary artery bypass graft versus medical management in such patients.

> **Key Points:** Echocardiography is needed to distinguish the two types of HF. Nearly all of the new therapies for the syndrome of HF have been targeted for systolic dysfunction.

Definition of Heart Failure

Congestive heart failure can be defined as a syndrome consisting of signs and symptoms of intravascular and interstitial volume overload (hypervolemia), including shortness of breath, rales, hepatomegaly, and edema; and manifestations of inadequate tissue perfusion, such as fatigue and poor exercise tolerance.

Chronic heart failure can be defined as the same syndrome that is either well compensated or appropriately treated so that the manifestations of acute hypervolemia are minimized.

> **Key Points:** HF is the major manifestation of left ventricular damage caused by systolic dysfunction and a dilated cardiomyopathy. Patients with systolic dysfunction usually have diastolic dysfunction, and the latter often remains after the systolic component is compensated. Left-sided failure can lead to right-sided failure.
>
> Diastolic dysfunction can exist independently and is frequently associated with a stiff, hypertrophied (but normal-sized) ventricle caused by chronic high blood pressure, congenital abnormalities, or both.
>
> Abnormalities in the periphery (anemia, beriberi heart disease, arteriovenous fistulas, and thyrotoxicosis) can cause high-output HF.

Prevalence and Prognosis in Heart Failure

HF, when caused by dilated cardiomyopathy, has a 15% to 25% annual cardiac mortality rate. Analysis of more than 30 years of follow-up from the Framingham Study data provides clinically relevant insights into the prevalence, incidence, secular trends, prognosis, and modifiable risk factors for the occurrence of HF in a general population sample.[3-5] HF occurs in about 2% of persons in their fifties and 10% of persons in their seventies, with the incidence approximately doubling with each decade of age. Women have a lower incidence at all ages. Male predominance is due to coronary heart disease, which confers a fourfold increased risk of HF. In the Framingham Study, once HF was present, one third of men and women died within 2 years of diagnosis. The 6-year mortality rate was 82% for men and 67% for women, which corresponded to a death rate fourfold to eightfold greater than that of the general population of the same age. Sudden death was common, accounting for 28% of the cardiovascular deaths in men with HF and 14% of the cardiovascular deaths in women with HF. Since the 1950s, survival after the onset of HF has improved about 12% per decade.[5] Hypertension and coronary disease were the predominant causes of HF and accounted for more than 80% of all clinical events. Factors reflecting deteriorating cardiac function were associated with a substantial increase in risk of overt HF. These include low vital capacity, sinus tachycardia, and left ventricular hypertrophy by electrocardiogram.

In 2004, more than 550,000 cases of HF were diagnosed in the United States,[6] and the prevalence of this condition is expected to double by 2037. Despite the high prevalence of HF, only about 2000 heart transplants are performed yearly. For the remainder, quality of life decreases, and less than 40% survive 4 years after diagnosis. In the following, we address the issue of whether exercise testing can improve risk stratification beyond clinical variables.[7-9]

> **Key Point:** Unlike other cardiovascular diseases, the incidence of HF is increasing. Although the mortality rate has improved with new treatments, it still remains high.

Clinical Risk Markers

Despite important advances in therapy for patients with chronic HF, the mortality rate for this condition remains high and continues to be one of the important challenges facing the clinician who manages these patients.[10] Cardiac transplantation has evolved into an important treatment option for patients with severe HF, but this option remains limited to a relatively small number of patients with end-stage disease because there continues to be a severe shortage of donor hearts. The high mortality rate and the widening gap between patients listed for transplantation and available donor hearts have magnified the need for reliable prognostic markers in HF. In addition, revascularization techniques for ischemic cardiomyopathies carry a risk that must be balanced against the benefits. The major risk markers for HF are listed in Table 7-1.

Consensus statements from the American Heart Association (AHA) and American College of Cardiology (ACC)[11] and a Bethesda Conference position statement[12] have helped establish guidelines for selection criteria among patients considered for transplantation. The major risk markers in HF include New York Heart Association (NYHA) functional class, reduced EF, reduced cardiac index, renal insufficiency (creatinine clearance <60 ml/min), persistent signs of congestion (orthopnea, jugular venous distention, edema, weight gain, or increased need for diuretics), persistent elevated filling pressure, and reduced exercise capacity. Since the early 1990s, more than 100 studies have demonstrated that peak VO_2 is a significant univariate or multivariate predictor of outcomes in patients with HF.

Increased reliance on the role of exercise testing for decision making in HF has occurred for several reasons. Since the early 1970s, workload achieved (i.e., METs), or exercise time, has been recognized as a significant prognostic marker. Expired gas analysis techniques are now much more widespread, in part because of computerization and increased automation,

TABLE 7-1   Variables Associated with Increased Risk in Chronic Heart Failure

Reduced ejection fraction (<25%)
Poor exercise capacity:
    NYHA functional class III or IV for 3 months
    Dyspnea on exertion
    Peak VO$_2$ <14 ml/kg/min
    Six-minute walk distance <300 m
    Dependency with activities of daily living
Heightened neurohormonal markers (BNP, ANP, endothelins, norepinephrine)
Complex ventricular ectopy
Reduced cardiac index (<2.0 L/min/m2)
Renal insufficiency (creatinine clearance <60 ml/min)
Persistent signs of hypervolemia (orthopnea, jugular venous distention, edema, weight
    gain, increased need for diuretics)
Left ventricular end-diastolic dimension >80 mm
Duration of heart failure
Hyponatremia (serum sodium <134 mEq/L)
High pulmonary capillary wedge pressure
Medical history: comorbid illness including anemia, chronic obstructive pulmonary
    disease, dementia, hepatic cirrhosis, cancer, cerebrovascular disease
Demographics: age >70 years
Vital signs: tachycardia, increased respiratory rate, hypotension

ANP, atrial natriuretic peptide ; *BNP,* brain natriuretic peptide; *NYHA,* New York Heart Association.

but also because of an appreciation for their applications to various cardiovascular and pulmonary disorders. Justification for their use in patients with HF has been strengthened by studies describing clinical applications of ventilatory and gas exchange abnormalities in HF.[8,13] Cardiopulmonary exercise testing is now part of the standard workup of the patient with HF, and the guidelines on transplantation consider this procedure an integral component of the decision-making process regarding transplantation.

Directly measured peak VO$_2$ has been shown to outperform clinical, hemodynamic, and other exercise test data in predicting 1- to 2-year mortality rates. Several investigators have reported that patients who achieve a peak VO$_2$ >14 ml/kg/min appear to have a prognosis similar to that among patients who receive transplantation (approximately 90% survival at 1 year). This cutpoint has emerged as a clinically practical prognostic marker in HF; a value ≤14 ml/kg/min or less is a relative indication for transplantation in the guidelines. It should be noted however, that many cutpoints for peak VO$_2$ in the clinically relevant range (10 to 17 ml/kg/min) have been used in studies to stratify risk in HF. This issue is addressed in more detail later. Despite the multitude of studies performed over the last 15 years, a number of issues related to the use of cardiopulmonary exercise testing and stratifying risk in HF require further clarification. These include the following:

- What is the place of cardiopulmonary exercise testing relative to clinical, hemodynamic, and other data in the risk paradigm in patients with HF?
- What is the optimal cutpoint for peak VO$_2$ when selecting patients for transplantation listing?

- Should peak VO_2 be expressed as an absolute value or corrected for age or body weight?
- How well do ventilatory gas exchange responses other than peak VO_2 (e.g., the ventilation [VE] versus VCO_2 slope, ventilatory threshold, rate of recovery of VO_2) predict risk?

Exercise Testing and Selection of Transplant Recipients

Because there are less than 2000 viable donor hearts available each year in the United States,[14] recipients must be carefully selected. In this regard, factors associated with 1- to 2-year survival rates among potential candidates are critical. These have included an EF less than 15%, complex ventricular ectopy, sympathetic nervous system activation, and impaired exercise capacity, although many other clinical markers have been associated with risk in HF (see Table 7-1). With advances in the treatment for HF, many patients once thought to have end-stage HF can be stabilized by aggressive medical therapy. Multidisciplinary HF management programs have been set up to manage and monitor patients, and these programs appear to improve survival.[15]

Increasing numbers of patients have undergone cardiac transplantation for end-stage HF, and approximately three quarters of these patients remain alive after 5 years. Because the transplant patient's heart is denervated, some intriguing hemodynamic responses to exercise are observed. The heart is not responsive to the normal parasympathetic and sympathetic control. The absence of vagal tone explains the high resting heart rates in these patients (100 to 110 beats per minute) and the relatively slow adaptation of the heart to a given amount of submaximal work. As a result, the delivery of oxygen to the working tissue is slower, contributing to earlier than normal metabolic acidosis and hyperventilation during exercise. Maximal heart rate is lower in transplant patients than in normal subjects, which contributes to a reduction in cardiac output and exercise capacity. Transplantation has been shown to partially, but not completely, normalize peak VO_2 and the ventilatory disturbances commonly seen in patients with severe HF.

> **Key Point:** The exercise test plays an important role in the selection of patients who are appropriate for transplantation. However, criteria for cardiac transplantation selection should be based on estimates from a number of clinical and exercise test variables rather than relying only on a threshold for peak VO_2. Transplantation partially restores exercise tolerance.

Cardiopulmonary Exercise Testing and Prognosis in Heart Failure

In a landmark study that provided an impetus for many others, Mancini and colleagues[16] followed three groups of patients referred for transplantation over 2 years. One group comprised patients accepted for transplantation on the basis of achieving a peak VO_2 <14 ml/kg/min; a second group comprised patients considered too well for transplantation (peak VO_2 < 14 ml/kg/min); and a third group comprised patients with a peak VO_2 <14 ml/kg/min but rejected from transplantation for noncardiac reasons. Patients with preserved exercise capacity (>14 ml/kg/min) had 1- and 2-year survival rates of 94% and 84%, respectively, roughly equivalent to those observed after transplantation. This was contrasted by patients with poor exercise capacity (peak VO_2 <14 ml/kg/min) who were rejected for transplantation, among whom 1- and 2-year survival rates were only 47% and 32%, respectively. It was suggested from these results that transplantation can be safely deferred for patients who achieve a peak VO_2 >14 ml/kg/min, and scarce donor hearts should be reserved for those patients unable to achieve this value. In addition, by both univariate and multivariate analysis, peak VO_2 was the best predictor of survival. This study fostered the concept that a single cutpoint, 14 ml/kg/min, provides a clinically applicable cutpoint between patients who require transplantation for survival benefit and those who do not.

Over the 15 years following the study of Mancini and colleagues,[16] more than 200 studies were published assessing the value of cardiopulmonary exercise variables to predict prognosis in HF. Some of the major studies are presented in Table 7-2. In virtually every one of these studies, peak VO_2 has been demonstrated to be a significant univariate or multivariate predictor of mortality (or other outcomes) in patients with HF. More recently, cardiopulmonary variables other than peak VO_2 have also been shown to be powerful risk markers in HF, in many cases outperforming peak VO_2 in predicting risk. The latter responses are generally expressions of the ventilatory inefficiency that are commonly observed in HF; these are discussed later. Although these studies varied widely in terms of severity of HF, endpoints used (e.g., change in listing status, hospitalization, and other outcomes have been used in addition to mortality), they provide the clear impression that measuring the cardiopulmonary response to exercise directly has a powerful impact on predicting risk in these patients. Currently, this procedure is an integral part of the workup for stratifying risk in patients with HF and is included in the various HF guidelines.

Until the mid-1990s, most studies in this area were not large enough to assess cardiopulmonary exercise variables multivariately with other established risk markers in HF. In the last few years, investigators have explored this issue using more robust data sets with longer follow-up periods that have permitted subgroup evaluations in addition to multivariate analyses including invasive hemodynamic data. In one such study, a detailed evaluation of clinical, hemodynamic, and exercise variables was performed during a 10-year period among patients referred for evaluation of HF at Stanford.[17] The longer follow-up period (mean, 4 years), the large number of deaths (187), and the inclusion of both measured and predicted VO_2 made it unique among the multivariate studies, and one of the more robust data sets to evaluate prognosis. Univariately, the most powerful predictors of death were from the exercise test; peak VO_2, VO_2 at the ventilatory threshold, VO_2 expressed as a percentage of the predicted value, peak systolic blood pressure lower than 130 mm Hg, and watts achieved were significant predictors of death.

TABLE 7-2   Sampling of Some of the Larger Studies Using Ventilatory Gas Exchange to Predict Outcomes in Chronic Heart Failure

Investigator	Year	No. of Subjects	Mean Age (Years)	Mean Follow-up (Months)	Annual Mortality Rate (%)*	Findings
Likoff[52]	1987	201	62 ± 10	28	23	Peak $VO_2 > 13$ ml/kg/min was independent predictor of increased mortality rate.
Stevenson[53]	1990	107	53 ± 11	6 ± 5	3	Ability to increase peak VO_2 by ≥ 2 ml/kg/min to a level ≥ 12 ml/kg/min) was an indication to defer transplantation in favor of more compromised candidates.
Mancini[16]	1991	122	50 ± 11	11 ± 9	—	Peak $VO_2 > 14$ ml/min/kg had 6% first-year mortality rate vs. 53% in patients with peak $VO_2 \leq 14$ ml/min/kg.
Saxon[54]	1993	528	50 ± 12	12 ± 14	24	By both univariate and multivariate analysis, peak $VO_2 < 11$ ml/kg/min was independent predictor of heart failure death but not of sudden death.
Cohn[55]	1993	V-HEFT I = 642, V-HEFT II = 804	59.5 ± 8	60	8	Peak VO_2 was highly significant univariate and multivariate predictor of survival.
Stevenson[56]	1995	265	52 ± 13	12	32	Peak $VO_2 \leq 10$ ml/kg/min was one of several predictors of death or urgent transplantation in patients with class IV symptoms.
Aaronson[57]	1995	272	52 ± 12	24 ± 18	33 ± 3	Peak $VO_2 \geq 14$ ml/kg/min predicted survival. Peak VO_2 was better predictor than percentage-predicted VO_2.
Chomsky[33]	1996	185	51.4 ± 10	10 ± 6	17	Peak VO_2 (dichotomized at 10 ml/kg/min) was independent predictor of survival both by univariate analysis and multivariate analysis.
Haywood[58]	1996	141	—	12	—	All deaths among patients on a transplant waiting list occurred in those with cardiac index <2 L/min/m² or peak $VO_2 < 12$ ml/kg/min.
Aaronson[59]	1997	Derivation sample = 268; validation sample = 199	51 ± 10	36	20	Noninvasive multivariate model outperformed invasive model in predicting risk.
Chua[60]	1997	102	58 ± 10	20 ± 14	12	Peak $VO_2 < 14$ ml/kg/min was one of several independent predictors of death in CHF patients.

*When not provided by investigator, number represents first-year mortality rate estimated from survival curve.

Continued

TABLE 7-2 Sampling of Some of the Larger Studies Using Ventilatory Gas Exchange to Predict Outcomes in Chronic Heart Failure—Cont'd

Investigator	Year	No. of Subjects	Mean Age (Years)	Mean Follow-up (Months)	Annual Mortality Rate (%)*	Findings
Cohen Solal[30]	1995	178	52	32	12	Both peak $VO_2 > 17$ ml/kg/min and age-predicted peak VO_2 (>63%) were predictors of survival by univariate analysis, but only age-predicted peak VO_2 was independent predictor of survival in multivariate analysis.
Myers[17]	1998	644	48 ± 11	47 ± 28	5.3	Peak VO_2 was better predictor of survival than clinical, hemodynamic, or other exercise variables.
Opasich[61]	1998	653	52 ± 9	17 ± 13	24	Peak VO_2 stratified by <10, 10 to 18, and >18 ml/kg/min identified high, medium, and low risk, respectively.
Osada[62]	1998	500	50 ± 10	25 ± 17	15	Peak $VO_2 \leq 14$ ml/kg/min was univariate and multivariate predictor of mortality. Peak exercise SBP < 120 mm Hg and percent predicted peak $VO_2 \leq 50\%$ predicted mortality in patients with peak $VO_2 \leq 14$ ml/min/kg.
Myers[32]	2000	644	48 ± 11	47 ± 28	5.3	Peak VO_2 was strongest predictor of survival among clinical and exercise test variables. Different cutoffs for peak VO_2 (between 10 and 17 ml/kg/min) all had roughly 20% differences in survival.
Cohen-Solal[63]	2002	175	53 ± 10	25 ± 10		Peak circulatory power (the product of systolic blood pressure and VO_2) was the only multivariate predictor of prognosis
Mezzani[64]	2003	570	60 ± 10	20 ± 14		Patients who achieve peak **RER** > 1.15 have markedly better survival even when peak VO_2 is ≤10 ml/kg/min.
deGroote[39]	2004	407	57 ± 11	26	≈8	B-natriuretic peptide, in combination with % age-predicted peak VO_2 achieved, was a strong predictor of survival.

CHF, congestive heart failure; *RER*, respiration exchange ratio; *SBP*, systolic blood pressure; *V-HEFT I*, vasodilator heart failure trial I; *V-HEFT II*, vasodilator heart failure trial II.

Age was the only predictor of death among clinical variables, and hemodynamic variables, including EF, pulmonary capillary wedge pressure, and left ventricular dimensions, were not important predictors of outcome. By multivariate analysis, peak VO_2 was the only significant predictor of death. This study provided the strongest evidence to date that directly measured peak VO_2 not only outperforms clinical and hemodynamic data but also is a better predictor of death than exercise duration or watts achieved.

Cardiopulmonary Markers of Risk Other than Peak VO$_2$

Although peak VO_2 defines the limits of the cardiopulmonary system, other responses also are important in defining the severity of HF and prognosis. These responses are to one extent or another related to the ventilatory response to exercise, the capacity of the cardiopulmonary system to adapt to the demands of a given work rate, or the ability of the cardiopulmonary system to recover from a bout of exercise. Responses such as the ventilatory threshold, the VE/VCO$_2$ slope, oxygen uptake kinetics, rate of recovery of VO_2, and the oxygen uptake efficiency slope (OUES) have been used with greater frequency to classify functional limitations and stratify risk in patients with heart disease. Examples of these are illustrated in Figure 7-1. Some of these responses have been demonstrated to have greater prognostic value than peak VO_2 and are summarized in Table 7-3.

Ventilatory Threshold

The ventilatory threshold, one important submaximal marker of cardiopulmonary function with a long history, has been employed in surprisingly few multivariate models to predict risk in HF. Studies that have included the ventilatory threshold have demonstrated that VO_2 at this point significantly predicts outcome. This point has the potential to be a particularly useful marker of outcome because for many patients with HF, "maximal" exercise is not achieved for various reasons or is difficult to define. In the aforementioned Stanford study, VO_2 at the ventilatory threshold was a significant univariate predictor of death in patients evaluated for HF, but in a multivariate analysis, peak VO_2 was a stronger predictor of death.[16] Gitt and colleagues[18] tested 223 consecutive patients with HF in Germany. They compared the prognostic power of peak VO_2, VO_2 at the ventilatory threshold, and the VE/VCO$_2$ slope in predicting all-cause death. Cutpoints for peak VO2 ≤14 ml/kg/min, VO_2 at the ventilatory threshold (VO$_2$AT) <11 ml/kg/min, and a VE/VCO$_2$ slope >34 were used as threshold values for high risk of death. Patients with a peak VO_2 ≤14 ml/kg/min had a greater than threefold increased risk, and a VO$_2$AT <11 ml/kg/min or a VE/VCO$_2$ slope >34 had a fivefold increased risk for early death. In patients with both VO$_2$AT <11 ml/kg/min and VE/VCO$_2$ slope >34, the risk of early death was tenfold higher. After correction for age, gender, EF, and NYHA class in a multivariate analysis, the combination of VO$_2$AT <11 ml/kg/min and VE/VCO$_2$ slope >34 was the best predictor of 6-month mortality risk (relative risk 5×).

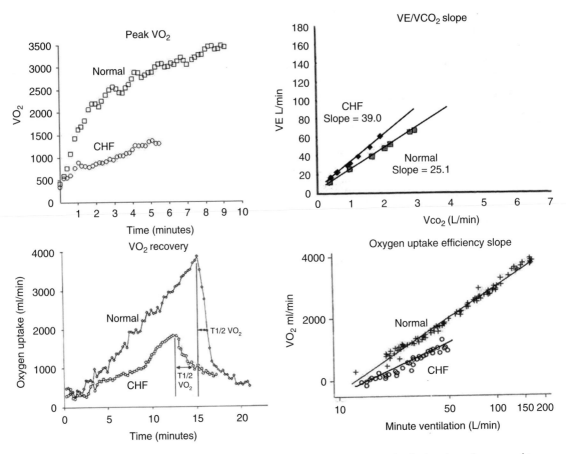

FIGURE 7-1 *Examples of four different cardiopulmonary exercise test methods that have been used to estimate prognosis in patients with cardiovascular disease. The peak VO_2 responses (upper left) are taken from a normal subject and a typical chronic heart failure (CHF) patient the same age. The VE/VCO_2 slope (upper right) is derived from the slope of the regression line between VE and VCO_2, excluding data points beyond the anaerobic threshold. VO_2 in recovery (lower left) shows a more graded recovery response in the CHF patient (i.e., longer recovery time) despite the lower exercise capacity. $T_{1/2}$ represents the time required for a 50% fall from the peak VO_2 value. The OUES (lower right) is derived by plotting VO_2 against the log of VE; a steeper slope reflects a lower VE for any given VO_2 (i.e., more efficient ventilation). (From Myers J: Applications of cardiopulmonary exercise testing in the management of cardiovascular and pulmonary disease, Int J Sports Med 26:S49-S55, 2005.)*

VE/VCO_2 Slope

Studies have shown that the VE/VCO_2 slope predicts mortality risk at least as well as, and independent from, peak VO_2. This response is usually expressed as the slope of the best-fit linear regression line relating VE and VCO_2 below the ventilatory compensation point for exercise lactic acidosis (see Figure 7-1). Whereas the slope of this relationship is normally between 20 and 30, values in the 30s are common in patients with mild to moderate HF, and values in the 40s are often observed in patients with more severe HF. An elevated VE/VCO_2 slope is a reflection of the pathophysiology of the abnormal

TABLE 7-3 Prognostic Studies on Ventilatory Gas Exchange Responses Other Than Peak VO_2

Study	Year	Subjects (n)	Mean Age (Years)	Mean Follow-up Period (Months)	Findings
VE/VCO_2 Slope					
Chua[60]	1997	CHF (173)	59 ± 12	—	VE/VCO_2 slope (>34) provided prognostic information; peak VO_2
Francis[65]	2000	CHF (303)	59 ± 11	47	Peak VO_2 and VE/VCO_2 slope similar in prognostic power
Robbins[66]	1999	CHF (470)	52 ± 11	18	VE/VCO_2 slope and low chronotropic index most powerful multivariate predictors of death
Gitt[18]	2002	CHF (223)	63 ± 11	21	VO_2 at the anaerobic threshold <11 ml/kg/min and VE/VCO_2 slope best predictors of risk
Kleber[67]	2000	CHF (142)	52 ± 10	16*	VE/VCO_2 slope outperformed peak VO_2 as predictor of death, Tx, or LVAD
Arena[20]	2003	CHF (213)	57 ± 13	32	VE/VCO_2 slope stronger predictor of cardiac mortality than peak VO_2
Corra[19]	2002	CHF (600)	57 ± 9	26	VE/VCO_2 slope was strongest predictor of death or Tx; peak VO_2 ≤10 ml/kg/min and VE/VCO_2 slope ≥35 had similar mortality rate
Bol[68]	2000	CHF (72)	63 ± 12	—	VE/VCO_2 slope was more powerful predictor of mortality than clinical variables or peak VO_2
VO_2 in Recovery					
de Groote[39]	1996	DCM (153)	50 ± 12	15*	VO_2 recovery significantly delayed in DCM vs. normals; ratio of exercise and recovery VO_2 independently predicted survival
VO_2 Kinetics					
Rickli[23]	2003	CHF (202)	52 ± 11	29	Mean response time >50 sec was strongest predictor of death or Tx, followed by predicted VO_2 <50%
Schlcher[24]	2003	CHF (146)	52 ± 10	25	Mean response time was strongest predictor of survival or freedom from Tx or hospitalization, followed by VE/VCO_2 slope
Brunner-LaRocca[25]	1999	CHF (48)	55 ± 10	22	Mean response time >60 seconds was significant predictor of mortality, and was more powerful than peak VO_2
Oxygen Uptake Efficiency Slope					
Pardaens[69]	2000	CHF (284)	52 ± 11	16*	Peak VO_2 was stronger predictor of death or cardiovascular events than OUES or VE/VCO_2 slope

*Median.
CHF, congestive heart failure; DCM, dilated cardiomyopathy; LVAD, left ventricular assist device implantation; OUES, oxygen uptake efficiency slope; Tx, transplantation.

ventilatory response to exercise in HF. Thus the VE/VCO$_2$ slope is elevated in the presence of early lactate accumulation, ventilation/perfusion mismatching in the lungs (e.g., poor cardiac output response to exercise), or the deconditioning that is commonly observed in HF.

Corra and colleagues[19] performed exercise tests on 600 patients with HF and followed them for death or urgent transplantation over a 2-year period. The VE/VCO$_2$ slope was the strongest independent predictor of a cardiac event (outperforming peak VO$_2$, EF, and other clinical and exercise test variables). The best cutpoint for predicting risk was 35 (relative risk 3×). The total mortality rate in patients with a VE/VCO$_2$ slope ≥35 was 30%, versus 10% in patients with a VE/VCO$_2$ slope <35. Patients with a VE/VCO$_2$ slope ≥35 had a similar mortality rate as those with a peak VO$_2$ ≤10 ml/kg/min.

Arena and colleagues[20] from our laboratory compared the prognostic power of peak VO$_2$ and the VE/VCO$_2$ slope in 213 patients with HF. Peak VO$_2$ and the VE/VCO$_2$ slope were demonstrated with univariate Cox regression analysis both to be significant predictors of cardiac-related mortality and hospitalization ($P < 0.01$). Multivariate analysis revealed that peak VO$_2$ added additional value to the VE/VCO$_2$ slope in predicting cardiac-related hospitalization but not cardiac mortality. Patients who exhibited a VE/VCO$_2$ slope ≥34 had a particularly high probability of hospitalization (>50% 1 year after evaluation) (Figure 7-2). The VE/VCO$_2$ slope was demonstrated with receiver operating characteristic (ROC) curve analysis to be significantly better than peak VO$_2$ in predicting cardiac-related mortality.

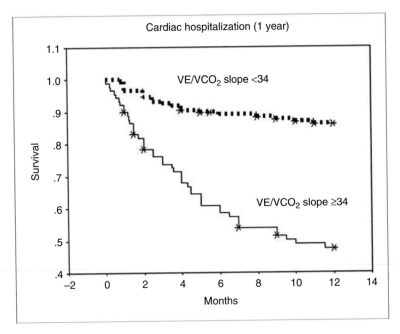

FIGURE 7-2　Kaplan-Meier survival curves for 1-year cardiac-related hospitalization using a VE/VCO$_2$ slope threshold <34 versus ≥34 (p < 0.0001).
(From Arena R et al: Peak VO$_2$ and VE/VCO$_2$ slope in patients with heart failure: a prognostic comparison, Am Heart J 147:354-360, 2004.)

Kleber and co-workers[21] evaluated the cardiopulmonary response to exercise in 142 patients with HF and followed them for a mean of 16 months. Forty-four events (37 deaths and 7 instances of heart transplantation, cardiomyoplasty, or left ventricular assist device implantation) occurred. Among peak VO_2, NYHA class, EF, total lung capacity, and age, the most powerful predictor of event-free survival was the VE/VCO_2 slope; patients with a VE/VCO_2 slope ≤130% of age- and gender-adjusted normal values had a significantly better 1-year event-free survival rate (88%) than patients with a slope >130% of the adjusted value (55%).

Several groups have demonstrated that the peak exercise VE/VCO_2 ratio predicts risk in HF. Robbins and colleagues[22] studied 470 consecutive patients with HF who were not taking beta blockers. There were 71 deaths in 1.5 years of follow-up. In univariate analyses, predictors of death included high peak VE/VCO_2 ratio, low chronotropic index, low peak VO_2, low resting systolic blood pressure, and older age. Nonparametric Kaplan-Meier plots demonstrated that by dividing the population according to peak VE/VCO_2 and peak VO_2, it was possible to identify groups at low, intermediate, and very high risk. In multivariate analyses, the only independent predictors of death were high VE/VCO_2 (adjusted relative risk 3×) and low chronotropic index (2×).

> **Key Points:** The VE/VCO_2 slope appears to have greater prognostic power than peak VO_2. It is likely that an abnormal VE/VCO_2 slope reflects many of the physiologic processes that lead to hyperventilation during exercise and thus are associated with disease severity (e.g., early lactate accumulation and ventilation/perfusion mismatching in the lungs caused by a poor cardiac output response to exercise). Importantly, the most useful risk stratification paradigm includes the VE/VCO_2 slope in addition to peak VO_2 and other clinical or exercise test variables in a multivariate model.

VO_2 Kinetics

The rate at which oxygen uptake responds to a given level of work, often expressed as oxygen uptake kinetics, has also been shown to have prognostic value. Indices of oxygen kinetics are easy to determine with current automated gas exchange technology, and offer promise as supplemental indices to more precisely stratify risk in patients with HF. Because these measures can be derived when exercise is submaximal, they may be particularly useful in HF patients unable to exercise maximally.

The mean response time (MRT), defined as the time required to reach 63% of the steady state VO_2, in patients with HF has been reported. Rickli and colleagues[23] observed that the MRT was the strongest univariate and multivariate predictor of cardiac mortality risk, and for patients who exhibited an abnormal MRT, a peak VO_2 <50% of the age-predicted value, and resting systolic blood pressure <105 mm Hg, the 1-year event rate was 59%. Schalcher and co-workers[24] studied 146 patients with HF and reported that, over a mean follow-up period of 25 months, the MRT more powerfully predicted death, need for urgent cardiac transplantation, or hospitalization than peak VO_2, as well as other exercise test and clinical variables. In an additional study from this group, VO_2 kinetics at exercise onset, expressed as a mean response time >60 seconds to a standardized protocol, was a stronger predictor of survival than peak VO_2, the VE/VCO_2 slope, and various clinical and laboratory markers known to be related to HF mortality rate.[25]

Although the measurement of VO_2 kinetics has been expressed different ways, all reflect the capacity of the cardiopulmonary system to adapt to the demands of a given work rate. This measurement appears to have important prognostic value and has an advantage in that it does not require judgment about the patient's maximal effort.

Oxygen Uptake Efficiency Slope

Another proposed index of ventilatory efficiency, the OUES, has been suggested as a useful measure to stratify the functional reserve of patients undergoing exercise testing, and this index has also been shown to have prognostic value. The OUES is determined by regressing oxygen uptake against the logarithm of total ventilation; thus it reflects the ventilatory requirement for work performed (VO_2) throughout exercise. Baba and colleagues[26] reported that the OUES was as effective as peak VO_2 for discriminating between HF functional classifications and that it was strongly correlated to peak VO_2. The purported advantages of the OUES are that it does not require maximal effort; it has been shown to be reproducible; and it has been suggested to reflect the combination of cardiovascular, musculoskeletal, and pulmonary influences that result in inefficient breathing, which are characteristic of HF and pulmonary disease.[27] However, other studies have suggested that the OUES has limited clinical utility.[28]

Oxygen Uptake in Recovery

The time required for oxygen uptake to return to the resting state in recovery from exercise (oxygen uptake recovery kinetics) has also been shown to be an important functional and prognostic marker.[29] A delay in the rate of recovery of VO_2 has been explained by a delay in the recovery of energy stores in the muscle, with skeletal muscle metabolic abnormalities, microcirculatory changes, and a prolongation of elevated cardiac output contributing.[30] Importantly, the recovery response does not appear to be affected by the exercise level achieved.[31]

Cutpoints for Peak VO_2

Although the cutpoint of 14 ml/kg/min for peak VO_2 has become well established as a marker of high risk, many studies have reported that other cutpoints effectively stratify risk, either chosen arbitrarily or using ROC curve analysis. Various cutpoints in the clinically relevant range (10 to 17 ml/kg/min) were evaluated in a large follow-up study at Stanford.[32] After pharmacologic stabilization at entrance into the study, all participants underwent cardiopulmonary exercise testing. Survival analysis was performed with death as the endpoint. Transplantation was considered a censored event. Four-year survival was determined for patients who achieved peak oxygen uptake values greater than and less than 10, 11, 12, 13, 14, 15, 16, and 17 ml/kg/min. Follow-up information was complete for 98.3% of the cohort. During a mean

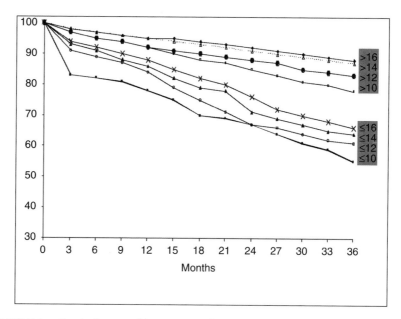

FIGURE 7-3 *Survival curves for patients achieving above versus below 12, 14, and 16 ml/kg/min for peak oxygen uptake. (From Myers J et al: Cardiopulmonary exercise testing and prognosis in severe heart failure: 14 mL/kg/min revisited, Am Heart J 139:78-84, 2000.)*

follow-up period of 4 years, 187 patients (29%) died and 101 underwent transplantation. Actuarial 1- and 5-year survival rates were 90.5% and 73.4%, respectively. Peak VO_2 was an independent predictor of survival and was a stronger predictor of mortality risk than work rate achieved and other exercise and clinical variables. A difference in survival of approximately 20% was achieved by dichotomizing patients above versus below each peak VO_2 value ranging between 10 and 17 ml/kg/min. These results are illustrated in Figure 7-3. Survival rate was significantly higher among patients achieving a peak VO_2 above than among those achieving a peak VO_2 below each of these values, but each cutpoint was similar in its ability to separate survivors from nonsurvivors.

> **Key Point:** Although 14 ml/kg/min is widely applied to stratify risk in patients with HF, an "optimal" cutpoint is likely to vary with the population studied. It appears better to apply peak VO_2 as a continuous variable in multivariate models to predict prognosis.

Interaction between Peak VO_2 and Hemodynamic Variables in Stratifying Risk

Survival is most accurately predicted when exercise variables are combined with other clinical and hemodynamic data.[7,16,17,33,34] Reduced left ventricular performance has been a common reason for referring a patient to an HF management clinic, and many studies have identified EF as a predictor of survival. However, EF by itself is an inadequate reflection of left ventricular performance and a patient's degree of hemodynamic compromise. Although EF has been reported to lose its prognostic value in the very low range,[35] others have shown that EF is associated with a marked increase in mortality risk once it is below 20%. Adding further confusion to this issue is the fact that EF, other measures of hemodynamic function, and peak VO_2 are poorly related.[36,37] Right-sided heart catheterization has been performed in HF patients to more directly assess cardiovascular performance and stratify risk. Variables such as low resting cardiac output and high intrapulmonary pressures have been associated with higher risk. However, some patients remain markedly symptomatic despite normalization of cardiac output and left ventricular filling pressures. The level of exercise intolerance perceived by patients with HF has a questionable relation to objective measures of circulatory, ventilatory, or metabolic dysfunction during exercise. In addition, these hemodynamic variables have not consistently been shown to be useful in prognosis. Peak VO_2 has functioned synergistically with hemodynamic responses in some of the studies discussed earlier.

Chomsky and colleagues[33] measured the cardiac output response to exercise along with gas exchange responses in 185 patients referred for evaluation for transplantation. The cardiac output response to exercise was considered normal in 83 patients and reduced in 102. By univariate analysis, patients with normal cardiac output responses had a better 1-year survival rate (95%) than did those with reduced cardiac output responses (72%). Survival in patients with a peak VO_2 >14 ml/kg/min (88%) was not different from that of patients with a peak VO_2 ≤14 ml/kg/min (79%). However, survival was worse in patients with a peak VO_2 ≤10 ml/kg/min (52%) versus those with a peak VO_2 >10 ml/kg/min (89%). By Cox regression analysis, the cardiac output response to exercise was the strongest independent predictor of survival (risk ratio 4×), with peak VO_2 dichotomized at 10 ml/kg/min (risk ratio 3×) as the only other independent predictor. Patients with reduced cardiac output responses and peak VO_2 ≤10 had an extremely poor 1-year survival rate (38%).

Metra and colleagues[34] performed cardiopulmonary exercise testing and direct hemodynamic monitoring in 219 consecutive patients with HF and followed them for mean of 19 months. During the follow-up period, 32 patients died and 6 underwent urgent transplantation, resulting in a 71% cumulative major event-free 2-year survival. Peak exercise stroke work index (SWI) was the most powerful prognostic variable selected by Cox multivariate analysis, followed by serum sodium and left ventricular EF for 1-year survival. However, peak VO_2 and serum sodium were the strongest determinants of 2-year survival. Two-year survival was 54% in the patients with a peak exercise SWI ≤30 g/m² versus 91% in those with an SWI >30 g/m² ($p < 0.0001$). A significant percentage of patients (41%) had a normal cardiac output response to exercise with an excellent 2-year survival rate (87% vs. 58% in the others) despite a relatively low peak VO_2 (15.1 ± 4.7 ml/kg/min).

> **Key Points:** Studies including direct hemodynamic measurements in addition to cardiopulmonary exercise responses have shown that they add independent prognostic information. However, invasive hemodynamic exercise testing in all patients with HF is not widely recommended. Cardiopulmonary exercise test variables have been shown to be stronger predictors of risk, suggesting that invasive hemodynamic measurements are usually not necessary for risk stratification in HF.

Peak VO$_2$ Combined with Plasma Biomarkers in Predicting Risk

The degree of neurohumoral activation assessed by plasma levels of norepinephrine, natriuretic peptides, and endothelins has been recognized as a marker of increased risk in HF.[38,39] Some investigators have suggested the application of neurohormones in combination with cardiopulmonary exercise testing to optimize predicting risk in patients with HF. The potential advantages of including these markers in multivariate risk models include the fact that they are more objective than peak VO$_2$ (e.g., peak VO$_2$ can be difficult to define in some patients), and as discussed earlier, many patients have a peak VO$_2$ that falls within the "gray zone" of intermediate risk.

Summary of Cardiopulmonary Exercise Testing and Risk Stratification in Heart Failure

Directly measured VO$_2$ has an established place in predicting outcomes in patients with HF. Peak VO$_2$ has been demonstrated in numerous studies to be an independent marker for risk of death or other endpoints. Increased automation of gas exchange systems has made these data easier to obtain, and this objective information is replacing the former dependence on subjective measures of clinical and functional status. Peak VO$_2$ is now a recognized criterion for selecting patients who could potentially benefit from heart transplantation. It is often a more powerful predictor of death when combined with other clinical, hemodynamic, and exercise data.

The commonly used cutpoint for peak VO$_2$ of 14 ml/kg/min to separate survivors from nonsurvivors, and thus help select patients for transplantation listing, is too simplistic. The combination of cardiopulmonary exercise data and other clinical and hemodynamic responses in multivariate scores has been shown to more powerfully stratify risk. It is also important to note that peak VO$_2$ is influenced by age, gender, body weight, and mode of exercise, and some studies have demonstrated that peak VO$_2$ expressed as a percentage of the predicted value (taking these variables into account) is a more powerful predictor of outcome than absolute peak VO$_2$ and gender and age. This approach is complicated by the fact that there are many age- and gender-predicted "standards" for peak VO$_2$.[40]

Cardiopulmonary exercise variables other than peak VO$_2$ have important prognostic value in HF. The focus of these studies has centered on the VE/VO$_2$ slope, although other expressions of ventilatory efficiency, including the maximal ventilatory equivalent for CO$_2$, the OUES, various measures of oxygen kinetics, and oxygen uptake in recovery, have all been shown to be strong prognostic markers. Summary reports from metabolic systems should be configured to provide both the VE/VCO$_2$ slope and peak VO$_2$, and consideration should be given to including the VE/VCO$_2$ slope in the HF and transplantation guidelines.

Relative to peak VO$_2$ or other cardiopulmonary exercise variables, hemodynamic variables are inconsistent in their ability to predict risk of death or clinical deterioration. The dissociation between hemodynamic observations and exercise responses underscores the complexity of HF. Exertional symptoms and hemodynamic variables should be treated as separate entities; the former is influenced by musculoskeletal metabolism and strength, body composition, and motivation in addition to cardiac function, whereas the latter is influenced largely by the degree of pump dysfunction. Nevertheless, more powerful estimates of risk have been demonstrated when peak VO$_2$ is combined with one or more hemodynamic variables.

Evaluation of Therapies for Heart Failure

The studies of drug efficacy in HF have focused on decreasing hospitalizations and improving survival. However, as one of the components of quality of life, exercise capacity has been studied to demonstrate at least that it is not decreased by therapy. The medications indicated for improved survival in patients with systolic dysfunction that have been studied with exercise testing include the renin-angiotensin-aldosterone system (RAAS) blocking drugs[41,42] and beta-blocking agents.[43-45] Table 7-4 summarizes the major exercise testing studies evaluating beta blockers in HF. Overall, the beta blockers have had minimal effects on exercise capacity. Cardiopulmonary exercise testing is more reproducible and accurate than the 6-minute walk test for demonstrating the effect of interventions on exercise capacity and, as outlined previously, is a powerful tool for deciding who will benefit from cardiac transplantation. Available evidence, although limited, suggests that beta blockade does not interfere with the prognostic value of cardiopulmonary exercise responses. With the evolution of cardiac-resynchronization therapy (CRT) using pacemakers as an important therapy in selected HF patients, the exercise test has been used to document the improvement in cardiovascular hemodynamics afforded by CRT.[46,47] A summary of some of the major studies evaluating exercise test responses to CRT is presented in Table 7-5.

Summary

HF represents the one category of patients with cardiovascular disease that is increasing in prevalence. Although the exercise test was once considered only a tool to diagnose coronary disease, it is now recognized that it has major applications for assessing functional capabilities, therapeutic interventions, and estimating prognosis in HF. Numerous hemodynamic abnormalities underlie the reduced exercise capacity commonly observed in chronic HF, including impaired heart rate responses, inability to distribute

TABLE 7-4   Effect of Beta Blockers on Exercise Test Responses in Chronic Heart Failure

Study	Year	No. of Subjects	Beta Blocker	Model/Protocol	Effect on Exercise Response vs. Placebo
Dubach[45]	2002	28	Bisoprolol	Ramp bicycle	No difference in peak VO_2, but trend for higher work rate and exercise time on bisoprolol.
CIBIS[70]	1994	641	Bisoprolol	Bicycle	21% improved NYHA class on bisoprolol vs. 15% on placebo.
MERIT-HF[71]	2000	3991	Metoprolol	Treadmill	No increase in peak VO_2, but improvement in submaximal exercise performance. Exercise time and HF-related symptoms improved with metoprolol.
RESOLVD[72]	2000	426	Metoprolol	6MW	No increase in peak VO_2, or submaximal exercise performance while on metoprolol, but exercise time and HF-related symptoms improved.
MDC[73]	1993	383	Metoprolol	Bicycle	No change in peak VO_2, but improvement in submaximal exercise performance, exercise duration, and HF-related symptoms on metoprolol.
ANZ[74]	1997	415	Carvedilol	Treadmill	No effect on treadmill performance.
PRECISE[75]	1996	278	Carvedilol	6MW, 9MTM	No improvement in exercise performance using 9MTM.
Colucci et al[76]	1996	366	Carvedilol	9MTM	No improvement in exercise performance using 9MTM.
MOCHA[77]	1996	345	Carvedilol	6MW, 9MTM	No effect on exercise performance.
Metra et al[34]	2000	150	Metoprolol vs. carvedilol	6MW	No difference in exercise tolerance, QOL, or submaximal exercise performance.

HF, heart failure; *6MW*, 6-minute walk test; *9MTM*, 9-minute treadmill; *NYHA*, New York Heart Association; *QOL*, quality of life.

TABLE 7-5 Summary of Studies on the Effects of Cardiac Resynchronization Therapy (CRT) on Exercise Capacity in Patients with Heart Failure

Study (Year)	N	Inclusion Criteria	Effect on Exercise Capacity
Auricchio (2004)[78]	86	NYHA class II QRS > 150 msec	Improved peak VO_2 Higher ventilatory threshold Improved 6-minute walk distance
Chan (2003)[79]	63	Consecutive CRT Patients with HF	Improved NYHA class Improved 6-minute walk distance Reduced LVEDD Improved LVEF
MIRACLE-ICD (2003)[80]	636	NYHA class 2-4 LVEF < 35% QRS > 120 msec	Improved 6-minute walk distance
MUSTIC (2003)[81]	58	NYHA class 3 LVEF < 35% QRS > 150 msec	Improved peak VO_2 Improved 6-minute walk distance Elevated AT Reduction in VE/VCO_2 Improved QOL
Gras (2002)[82]	103	Consecutive CRT Patients with HF	Improved NYHA class Improved QOL Improved 6-minute walk distance Improved LVEDD

Improved mitral regurgitation and LV filling time

INSYNC (2002)[83]	81	Symptomatic HF EF <35% QRS > 130 msec	Improved NYHA class Improved 6-minute walk distance Improved LV dimensions Improved fractional shortening
MIRACLE (2002)[47]	453	NYHA class 3-4 LVEF > 35% QRS > 130 msec	Improved peak VO_2 Improved 6-minute walk distance Improved QOL
Molhoek (2002)[84]	40	NYHA class III or IV EF < 35% QRS > 120 msec	Improved NYHA class Improved QOL Improved 6-minute walk distance

Study Year	N	Inclusion	Changes in Exercise Capacity with CRT
PATH-CHF (2002)[85]	53	NYHA class 3-4 QRS > 120 msec "Severe cardiomyopathy" PR interval > 150 msec	Improved peak VO_2 Improved 6-minute walk distance Elevated AT Reduction in VE/VCO_2 Improved QOL Effect greater with lower baseline VO_2
CONTAK CD (2001)[86]	490	NYHA class 2-4 LVEF > 35% QRS <120 msec	Improved peak VO_2 Improved 6-minute walk distance Improved QOL

AT, anaerobic threshold; CM, cardiomyopathy; CRT, cardiac resynchronization therapy; HF, heart failure; LVEDD, left ventricular end-diastolic dimension; LVEF, left ventricular ejection fraction; NYHA, New York Heart Association; QOL, quality of life; VE/VCO_2, slope of minute ventilation/CO_2 production; VO_2, oxygen uptake.

cardiac output normally, abnormal arterial vasodilatory capacity, abnormal cellular metabolism in skeletal muscle, higher than normal systemic vascular resistance, higher than normal pulmonary pressures, and ventilatory abnormalities that increase the work of breathing and cause exertional dyspnea.[48] Intervention with angiotensin-converting enzyme (ACE) inhibitors, beta blockade, CRT, or exercise training can improve many of these abnormalities. However, although ACE inhibitors and beta blockers are now widely used in HF because of their well-documented effects on survival, their effect on exercise capacity has been inconsistent. This is in part due to differences in methodology (e.g., differences in study design, exercise protocols, functional endpoints used, and absence of gas exchange data). Submaximal exercise responses (e.g., ventilatory threshold, VE/VCO_2 slope, 6-minute walk performance) have shown marked improvements with training or other interventions, but these responses are underused among studies assessing these interventions.

Over the last 15 years, exercise testing with ventilatory gas exchange responses has been demonstrated to have a critical role in the risk paradigm in HF. In many studies, peak VO_2 has been shown to be a stronger predictor of risk than established clinical markers such as symptoms, clinical signs, EF, and other invasive hemodynamic data. However, these studies have also been confounded by differences in the approach to the exercise test, in addition to the use of different endpoints in the various studies (e.g., transplant listing, change in listing status, and hospitalization, in addition to mortality). Recent studies have been consistent in the demonstration that the VE/VCO_2 slope is an even stronger predictor of risk than peak VO_2. These studies have also suggested that other cardiopulmonary exercise test responses, such as oxygen kinetics, oxygen uptake in recovery, and the OUES, are important risk markers, and these may evolve to have a greater role in establishing risk in HF. Recent studies have considered other exercise test responses including heart rate recovery[49,50] and ectopy[51] and found both to have independent prognostic power in patients with HF. These exercise test responses have not yet been combined or compared with expired gas analysis results and could improve risk stratification.

References

1. Zile MR, Baicu CF, Gaasch WH: Diastolic heart failure—abnormalities in active relaxation and passive stiffness of the left ventricle, *N Engl J Med* 350:1953-1959, 2004.
2. Gottdiener JS et al: Outcome of congestive heart failure in elderly persons: influence of left ventricular systolic function. The Cardiovascular Health Study, *Ann Intern Med* 137:631-639, 2002.
3. Kannel WB, Belanger AJ: Epidemiology of heart failure, *Am Heart J* 121:951-957, 1991.
4. Lloyd-Jones DM et al: Lifetime risk for developing congestive heart failure: the Framingham Heart Study, *Circulation* 106:3068-3072, 2002.

5. Levy D et al: Long-term trends in the incidence of and survival with heart failure, *N Engl J Med* 347:1397-1402, 2002.

6. *2004 heart and stroke statistical update,* Dallas, 2004, American Heart Association.

7. Myers J, Gullestad L: The role of exercise testing and gas exchange measurement in the prognostic assessment of patients with heart failure, *Curr Opin Cardiol* 13:145-155, 1998.

8. Myers J: Applications of cardiopulmonary exercise testing in the management of cardiovascular and pulmonary disease, *Int J Sports Med* 26:S49-S55, 2005.

9. Corra U, Mezzani A, Bosimini E, Giannuzzi P: Cardiopulmonary exercise testing and prognosis in chronic heart failure; a prognosticating algorithm for the individual patient, *Chest* 126:942-950, 2004.

10. Hunt SA et al: ACC/AHA 2005 guideline update for the diagnosis and management of chronic heart failure in the adult: a report of the American College of Cardiology/American Heart Association Task Force on Practice Guidelines, *Circulation* 112(12):154-235, 2005.

11. Costanzo MR et al: Selection and treatment of candidates for heart transplantation. A statement for health professionals from the Committee on Heart Failure and Cardiac Transplantation of the Council on Clinical Cardiology, American Heart Association, *Circulation* 92:3593-3612, 1995.

12. Mudge GH et al: Twenty-fourth Bethesda conference: cardiac transplantation: Task Force 3: recipient guidelines/prioritization, *J Am Coll Cardiol* 22:21-31, 1993.

13. Guazzi M: Exercise testing to monitor heart failure treatment. In Wasserman K, ed: *Cardiopulmonary exercise testing and cardiovascular health,* Armonk, NY, 2002, Futura.

14. Pierson RN et al: Thoracic organ transplantation, *Am J Transplant* 4: 93-105, 2004.

15. Stewart S, Marley JE, Horowitz JD: Effects of a multidisciplinary, home-based intervention on planned readmissions and survival among patients with chronic congestive heart failure: a randomized controlled trial, *Lancet* 354:1077-1083, 1999.

16. Mancini DM et al: Value of peak exercise oxygen consumption for optimal timing of cardiac transplantation in ambulatory patients with heart failure, *Circulation* 83:778-786, 1991.

17. Myers J et al: Clinical, hemodynamic, and cardiopulmonary exercise test determinants of outcome in patients referred for evaluation of heart failure, *Ann Intern Med* 129:286-293, 1998.

18. Gitt A et al: Exercise anaerobic threshold and ventilatory efficiency identify heart failure patients for high risk of early death, *Circulation* 106:3079-3084, 2002.

19. Corra U et al: Ventilatory response to exercise improves risk stratification in patients with chronic heart failure and intermediate functional capacity, *Am Heart J* 143:418-426, 2002.

20. Arena R et al: Peak VO_2 and VE/VCO_2 slope in patients with heart failure: a prognostic comparison, *Am Heart J* 147:354-360, 2004.

21. Kleber FX et al: Impairment of ventilatory efficiency in heart failure: prognostic impact, *Circulation* 101:2803-2809, 2000.
22. Robbins M et al: Ventilatory and heart rate responses to exercise: better predictors of heart failure mortality than peak oxygen consumption, *Circulation* 100:2411-2417, 1999.
23. Rickli H et al: Combining low-intensity and maximal exercise test results improves prognostic prediction in chronic heart failure, *J Am Coll Cardiol* 42:116-122, 2003.
24. Schalcher C et al: Prolonged oxygen uptake kinetics during low-intensity exercise are related to poor prognosis in patients with mild-to-moderate congestive heart failure, *Chest* 124:580-586, 2003.
25. Brunner-La Rocca HP et al: Prognostic significance of oxygen uptake kinetics during low level exercise in patients with heart failure, *Am J Cardiol* 84:741-744, 1999.
26. Baba R et al: Oxygen uptake efficiency slope as a useful measure of cardiorespiratory functional reserve in adult cardiac patient, *Eur J Appl Physiol* 80:397-401, 1999.
27. Van Laethem C et al: Oxygen uptake efficiency slope, a new submaximal parameter in evaluating exercise capacity in chronic heart failure patients, *Am Heart J* 149:175-180, 2005.
28. Mourot L, Perrey S, Tordi N, Rouillon JD: Evaluation of fitness level by the oxygen uptake efficiency slope after a short-term intermittent endurance training, *Int J Sports Med* 25:85-91, 2004.
29. Pavia L, Myers J, Cesare R: Recovery kinetics of oxygen uptake and heart rate in patients with coronary artery disease and heart failure, *Chest* 116:808-813, 1999.
30. Cohen-Solal A et al: Prolonged kinetics of recovery of oxygen consumption after maximal graded exercise in patients with chronic heart failure, *Circulation* 91:2924-2932, 1995.
31. Scrutinio D et al: Percent achieved of predicted peak exercise oxygen uptake and kinetics of recovery of oxygen uptake after exercise for risk stratification in chronic heart failure, *Int J Cardiol* 64:117-124, 1998.
32. Myers J et al: Cardiopulmonary exercise testing and prognosis in severe heart failure: 14 mL/kg/min revisited, *Am Heart J* 139:78-84, 2000.
33. Chomsky DB et al: Hemodynamic exercise testing: a valuable tool in the selection of cardiac transplantation candidates, *Circulation* 94:3176-3183, 1996.
34. Metra M et al: Use of cardiopulmonary exercise testing with hemodynamic monitoring in the prognostic assessment of ambulatory patients with chronic heart failure, *J Am Coll Cardiol* 33:943-950, 1999.
35. Dec GW, Fuster V: Idiopathic dilated cardiomyopathy, *N Engl J Med* 331:1564-1575, 1994.
36. Myers J, Froelicher VF: Hemodynamic determinants of exercise capacity in chronic heart failure, *Ann Intern Med* 115:377-386, 1991.

37. Wilson JR, Rayos G, Keoh TK, Gothard P: Dissociation between peak exercise oxygen consumption and hemodynamic dysfunction in potential heart transplantation candidates, *J Am Coll Cardiol* 26:429-435, 1995.

38. Isnard R et al. Combination of B-type natriuretic peptide and peak oxygen consumption improves risk stratification in outpatients with chronic heart failure, *Am Heart J* 146:729-735, 2003.

39. de Groote P et al: B-type natriuretic peptide and peak exercise oxygen consumption provide independent information for risk stratification in patients with stable congestive heart failure, *J Am Coll Cardiol* 43:1584-1589, 2004.

40. Myers J: *Essentials of cardiopulmonary exercise testing,* Champaign, IL, 1996, Human Kinetics.

41. Abdulla J et al, TRACE Study Group: The angiotensin converting enzyme inhibitor trandolapril has neutral effect on exercise tolerance or functional class in patients with myocardial infarction and reduced left ventricular systolic function, *Eur Heart J* 24:2116-2122, 2003.

42. Kiowski W, Sutsch G, Dossegger L: Clinical benefit of angiotensin-converting enzyme inhibitors in chronic heart failure, *J Cardiovasc Pharmacol* 27:S19-24, 1996.

43. Russell SD et al: Rationale for use of an exercise end point and design for the ADVANCE (a dose evaluation of a vasopressin antagonist in HF patients undergoing exercise) trial, *Am Heart J* 145:179-186, 2003.

44. Narang R, Swedberg K, Cleland JG: What is the ideal study design for evaluation of treatment for heart failure? Insights from trials assessing the effect of ACE inhibitors on exercise capacity, *Eur Heart J* 17:120-134, 1996.

45. Dubach P et al: Effects of bisoprolol fumarate on left ventricular size, function, and exercise capacity in patients with heart failure: analysis with magnetic resonance myocardial tagging, *Am Heart J* 143:676-683, 2002.

46. Abraham WT et al, Multicenter InSync ICD II Study Group: Effects of cardiac resynchronization on disease progression in patients with left ventricular systolic dysfunction, an indication for an implantable cardioverter-defibrillator, and mildly symptomatic chronic heart failure, *Circulation* 110:2864-2868, 2004.

47. Abraham WT et al, MIRACLE Study Group: Multicenter InSync Randomized Clinical Evaluation. Cardiac resynchronization in chronic heart failure, *N Engl J Med* 346:1845-1853, 2002.

48. Pina IL et al, American Heart Association Committee on Exercise, Rehabilitation, and Prevention: Exercise and heart failure: a statement from the American Heart Association Committee on Exercise, Rehabilitation, and Prevention, *Circulation* 107:1210-1225, 2003.

49. Lipinski MJ, Vetrovec G, Gorelik D, Froelicher V: The importance of heart rate recovery in patients with heart failure or left ventricular systolic dysfunction, *Journal of Cardiac Failure* 11:624-630, 2005.

50. Arena R et al: Prognostic value of heart rate recovery in patients with heart failure, *Am Heart J* 151:851.e7-851.e13, 2006.

51. O'Neill JO, Young JB, Pothier CE, Lauer MS: Severe frequent ventricular ectopy after exercise as a predictor of death in patients with heart failure, *J Am Coll Cardiol* 44(4):820-826, 2004.

52. Likoff MJ, Chandler SL, Kay HR: Clinical determinants of mortality in chronic congestive heart failure secondary to idiopathic dilated or to ischemic cardiomyopathy, *Am J Cardiol* 59:634-638, 1987.

53. Stevenson LW et al: Exercise capacity for survivors of cardiac transplantation or sustained medical therapy for stable heart failure, *Circulation* 81:78-85, 1990.

54. Saxon LA et al: Predicting death from progressive heart failure secondary to ischemic or idiopathic dilated cardiomyopathy, *Am J Cardiol* 72: 62-65, 1993.

55. Cohn JN et al: Ejection fraction, peak exercise, oxygen consumption, cardiothoracic ratio, ventricular arrhythmias, and plasma norepinephrine as determinants of prognosis in heart failure, *Circulation* 87:vi-16, 1993.

56. Stevenson LW et al: Target heart failure populations for newer therapies, *Circulation* 92:II-174–II-181, 1995.

57. Aaronson KD, Mancini DM: Is percentage of predicted maximal exercise oxygen consumption a better predictor of survival than peak exercise oxygen consumption for patients with severe heart failure? *J Heart Lung Transplant* 14:981-989, 1995.

58. Haywood GA et al: Analysis of deaths in patients awaiting heart transplantation: impact on patient selection criteria, *Heart* 75:455-462, 1996.

59. Aaronson KD et al: Development and prospective validation of a clinical index to predict survival in ambulatory patients referred for cardiac transplant evaluation, *Circulation* 95:2660-2667, 1997.

60. Chua TP et al: Clinical correlates and prognostic significance of the ventilatory response to exercise in chronic heart failure, *J Am Coll Cardiol* 29:1585-1590, 1997.

61. Opasich C et al: Peak exercise oxygen consumption in chronic heart failure: toward efficient use in the individual patient, *J Am Coll Cardiol* 31:766-775, 1998.

62. Osada N et al: Cardiopulmonary exercise testing identifies low risk patients with heart failure and severely impaired exercise capacity considered for heart transplantation, *J Am Coll Cardiol* 31:577-582, 1998.

63. Cohen Solal A et al: A non-invasively determined surrogate of cardiac power (circulatory power) at peak exercise is a powerful prognostic factor in chronic heart failure, *Eur Heart J* 23:806-814, 2002.

64. Mezzani A et al: Contribution of peak respiratory exchange ratio to peak VO_2 prognostic reliability in patients with chronic heart failure and severely reduced exercise capacity, *Am Heart J* 145:1102-1107, 2003.

65. Francis DP et al: Cardiopulmonary exercise testing for prognosis in chronic heart failure: continuous and independent prognostic value from VE/VCO_2 slope and peak VO_2, *Eur Heart J* 21:154-161, 2000.

66. Robbins M et al: Ventilatory and heart rate responses to exercise: better predictors of heart failure mortality than peak oxygen consumption, *Circulation* 100:2411-2417, 1999.

67. Kleber FX et al: Impairment of ventilatory efficiency in heart failure: prognostic impact, *Circulation* 101:2803-2809, 2000.

68. Bol E et al: Cardiopulmonary exercise parameters in relation to all-cause mortality in patients with chronic heart failure, *Int J Cardiol* 72:255-263, 2000.

69. Pardaens K, Van Cleemput J, Vanhaecke J, Fagard RH: Peak oxygen uptake better predicts outcome than submaximal respiratory data in heart transplant candidates, *Circulation* 101:1152-1157, 2000.

70. CIBIS Investigators and Committees: A randomized trial of beta-blockade in heart failure. The Cardiac Insufficiency Bisoprolol Study (CIBIS), *Circulation* 90:1765-1773, 1994.

71. Hjalmarson A, Fagerberg B: MERIT-HF mortality and morbidity data, *Basic Res Cardiol* 95:I98-I103, 2000.

72. Prakash A, Markham A: Metroprolol: a review of its use in chronic heart failure, *Drugs* 60:647-678, 2000.

73. Waagstein et al: Beneficial effects of metroprolol in idiopathic dilated cardiomyopathy. Metroprolol in Dilated Cardiomyopathy (MDC) Trial Study Group, *Lancet* 342:1441-1446, 1993.

74. Hjalmarson A, Kneider M, Waagstein F: The role of beta-blockers in left ventricular dysfunction and heart failure, *Drugs* 54:501-510, 1997.

75. Packer M et al: Double-blind, placebo-controlled study of the effects of carvedilol in patients with moderate to severe heart failure. The PRECISE Trial, *Circulation* 94:2793-2799, 1996.

76. Colucci WS et al: Carvedilol inhibits clinical progression in patients with mild symptoms of heart failure. US Carvedilol Heart Failure Study Group, *Circulation* 94:2800-2806, 1996.

77. Bristow MR et al: Carvedilol produces dose-related improvements in left ventricular function and survival in subjects with chronic heart failure. MOCHA Investigators, *Circulation* 94:2807-2816, 1996.

78. Auricchio A et al: Pacing Therapies in Congestive Heart Failure II Study Group; Guidant Heart Failure Research Group. Clinical efficacy of cardiac resynchronization therapy using left ventricular pacing in heart failure patients stratified by severity of ventricular conduction delay, *J Am Coll Cardiol* 42:2125-2127, 2003.

79. Chan KL et al: Functional and echocardiographic improvement following multisite biventricular pacing for congestive heart failure, *Can J Cardiol* 19:387-390, 2003.

80. Young JB et al: Multicenter InSync ICD Randomized Clinical Evaluation (MIRACLE ICD) Trial Investigators. Combined cardiac resynchronization and implantable cardioversion defibrillation in advanced chronic heart failure: the MIRACLE ICD Trial, *JAMA* 289:2685-2694, 2003.

81. Alonso C et al: MUSTIC Study Group. Effects of cardiac resynchronization therapy on heart rate variability in patients with chronic systolic heart failure and intraventricular conduction delay, *Am J Cardiol* 91:1144-1147, 2003.

82. Gras D et al: Cardiac resynchronization therapy in advanced heart failure the multicenter InSync clinical study, *Eur J Heart Fail* 4:311-320, 2002.

83. Kuhlkamp V: InSync 7272 ICD World Wide Investigators. Initial experience with an implantable cardioverter-defibrillator incorporating cardiac resynchronization therapy, *J Am Coll Cardiol* 39:790-797, 2002.

84. Molhoek SG et al: Effectiveness of resynchronization therapy in patients with end-stage heart failure, *Am J Cardiol* 90:379-383, 2002.
85. Auricchio A et al: The Pacing Therapies for Congestive Heart Failure (PATH-CHF) study: rationale, design, and endpoints of a prospective randomized multicenter study, *Am J Cardiol* 83:130D-135D, 1999.
86. Higgins SL et al: Cardiac resynchronization therapy for the treatment of heart failure in patients with intraventricular conduction delay and malignant ventricular tachyarrhythmias, *J Am Coll Cardiol* 42:1454-1459, 2003.

8   Exercise Testing of Patients Recovering from Myocardial Infarction

Introduction

Though the death rate for coronary heart disease (CHD) has been decreasing steadily since the mid-1960s, it still remains the leading cause of death in the United States.[1] Four deaths in every 10 are due to cardiac disorders, and of these, 90% can be attributed to CHD. The four distinct clinical manifestations of CHD are primary cardiac arrest, stable angina pectoris, acute coronary syndromes (ACSs),[2] and acute myocardial infarction (MI). The resting electrocardiogram (ECG) is critical to guiding therapy, with ST elevation indicating the prompt application of thrombolysis or percutaneous coronary intervention (PCI), and ST depression necessitating antiplatelet drugs (Figure 8-1).

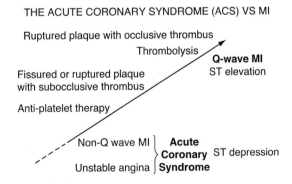

THE ACUTE CORONARY SYNDROME (ACS) VS MI

FIGURE 8-1   *Comparison of the pathophysiology and treatment of acute coronary syndrome (ACS) vs. ST-elevation MI. They are on a continuum of the mechanisms of coronary atherosclerosis. The resting ECG is critical to guiding therapy: ST elevation indicates the need for prompt application of thrombolysis or PCI, and ST depression requires antiplatelet drugs. When available, direct PCI is recommended for acute MI rather than thrombolysis.*

Each year 900,000 people in the United States experience acute MI. Of these, roughly 225,000 die, including 125,000 who die before obtaining medical care. The case fatality rate in MI patients is temporally related to onset. The risk of death is highest within the first 24 hours of onset of signs or symptoms and declines throughout the following year. Following the onset of a first MI in middle-aged men, 30% to 50% are dead within 30 days and 85% of these deaths occur within the first 24 hours. Those patients with a first MI who actually reach a hospital alive have a 10% to 18% risk of dying before discharge. The mortality rate thereafter falls from an annualized rate of 9% over months 2 through 6, to 4% for months 7 through 30, to 3% over the next 3 years. Other studies have suggested a mortality rate of 11% in the first 3 months after hospital discharge and then lower rates thereafter. In comparison with standard medical therapy, thrombolytic therapy exerts a highly significant 20% reduction in 35-day mortality rate among patients with acute MI and ST elevation, corresponding to an overall reduction of 21 deaths per 1000 patients treated. Temporal comparison studies have suggested a reduction in mortality rate that is due to modern therapies and prevention.[3,4] The impact of the 30% reduction in mortality rate with implantable defibrillators in post-MI patients with left ventricular dysfunction has not been factored in yet.

The pathophysiologic determinates of prognosis following MI are the amount of viable myocardium and the amount of myocardium in jeopardy. Inferences can be made regarding these two determinants clinically if a patient has had heart failure (HF) or cardiogenic shock and continued chest pain or ischemia. Using cardiac catheterization, they can be assessed by ejection fraction and the number of vessels occluded. The clinical findings manifested by abnormalities of these two determinants are the basis for several indices that have been used to predict risk. Clinical data have also been useful in triaging patients in regard to the necessary length of stay in the hospital. The criteria for a complicated MI are listed in Table 8-1. Patients without these criteria (i.e., those with uncomplicated MIs) can be discharged within 3 to 5 days, whereas those with these criteria require longer hospitalization and closer observation.

Health care professionals must be able to advise post-MI patients as to what they should or should not do to improve their prognosis. One strategy has been to identify high-risk patients by using various clinical markers and test results.[7] Clinical markers that have indicated high risk include prior MI, congestive heart failure, cardiogenic shock, tachycardia, continued chest pain, older age, stroke or transient ischemic attack, and complicating illnesses.

TABLE 8-1   Characteristics That Lead to the Classification of an MI as Being Complicated

CHF
Cardiogenic shock
Large MI—as determined by CPK, troponin, or ECG
Pericarditis
Dangerous arrhythmias, including conduction abnormalities
Concurrent illnesses
Pulmonary embolus
Continued ischemia
Stroke or TIA

CHF, congestive heart failure; *CPK,* creatine phosphokinase; *ECG,* electrocardiogram; *MI,* myocarcial infarction; *TIA,* transient ischemic attack.

Procedures used to determine risk with some success have included the chest x-ray, routine ECG, ambulatory monitoring, radionuclide cardiac tests, and exercise testing. The assumption has been that patients at high risk should be considered for intervention; these interventions usually are coronary artery bypass surgery (CABS) and PCI. Because of easy access to these procedures, nearly all post-MI patients undergo cardiac catheterization before discharge, particularly since PCI is superseding thrombolysis.[8] Exercise testing is now less used to decide who needs cardiac catheterization because it is the clinical norm to have one. Furthermore, successful PCI is being promoted as obviating exercise testing and clinical risk assessment for decisions regarding early discharge after MI.[9]

> **Key Point:** Exercise testing is now less relied on to determine who needs cardiac catheterization because it is the clinical norm to have a cardiac catheterization. However, exercise testing continues to have important applications in MI patients for both diagnosis and prognosis.

American College of Cardiology/American Heart Association Exercise Testing Guidelines: Recommendations for Exercise Testing after Myocardial Infarction

The following is a synopsis of the American College of Cardiology/American Heart Association (ACC/AHA) guidelines for the use of the standard exercise test after myocardial infarction.[10] The updates for 2002 are included. Specifically in regard to post-MI testing, the issue of the effects of new therapies, particularly thrombolysis and PCI, were addressed.[11]

   Class I (definitely appropriate)—conditions for which there is evidence and/or general agreement that the standard exercise test is useful and helpful in patients recovering from an MI

1. Before discharge for prognostic assessment, activity prescription, evaluation of medical therapy (submaximal at about 4 to 6 [rather than 7] days)
2. Early after discharge for prognostic assessment, activity prescription, evaluation of medical therapy, and cardiac rehabilitation, if the predischarge exercise test was not done (symptom-limited at about 14 to 21 days)
3. Late after discharge for prognostic assessment, activity prescription, evaluation of medical therapy, and cardiac rehabilitation if the early exercise test was submaximal

Class IIa (probably appropriate)—conditions for which there is conflicting evidence and/or a divergence of opinion that the standard exercise test is useful and helpful in patients recovering from an MI but the weight of evidence for usefulness/efficacy is in favor of the exercise test

1. After discharge for activity counseling and/or exercise training as part of cardiac rehabilitation in patients who have undergone a coronary revascularization procedure

Class IIb (possibly appropriate)—conditions for which there is conflicting evidence and/or a divergence of opinion that the standard exercise test is useful and helpful in patients recovering from an MI but the usefulness/efficacy is less well established

1. In patients with an abnormal resting ECG due to left bundle branch block, interventricular conduction delay, electronically paced, left ventricular hypertrophy, digoxin therapy, or those demonstrating major ST-segment depression (>1 mm) in several leads
2. Periodic follow-up exercise testing in patients who continue to participate in exercise training or as part of supervised or unsupervised cardiac rehabilitation

Class III (not appropriate)*—conditions for which there is evidence and/or general agreement that the standard exercise test is not useful and helpful in patients recovering from an MI and in some cases may be harmful

1. Severe comorbidity likely to limit life expectancy and/or candidacy for revascularization
2. At any time to evaluate patients with acute MI who have uncompensated HF, arrhythmia, or cardiac conditions that severely limit their ability to exercise (level of evidence C)
3. Before discharge to evaluate patients who have already been selected for, or undergone, cardiac catheterization. Although a stress test may be useful before or after catheterization to evaluate or identify ischemia in the distribution of a coronary lesion of borderline severity, stress imaging tests are recommended (level of evidence C)

---

*Exceptions are noted under classes IIb and III.

Clinical experience has demonstrated the benefits of the treadmill test in patients after an MI for the following two reasons:

1. Demonstration of exercise capacity for activity prescription after hospital discharge; this includes domestic and occupational work evaluation, and exercise training as part of comprehensive cardiac risk reduction and rehabilitation
2. Evaluation of the adequacy of medical therapy and the need to employ other diagnostic or treatment options

---

Key Point: Exercise testing continues to have important applications in MI patients, including prognostication, functional assessment, and evaluation of the adequacy of interventions.

Methodologic Studies

Safety of Exercise Testing Early after Myocardial Infarction

The risk of death or major arrhythmias by performing an exercise test early after MI is very small. However, the major experience is based on clinically selected MI patients—those without major complications such as heart failure, severe arrhythmia or ischemia, left ventricular dysfunction, or other severe diseases. Risk is highest in those rejected for testing for these clinical reasons. The incidence of fatal cardiac events, including fatal MI and cardiac rupture, is 0.03%; nonfatal MI and unsuccessfully resuscitated cardiac arrest is 0.09%; and complex arrhythmias including ventricular tachycardia is 1.4%. Symptom-limited protocols have an event rate that is twice that of submaximal tests, although the overall fatal event rate is quite low.[12-14] Submaximal testing can be performed at 4 to 6 days, and a symptom-limited test is typically recommended 3 to 6 weeks later.

Key Point: Exercise testing early after MI is safe and clinically helpful.

Effect of Q-Wave Location on ST-Segment Shifts

The association between ST elevation and myocardial damage was studied in 97 patients with a prior transmural MI who underwent coronary angiography and treadmill testing.[15] In patients with a previous inferior wall infarction, the ST-segment response had a high degree of sensitivity and specificity (approximately 90%) in detecting additional coronary disease. However, in patients with a previous anteroseptal MI, the ST response had much less sensitivity. It was thought that the aneurysm generated an ischemic vector, canceling ST-segment changes and producing a false-negative treadmill test. If the anterior infarction extended beyond V4, the sensitivity rate of treadmill testing dropped even further. We used perfusion scans and computerized

ST-vector shifts to evaluate the effect of Q-wave location on the relationship of ST shifts to ischemia.[16] Anterolateral MIs had large ST-segment spatial shifts that did not indicate ischemia; when shifts occurred in patients with inferior or subendocardial MIs, ischemia was detected by thallium defects. It appeared that large anterior MIs behave as if left bundle branch block was present and the ST shifts have a very low specificity for ischemia. However, in a subsequent study, we demonstrated that severe angiographic disease could be recognized despite Q waves using ST depression.[17]

> **Key Point:** The resting ECG is critical to consider in the evaluation of the ST response to exercise in all patient groups including those post-MI.

Results of Exercise Testing and Coronary Angiography following Myocardial Infarction

Exercise testing after MI has been used to decide who has multivessel disease. The angiographic studies evaluating its efficacy for this are summarized in Table 8-2.[18-24] These angiographic studies involve populations that are much selected, often containing a higher prevalence of patients with angina than the usual post-MI population because they are more likely to undergo angiography. Review of the studies demonstrates a limited sensitivity and specificity for multivessel disease in post-MI patients.

> **Key Point:** Exercise testing has limited sensitivity and specificity for multivessel disease in post-MI patients.

Prognostic Studies

The prognostic studies of exercise testing after MI have been well summarized in two meta-analyses. The first meta-analysis considered reports published between 1972 and 1987 of longitudinal studies using exercise testing in the early post-MI period with a follow-up for cardiac events.[25] The five exercise test variables suggested to have prognostic importance are ST-segment depression (and ST elevation), exercise test–induced angina, poor exercise capacity or excessive heart rate response to a low workload, a blunted systolic blood pressure (SBP) response (or exertional hypotension), and premature ventricular contractions (PVCs).

The VA-UC Meta-Analysis of Exercise Testing after Myocardial Infarction

Exercise-Induced ST-Segment Shifts

ST Depression   Nine out of the 28 centers reporting appropriate studies found ST segment depression to be significantly predictive of subsequent

TABLE 8-2 Studies in Which Results of Exercise Testing Were Used to Predict Results of Coronary Angiography after Acute Myocardial Infarction

			Exercise Test Characteristics				
Investigator	Year Published	Patients Tested	Endpoints for Testing	ECG Leads	Protocol	Time after MI	Angiography Time after MI
Weiner[18]	1978	154	SS, SBPd, >4 mm, RVA	12LD	Bruce	2-36 mo	2-36 mo
Paine[19]	1978	100	90% MHR, SS, IVCD, 1 mm	V_{4-6}	Bruce	4 mo	4 mo
Dillahunt[20]	1979	28	SS, 1 mm, >3PVC/min, 5 min	CM_5, V_2	Naughton	10-18 days	4-20 wk
Sammel[26]	1980	77	SS, 6 METs	12LD	Green Lane	1 mo	1 mo
Fuller[27]	1981	40	HR 120, SS, 1 mm, >5 PVCs	12LD	Low Bruce	9-18 days	5-12 wk
Starling[23]	1981	57	SS, VT, SBPd, HBP	12LD	Naughton	9-21 days	3-12 wk
Boschat[21]	1981	65	85% MHR, 1 mm	12LD	Bruce	2-12 mo	2-12 mo
Schwartz[22]	1981	48	SS, SBPd VT, 2mm, 75% MHR	12LD	Low Bruce	18-22 days	3 wk
De Feyter[24]	1982	179	SS, VT	12LD	Bruce	6-8 wk	6-8 wk
Akhras[28]	1984	119	SS	12LD	Bruce	2 wk	6 wk
Morris[29]	1984	110	SS	12LD	UPR Bike	>6 wk	<3 mo
van der Wall[30]	1985	176	SS	12LD	Bruce/TH	6-8 wk	6-8 wk

Exercise test characteristic columns: CM$_5$, A bipolar lead; *HBP,* high blood pressure; *HR,* heart rate; *IVCD,* intraventricular conduction defect; *MET,* a maximal exercise level allowed to be reached as estimated from workload; *MHR,* heart rate at maximal effort; *mm,* amount in millimeters of ST shift taken as an endpoint; *(percent heart rate),* percentage of age-predicted maximal heart rate chosen as a limit; *SPBd,* systolic blood pressure drop; *SS,* signs or symptoms, or both; *12LD,* the full set of 12 leads; *V$_5$,* fifth precordial lead; *VT,* ventricular tachycardia. *Protocol,* type of exercise study done: *Bruce,* Bruce protocol stopped at 85% of the age-predicted maximal heart rate; *low Bruce,* Bruce protocol with 0 and 1/2 stages, which are 0% and 5% grade at 1.7 miles per hour before stage 1 (10% grade at 1.7 miles per hour); *Bruce/TH,* Bruce protocol with thallium imaging; *Green Lane,* Green Lane Hospital treadmill protocol; *Naughton,* Naughton treadmill test; *UPR,* upright bicycle combined with radionuclide testing.
Time after MI, Mean time after myocardial infarction that the exercise test or angiography was done.

death; an additional six centers reported a positive but insignificant association. Nine centers reported a null effect, with four failing to report data on ST-segment depression.

ST Elevation   These results are too inconsistent to make a conclusion.

Exercise-Induced Arrhythmias
Only 5 out of 24 centers reported exercise test–induced PVCs to indicate a significant increase in risk. Four centers did not include results regarding PVCs; nine centers reported null or negative associations of PVCs with mortality.

Exercise Capacity

Nine centers out of 24 reported that a low exercise capacity and/or an excessive heart rate response to exercise indicated a high-risk group. Five additional centers reported nonsignificant positive associations, Stanford reported a positive association in only one of three studies, and 10 centers failed to report sufficient data on this variable to assess its effect.

Exercise-Induced Angina

Only 5 of 24 centers reported exercise test–induced angina to indicate a significantly increased risk group. Eight centers failed to report angina data. Seven of the remaining 11 reported nonsignificant positive associations.

Systolic Blood Pressure Response to Exercise

Nine of 24 centers found that inadequate or abnormal SBP response to exercise significantly identified a high-risk group; 11 of the centers failed to report data, and four of the remaining six reported a nonsignificant positive association.

> **Key Point:** The most consistent prognostic indicators from the exercise test in the post-MI patient include exercise capacity and the SBP response.

Clinical Design Features

Exercise Protocol   Bicycle protocols, especially a supine protocol, can give different responses than a treadmill. Most protocols were continuous, but some were not progressive in workload increments. The standard Bruce protocol was used in most studies, but the fact that it starts at a relatively high workload (5 METs) could result in a reduced exercise tolerance for some post-MI patients. The protocol, as well as beta blockade, fitness, and anxiety, can affect heart rate responses at submaximal levels.

Endpoints of Exercise Test   If the test is stopped at a certain amount of ST-segment shift, MET level, or heart rate, the response may not be appropriate to be considered as a continuous variable. In addition, higher values, which might be more discriminating, might not be reached.

ECG Leads Monitored   Use of different electrode placements can make comparisons between studies difficult, but probably does not have a great impact.

Time after MI When Exercise Test Was Performed   "Stunned" myocardium and deconditioning affect predischarge testing more than they affect hemodynamic responses later. ST-segment responses appear to be more labile early after MI. The responses differ at various times after MI as well, with a spontaneous improvement in hemodynamics occurring by 2 months. The spontaneous improvement in both ejection fraction and exercise capacity and their failure to correlate with each other makes them difficult to interpret. The studies that included exercise testing at multiple times found the same responses to have a different predictive value depending on the specific times when the tests were performed. There is a spontaneous improvement during the first year after MI in the blunted blood pressure response to exercise that occurs particularly in large anterior MIs.

Q-Wave Location Different MI locations affect prognosis differently, and have a different "normal" response to exercise. Exercise predictors may be different in each type of MI.

Inclusion of Non–Q-Wave MIs After much controversy regarding the risk of having a "subendocardial" MI, a study from Mayo Clinic appears to clarify the situation.[31] From 1960 to 1979, 1221 residents of Rochester, Minnesota, had an MI as the first manifestation of CHD; 784 had a transmural (Q-wave) MI and 353 had a non–Q-wave MI. The 30-day fatality rate was 18% among transmural MIs and 9% among subendocardial MIs. No significant difference was found in the rates of reinfarction, CABS, or mortality over the next 5 years. HF was more common among patients with transmural MIs, and angina was more common among patients with non–Q-wave MIs. This review and other data support the concept that ST depression at rest and with exercise effectively stratifies patients after non–Q-wave MI. This group is now considered in the ACS category with unstable angina requiring antiplatelet agents rather than thrombolysis.

The failure of exercise-induced ST-segment depression to consistently be associated with increased risk in patients after MI has been hard to explain. This failure could be a result of population differences and the resting ECG. To test this, we studied 198 men who survived an MI, underwent a submaximal predischarge treadmill test, and were followed for cardiac events for 2 years.[32] Abnormal ST-segment depression was associated with twice the risk for death, and the risk increased to 11 times in patients without diagnostic Q waves, similar to the results obtained by Krone and colleagues[33] in patients with an initial non–Q-wave MI. These results suggest that the difference in the prognostic value of the post-MI exercise ECG between studies is due to variations in the prevalence of the patterns of the resting ECG among study populations. Angiographic studies, however, have demonstrated that exercise-induced ST depression is associated with severe coronary artery disease whether or not Q waves are present. The conflicting results from follow-up and angiographic studies most probably relate to the fact that early mortality is strongly associated with left ventricular damage whereas later mortality is associated with ischemia and severe coronary artery disease.

Thoroughness and Length of Follow-up Patients lost to follow-up most likely have a higher percentage of deaths. Also, follow-up affects the analysis if censored data cannot be handled adequately with the statistical program. Mortality changes over time, and predictors change.

Percentage of Patients Undergoing CABS (or PCI) during Follow-up CABS could alter mortality and affect outcome prediction. Also, patients with ischemic predictors would be selected to have this procedure more frequently. These patients should be censored at the time of the intervention, but such censoring should not be random.

Cardiac Events Considered as Endpoints   The only hard endpoints that should be considered, from an epidemiologic point of view, are death and reinfarction. Separation or distinction of sudden death makes little sense and may confuse the analysis, particularly if those with sudden death are compared with all others (including nonsudden cardiac death). Noncardiac deaths are often difficult to distinguish and lead to biased results but may play a confusing role, particularly in older populations. CABS and PCI are not valid endpoints and should be considered as a censored outcome; it is clearly related to certain exercise test results that physicians feel motivated to "fix" with that procedure. "Instability" or progression of symptoms (HF or angina) is a soft endpoint that should not be used for epidemiologic purposes.

Mortality Rate during Follow-up   If there is a low mortality rate, more patients are needed to find a statistical difference between those with or without certain variables. Some studies have compensated for this by using soft endpoints and combining endpoints.

Prior MI Patients Included or Not   Prior MI is an important predictive variable that depends on the severity of the prior MI or MIs. Patients with prior large MIs are biased toward being admitted with non–Q-wave MIs because another transmural MI increases their likelihood of dying before hospitalization. Few studies have accounted for the number or severity of prior MIs.

Exclusion Criteria   Clearly, clinical judgment applied to the post-MI population to exclude patients from exercise testing identifies the highest risk group.

Age Range and Gender   Women are thought to have a higher MI mortality risk and are known to respond differently than men to exercise testing. Because of this they should be considered separately, but the studies do not contain a sufficient number for valid analysis. Death rates are directly related to age.

Medications Taken after Discharge from Hospital and at the Time of the Test   Digoxin causes ST depression, but it is usually taken for HF, thus implicating an ischemic etiology for potential death due to dysfunction. Digoxin administration after MI may actually be an independent risk predictor and act by predisposing to ventricular dysrhythmias. Beta blockers affect blood pressure and heart rate responses and improve survival but do not seem to affect the value of the exercise test.[34-36] Although beta-adrenergic blockade attenuates the ischemic response, two long-term follow-up studies have demonstrated that these agents do not interfere with poor exercise capacity as a marker of adverse prognosis.[37,38] Patients taking beta blockers after MI should continue to do so at the time of exercise testing. Because patients will be taking these medications for an indefinite period after infarction, the exercise test response while on beta blockers would provide information regarding the adequacy of medical therapy in preventing ischemia and arrhythmias, as well as controlling the heart rate and blood pressure response during exercise. Moreover, discontinuation of beta blockers solely for the purpose of exercise testing may expose the patient to the unnecessary risks of recurrent ischemia, arrhythmia, and exaggerated hemodynamic responses during exercise.

Later Studies

Two studies from the pre-thrombolytic era were not included in our meta-analysis because they were only reported after a long follow-up period. Between 1979 and 1983, 1773 consecutive patients were admitted to Glostrup County Hospital in Denmark with an acute MI. Of 1430 patients who were alive after 3 weeks, 718 performed an exercise test.[39] Survival data were available after 15 years for all patients. Performing an exercise test was associated with a mortality reduction of one half when adjusting for known differences between the groups. Among patients who performed the test, most indicators of ischemia were without prognostic information. Exercise capacity was the best predictor of future mortality. Only ST-segment depression of 2 mm or more could identify a population with an increased risk of death. In the United Kingdom, 255 consecutive patients (210 men) age 55 years or less (mean 48 years) admitted to hospital for an MI (1981–1985) were eligible.[40] Of these, 150 patients (130 men) were able to undergo an exercise test and coronary angiography within 6 months; they were followed up for up to 15 years. Survival at a median of 16 years was 52% for the whole cohort, 62% for the study group, and 48% for the excluded group. From 9 years onward survival deteriorated significantly in the study group compared with an age-matched control population. Fifteen years after MI, 121 patients (81%) in the study group had had at least one cardiovascular event, leaving 29 (19%) event free. The number of diseased vessels was the major determinant of time to first event and event-free survival, but exercise capacity was also important in the prediction of time to first event.

Duke Meta-Analysis of Stress Testing Modalities after Acute Myocardial Infarction

The previously described meta-analysis summarizes the experience in the pre-thrombolytic era; an excellent report from Duke presents a meta-analysis of the exercise ECG, stress myocardial perfusion imaging, and stress ventricular function imaging reports published from 1980 to 1995.[41] The study's authors described the predictive values of ECG, radionuclide, and echocardiographic markers for cardiac death or nonfatal MI.

Quality Assessment

Study quality was evaluated (independent of outcome assessment) according to criteria defined within the heart failure guidelines revised for use with noninvasive testing literature.[42] Specific methodologic flaws included the following: (1) patient selection: nonconsecutive or referral patient series; (2) study administration: providing a limited description of the testing protocol and abnormal test/image interpretation criteria; (3) withdrawals/dropouts: no description of patient loss during follow-up or a low follow-up rate; (4) outcome measurements: use of combined "hard" and "soft" endpoints, including recurrent angina or coronary surgery or less than 2-month duration of follow-up; and (5) statistical analysis: no attempt to control for or stratify by significant confounding variables. Of the initial 115 articles identified by literature review, the Duke investigators rejected 53%.

Summary Odds Ratio for Cardiac Death and Death or Reinfarction

Exercise ECG   The summary odds ratio (OR) for cardiac death was significantly higher for patients with 1 mm of ST depression (OR 2), impaired systolic blood pressure (OR 4), or limited exercise capacity (OR 4). A similar pattern was noted for the combined endpoint. Although not as predictive of cardiac death, exercise-induced chest pain did better predicting death or reinfarction (OR 2).

Exercise and Pharmacologic Stress Myocardial Perfusion Imaging   Among the 1247 patients who underwent exercise myocardial perfusion imaging, the occurrence of a reversible defect (either within or remote from the infarction site) was associated with a 1-year cardiac death rate of 7.1% and a death or nonfatal MI rate of 15.8%. Similar rates were reported for multiple perfusion defects. For a reversible perfusion defect, the summary odds of cardiac death were 3 and, for death or reinfarction, 4.

For pharmacologic stress perfusion imaging, the summary OR for cardiac death with a reversible perfusion defect was only 1.2 times higher. Patients who had a dipyridamole-induced reversible perfusion defect had a two-times higher risk of 1-year cardiac death or MI.

Exercise and Pharmacologic Ventricular Function Imaging   Rates of cardiac death (27%) and combined events (31%) were highest for patients who had a peak exercise ejection fraction < 40%. Summary ORs of cardiac death were 3.2, 4.2, and 1.2 times for ejection fraction < 40%, ejection fraction change <5%, and a new echocardiographic wall motion abnormality, respectively. For the same markers, summary ORs of cardiac death or MI were 4.4, 3.6, and 1.7 times higher. Rates of cardiac events were lower (5.4% to 8.4%) for patients with a pharmacologically induced new or worsening wall motion abnormality.

Comparative Predictive Value in the Thrombolytic Era
The average cardiac death rates were lower in studies including thrombolytic-treated patients than in those that did not (4% vs. 7%). Positive predictive values were usually decreased in patients receiving thrombolytic therapy.

Effect of Low Prevalence (e.g., the Reperfusion Era)   The positive predictive values of noninvasive risk markers for cardiac death and combined cardiac death or nonfatal MI are low in studies with low mortality rates. The therapy clinicians apply as a result of an abnormal predischarge test should subsequently lower a patient's posttest likelihood for events. A significant proportion of acute MI survivors have single-vessel disease and, even with an abnormal test for ischemia, have a good prognosis, making prediction difficult. This can be seen in cohorts where sensitivity is high but specificity is low. An example of lower positive predictive values in lower-risk groups was observed in reports of patients treated with thrombolytics. Predischarge testing after reperfusion therapy may have a limited predictive value for several reasons. Successful reperfusion results in less myocardial damage and may leave patients with nonsignificant angiographic lesions and a negative stress test who still have an increased likelihood of reinfarction. Additionally, patients who receive thrombolytic agents are generally lower risk than other post-MI patients because they are younger and less likely to have complicating illnesses.

The Duke researchers observed little improvement in the quality of the data since our similar meta-analysis published 10 years earlier.[43]

Key Point: The Duke scholarly meta-analysis provides the best synopsis of the knowledge regarding noninvasive stress testing for risk stratification after MI.

The Reperfusion Era

Contemporary management of the patient with acute MI includes one or more of the following: medical therapy, thrombolytic agents, and coronary revascularization. The first striking improvement in survival in all subsets is with beta blockers (25% reduction in the first year after MI). The next dramatic change in treatment of patients with acute MI was the broad use of thrombolytic therapy beginning in 1988. Equally important has been the widespread use of aspirin, beta-adrenergic blocking agents, and vasodilator therapy; common use of angiotensin-converting enzyme (ACE) inhibitors; and a far more aggressive use of revascularization therapy in patients who have clinical markers of a poor prognosis. It is this constellation of new therapies and not solely the administration of thrombolytic therapy that marks what is generally referred to as the "reperfusion era." This period has witnessed an impressive reduction in early and 1-year mortality rates for acute MI patients, which is particularly striking in patients who have received thrombolytic therapy and revascularization during hospitalization. The 1990s brought the widespread application of cardiac catheterization, largely negating the use of the exercise test to select patients for this procedure as had been the situation earlier. Currently, the evidence supports the use of angiography when possible instead of thrombolysis and even "facilitated" PCI where thrombolysis is only used to hold the patient until angiography is possible. In any circumstance, once the coronary arteries are visualized it is hard for the angiographer not to open closed arteries with drug-eluting stents. CABS remains only for patients with difficult lesions. The majority of patients recover from their MI with minimal loss of myocardium and reperfused myocardium as well. Thus the exercise test plays a different role than it did in the past.

Shorter hospital stays, widespread use of thrombolytic agents, greater use of revascularization strategies, implantable cardiac defibrillators, and increased use of beta-adrenergic blocking agents and ACE inhibitors or angiotensin-receptor blockers continue to change the clinical presentation of the post-MI patient. Not all patients will have received each of these various therapies; hence survivors of MI are quite heterogeneous. The Canadian Assessment of Myocardial Infarction (CAMI) study reported that among 3178 consecutive patients with acute MI, 45% received thrombolytic agents, 20% underwent PCI, and 8% had CABS.[44] Medications at the time of hospital discharge included beta blockers in 61%, ACE inhibitors in 24%, and aspirin in 86%.

Whereas exercise testing was helpful in the management of post-MI patients in the prethrombolytic era, the impact of thrombolytic therapies over the past decade has decreased the value of exercise testing.[45] The GISSI-2 database has enabled reevaluation of the prognostic role of exercise testing in patients who have received thrombolysis.[46] Exercise tests were performed on 6296 patients at an average of 28 days after randomization for thrombolysis after MI. The test was not performed on 3923 patients (40%) because of contraindications. The test was positive for ischemia in 26% of the patients, negative in 38%, and nondiagnostic in 36%. Among the patients with an ischemic test result, 33% had symptoms, whereas 67% had silent myocardial ischemia. The mortality rate was 7.1% among patients who did not have an exercise test and 1.7% for those with an ischemic test, 0.9% for those who had a normal test, and 1.3% for those with nondiagnostic tests. In an adjusted analysis, symptomatic ischemia, ischemia at a submaximal work load, low work capacity, and abnormal SBP were independent predictors of 6-month mortality risk (relative risks of 2 times for each). However, when these variables were considered simultaneously, only symptomatic induced ischemia and low work capacity were confirmed as independent predictors of mortality (Cox hazard ratio of 2 and 1.8, respectively). The Gruppo Italiano per lo Studio della Sopravvivenza nell' Infarto Miocardio (GISSI) investigators concluded that patients with a normal exercise response have an excellent medium-term prognosis and do not need further investigation as shown by others.[47] However, evaluation must be directed to the patients who cannot undergo exercise testing because the mortality rate was five to seven times greater in that group. The GISSI-2 researchers calculated the Duke Treadmill Score (DTS) and the Veterans Affairs Medical Centers Score (VAMCS) for each patient and used coefficients of a multivariate analysis to develop a simple predictive scoring system.[48] Six-month mortality rates in the subgroups of each scoring system were as follows: DTS— low risk 0.6%, moderate risk 1.8%, high risk 3.4%; VAMCS—low risk 0.6%, moderate risk 2%, high risk 5%; GISSI-2 Index—low risk 0.5%, moderate risk 2%, high risk 6%. The results of multivariate analysis were as follows: DTS— moderate risk 2.5 times, high risk 5 times; VAMCS—moderate risk 3 times, high risk 6 times; GISSI-2 Index—moderate risk 3 times, high risk 9 times.

The prognosis among survivors of MI continues to improve as newer treatment strategies are applied. The 1-year postdischarge mortality rate in the

CAMI study was 8.4%, and was distinctly lower in the 45% of patients who received thrombolytic therapy (4% mortality rate) and in the 28% who underwent coronary angioplasty (3% mortality rate) or coronary artery bypass surgery (3.7% mortality rate).[49] Data from the Global Utilization of Streptokinase and Tissue Plasminogen Activator for Occluded Coronary Arteries (GUSTO) trial demonstrate that 57% of the 41,021 patients who received thrombolytic therapy were uncomplicated (no recurrent ischemia, reinfarction, HF, stroke, or invasive procedures) at 4 days after MI.[50] The mortality rate at 1 month was 1% and at 1 year was 3.6%. Recurrent ischemia occurred in 7% of this group. These and other data from large thrombolytic trials demonstrate that those patients unable to perform an exercise test have the highest adverse cardiac event rate, whereas uncomplicated stable patients have a low cardiac event rate even before undergoing further risk assessment by exercise testing.[51,52]

In the second Danish trial in acute MI (DANAMI-2) study, patients with ST-elevation acute MI (STEMI) were randomized to PCI or fibrinolysis.[53] Of 1462 patients discharged alive, 80% performed an exercise test. Primary endpoint was a composite of death and reinfarction. Patients randomized to fibrinolysis developed ST depression to a greater extent than patients randomized to primary PCI (22% vs. 15%). Multivariable predictors of death and reinfarction included age, gender, diabetes, previous stroke, anterior acute MI, randomization to fibrinolysis, and exercise capacity. Exercise-induced ST depression was predictive of the clinical outcome in the fibrinolysis group (twofold relative risk) but not in the primary PCI group. Thus exercise testing after contemporary reperfusion therapies for STEMI confers important prognostic information. Exercise capacity is a strong prognostic predictor of death and reinfarction irrespective of treatment strategy, whereas the prognostic significance of ST depression seems to be strongest in the fibrinolysis-treated patients (probably because of more residual ischemia than with PCI).

> **Key Point:** Two meta-analyses of 30 studies including over 20,000 patients found that exercise capacity and abnormal SBP response were more predictive of adverse cardiac events after MI than measures of exercise-induced ischemia. Although the majority of the studies included were performed before the reperfusion era, similar results were found in the GISSI report that considered 6000 patients who received thrombolysis.

Activity Counseling

Exercise testing after MI is useful in counseling patients and their families regarding domestic, recreational, and occupational activities that can be safely performed after hospital discharge. Exercise capacity in METs derived from the exercise test can be applied to estimate an individual's tolerance for specific activities. Published charts that estimate energy requirements of various activities are available,[54] but should be used only as a guide, realizing that the intensity at which activities performed will directly influence the amount of energy required. Most domestic chores and activities require less than 5 METs, hence a submaximal test at the time of hospital discharge can be useful in counseling regarding the first several weeks after MI.

Follow-up symptom-limited testing performed at 3 to 6 weeks after MI can assist in further activity prescription and issues regarding return to work. Most occupational activities require less than 5 METs. In the 15% of individuals in the workforce whose work involves heavy manual labor,[55] the exercise test data should not be used as the sole criterion for recommendations regarding return to work. Energy demands of lifting heavy objects, temperature, environmental stressors, and psychologic stresses are not assessed by routine exercise tests and must be taken into consideration. In patients with low exercise capacity, left ventricular dysfunction, or exercise-induced ischemia, and those who are otherwise apprehensive about returning to a physically demanding occupation, simulated work tests can be performed.[56,57]

Exercise testing is essential in the development of the exercise prescription to establish a safe and effective training intensity for cardiac rehabilitation, for risk stratification of patients to determine the level of supervision and monitoring required during exercise training sessions, and in evaluation of training program outcome.[58] For these reasons, symptom-limited exercise testing before program initiation is needed for all patients in whom cardiac rehabilitation is recommended (recent MI, recent CABS, recent coronary angioplasty, chronic stable angina, controlled HF).[59] Although there are no available studies to assess its value, the stable cardiac patient who continues an exercise training program should have an exercise test performed after the initial 8 to 12 weeks of exercise training and at least yearly thereafter, or sooner as needed depending on changes in symptoms or medications that may affect the exercise prescription.

> **Key Point:** Exercise testing as part of cardiac rehabilitation is useful to develop the exercise prescription, evaluate improvement in exercise capacity, and provide feedback to the patient.

Summary

The benefits of performing an exercise test in post-MI patients are listed in Table 8-3. Submitting patients to exercise testing can expedite and optimize their discharge from the hospital. The patient's response to exercise, work capacity, and limiting factors at the time of discharge can be assessed by the exercise test. An exercise test before discharge is important for giving patients guidelines for exercise at home, reassuring them of their physical status, and determining the risk of complications. It provides a safe basis for advising the patient to resume or increase his or her activity level and return to work. The test can demonstrate to the patient, relatives, or employer the effect of the MI on the capacity for physical performance. Psychologically, it can cause an improvement in the patient's self-confidence by making the patient less anxious about daily physical activities. The test has been helpful in reassuring spouses of post-MI patients of their physical capabilities. The psychologic impact of simply performing the test can be important for many patients. Many patients increase their activity and actually rehabilitate themselves after being encouraged and reassured by their response to this test.

TABLE 8-3   Benefits of Exercise Testing after Myocardial Infarction

Predischarge Submaximal Test
Setting safe exercise levels (exercise prescription)
Optimizing discharge
Altering medical therapy
Triaging for intensity of follow-up
First step in rehabilitation—assurance, encouragement
Reassuring spouse
Recognizing exercise-induced ischemia and dysrhythmias

Maximal Test for Return to Normal Activities
Determining limitations
Prognostication
Reassuring employers
Determining level of disability
Triaging for invasive studies
Deciding on medications
Exercise prescription
Continued rehabilitation

Exercise testing is also useful in activity counseling after hospital discharge. It is also an important tool in exercise training as part of comprehensive cardiac rehabilitation, where it can be used to develop and modify the exercise prescription, assist in providing activity counseling, and assess the patient's response at the initiation of, and progress in, the exercise training program.

One consistent finding in the review of the post-MI exercise test studies that included a follow-up for cardiac endpoints is that patients who met whatever criteria set forth for exercise testing were at lower risk than patients not tested. This finding supports the clinical judgment of the skilled clinician. In the complete data set from the review, only an abnormal SBP response and a low exercise capacity were consistently associated with a poor outcome.

Two meta-analyses found that exercise incapacity and abnormal SBP response were more predictive of adverse cardiac events after MI than measures of exercise-induced ischemia. Although the majority of the studies included were performed before the reperfusion era, similar results were found in the GISSI report that considered 6000 patients who received thrombolysis. Thus the exercise test remains an important tool in the evaluation of patients following an MI.

References

1. Hunink MG et al: The recent decline in mortality from coronary heart disease, 1980-1990. The effect of secular trends in risk factors and treatment, *JAMA* 277(7):535-542, 1997.
2. Braunwald E et al, American College of Cardiology, American Heart Association, Committee on the Management of Patients with Unstable Angina: ACC/AHA 2002 guideline update for the management of patients

with unstable angina and non–ST-segment elevation myocardial infarction—summary article: a report of the American College of Cardiology/American Heart Association Task Force on Practice Guidelines (Committee on the Management of Patients with Unstable Angina), *J Am Coll Cardiol* 40(7):1366-1374, 2002.

3. Arciero TJ et al: Temporal trends in the incidence of coronary disease, *Am J Med* 117(4):228-233, 2004.

4. Goldman L et al: The effect of risk factor reductions between 1981 and 1990 on coronary heart disease incidence, prevalence, mortality and cost, *J Am Coll Cardiol* 38(4):1012-1017, 2001.

5. Dargie H: Myocardial infarction: redefined or reinvented? *Heart* 88(1): 1-3, 2002.

6. Dalby M, Bouzamondo A, Lechat P, Montalescot G: Transfer for primary angioplasty versus immediate thrombolysis in acute myocardial infarction: a meta-analysis, *Circulation* 108(15):1809-1814, 2003.

7. American College of Physicians: Guidelines for risk stratification after myocardial infarction, *Ann Intern Med* 126(7):556-560, 1997.

8. Cucherat M, Bonnefoy E, Tremeau G: Primary angioplasty versus intravenous thrombolysis for acute myocardial infarction, *Cochrane Database Syst Rev* 3:CD001560, 2003.

9. Heggunje PS et al: Procedural success versus clinical risk status in determining discharge of patients after primary angioplasty for acute myocardial infarction, *J Am Coll Cardiol* 44(7):1400-1407, 2004.

10. Gibbons RJ et al: ACC/AHA guidelines for exercise testing. A report of the American College of Cardiology/American Heart Association Task Force on Practice Guidelines (Committee on Exercise Testing), *J Am Coll Cardiol* 30(1):260-311, 1997.

11. Antman EM et al, American College of Cardiology, American Heart Association, Canadian Cardiovascular Society: ACC/AHA guidelines for the management of patients with ST-elevation myocardial infarction—executive summary. A report of the American College of Cardiology/American Heart Association Task Force on Practice Guidelines (writing committee to revise the 1999 guidelines for the management of patients with acute myocardial infarction), *J Am Coll Cardiol* 44(3):671-719, 2004.

12. Juneau M et al: Symptom-limited versus low level exercise testing before hospital discharge after myocardial infarction, *J Am Coll Cardiol* 20: 927-933, 1992.

13. Hamm LF, Crow RS, Stull A, Hannan P: Safety and characteristics of exercise testing early after myocardial infarction, *Am J Cardiol* 63: 1193-1197, 1989.

14. Jain A, Myers GH, Sapin PM, O'Rourke RA: Comparison of symptom-limited and low level exercise tolerance tests early after myocardial infarction, *J Am Coll Cardiol* 22:1816-1820, 1993.

15. Castellanet MJ, Greenberg PS, Ellestad MH: Comparison of S-T segment changes on exercise testing with angiographic findings in patients with prior myocardial infarction, *Am J Cardiol* 42:29-35, 1978.

16. Ahnve S et al: Can ischemia be recognized when Q waves are present on the resting electrocardiogram? *Am Heart J* 110:1016-1020, 1986.

17. Miranda C et al: Post MI exercise testing: non Q wave vs Q wave, *Circulation* 84:2357-2365, 1991.
18. Weiner DA: Prognostic value of exercise testing early after myocardial infarction, *J Cardiac Rehab* 3:114-122, 1983.
19. Paine TD et al: Relation of graded exercise test findings after myocardial infarction to extent of coronary artery disease and left ventricular dysfunction, *Am J Cardiol* 42:716-723, 1978.
20. Dillahunt PH, Miller AB: Early treadmill testing after myocardial infarction, *Chest* 76:150-155, 1979.
21. Boschat J et al: Treadmill exercise testing and coronary cineangiography following first myocardial infarction, *J Cardiac Rehab* 1:206-211, 1981.
22. Schwartz KM et al: Limited exercise testing soon after myocardial infarction. Correlation with early coronary and left ventricular angiography, *Ann Intern Med* 94:727-734, 1981.
23. Starling MR, Crawford MH, Richards KL, O'Rourke RA: Predictive value of early postmyocardial infarction modified treadmill exercise testing in multivessel coronary artery disease detection, *Am Heart J* 102:169-175, 1981.
24. De Feyter PJ, van den Brand M, Serruys PW, Wijns W: Early angiography after myocardial infarction: what have we learned? *Am Heart J* 109:194-199, 1985.
25. Froelicher VF, Perdue S, Pewen W, Risch M: Application of meta-analysis using an electronic spreadsheet to exercise testing in patients with myocardial infarction, *Am J Med* 83:1045-1054, 1987.
26. Sammel NL et al: Angiocardiography and exercise testing at one month after a first myocardial infarction, *Aust NZ J Med* 10:182-187, 1980.
27. Fuller CM et al: Early post-myocardial infarction treadmill stress testing. An accurate predictor of multivessel coronary disease and subsequent cardiac events, *Ann Intern Med* 94:734-739, 1981.
28. van der Wall EE et al: Thallium-201 exercise testing in patients 6-8 weeks after myocardial infarction: limited value for the detection of multivessel disease, *Eur Heart J* 6(1):29-36, 1985.
29. Akhras F et al: Early exercise testing and elective coronary artery bypass surgery after uncomplicated myocardial infarction. Effect on morbidity and mortality, *Br Heart J* 52(4):413-417, 1984.
30. Morris DD et al: Noninvasive prediction of the angiographic extent of coronary artery disease after myocardial infarction: comparison of clinical, bicycle exercise electrocardiographic, and ventriculographic parameters, *Circulation* 70(2):192-201, 1984.
31. Connolly DC, Elveback LR: Coronary heart disease in residents of Rochester, Minnesota. VI. Hospital and posthospital course of patients with transmural and subendocardial myocardial infarction, *Mayo Clin Proc* 60:375-381, 1985.
32. Klein J et al: Does the resting electrocardiogram after myocardial infarction determine the predictive value of exercise-induced ST depression? A two year follow-up in a veteran population, *J Am Coll Cardiol* 14:305-311, 1989.

33. Krone R et al: Risk stratification in patients with first non–Q wave infarction: limited value of the early low level exercise test after uncomplicated infarcts, *J Am Coll Cardiol* 14:31-37, 1989.
34. Ades PA et al: Effect of metoprolol on the submaximal stress test performed early after acute myocardial infarction, *Am J Cardiol* 60:963-966, 1987.
35. Curtis JL et al: Propranolol therapy alters estimation of potential cardiovascular risk derived from submaximal postinfarction exercise testing, *Am Heart J* 121:1655-1664, 1991.
36. Krone RJ, Miller JP, Gillespie JA, Weld FM, Multicenter Post-infarction Research Group: Usefulness of low level exercise testing early after acute myocardial infarction in patients taking beta blocking agents, *Am J Cardiol* 60:23-27, 1987.
37. Ronnevik PK, VonderLippe G: Prognostic importance of predischarge exercise capacity for long term mortality and nonfatal myocardial infarction in patients admitted for suspected acute myocardial infarction and treated with metoprolol, *Eur Heart J* 13:1468-1472, 1992.
38. Murray DP et al: Does beta adrenergic blockade influence the prognostic implications of post–myocardial infarction exercise testing? *Br Heart J* 60:474-479, 1988.
39. Dominguez H, Torp-Pedersen C, Koeber L, Rask-Madsen C: Prognostic value of exercise testing in a cohort of patients followed for 15 years after acute myocardial infarction, *Eur Heart J* 22(4):300-306, 2001.
40. Awad-Elkarim AA et al: A prospective study of long term prognosis in young myocardial infarction survivors: the prognostic value of angiography and exercise testing, *Heart* 89(8):843-847, 2003.
41. Shaw LJ et al: A metaanalysis of predischarge risk stratification after acute myocardial infarction with stress electrocardiographic, myocardial perfusion, and ventricular function imaging, *Am J Cardiol* 78(12): 1327-1337, 1996.
42. Baker DW et al: Management of heart failure. III. The role of revascularization in the treatment of patients with moderate or severe left ventricular systolic dysfunction, *JAMA* 272:1528-1534, 1994.
43. Chalmers TC: Problems induced by meta-analyses, *Stat Med* 10:971-979, 1991.
44. Rouleau JL et al: Myocardial infarction patients in the 1990's—their risk factors, stratification and survival in Canada: the Canadian Assessment of Myocardial Infarction (CAMI) study, *J Am Coll Cardiol* 27:1119-1127, 1996.
45. Stevenson R et al: Reassessment of treadmill stress testing for risk stratification in patients with acute myocardial infarction treated by thrombolysis, *Br Heart J* 70:415-420, 1993.
46. Villella A et al: Prognostic significance of maximal exercise testing after myocardial infarction treated with thrombolytic agents: the GISSI-2 data-base, *Lancet* 346(8974):523-529, 1995.
47. Piccalo G et al: Value of negative predischarge exercise testing in identifying patients at low risk after acute myocardial infarction treated by systemic thrombolysis, *Am J Cardiol* 70:31-33, 1992.
48. Villella M et al: Ergometric score systems after myocardial infarction: prognostic performance of the Duke Treadmill Score, Veterans

Administration Medical Center Score, and of a novel score system, GISSI-2 Index, in a cohort of survivors of acute myocardial infarction, *Am Heart J* 145(3):475-483, 2003.

49. Rouleau JL et al: Myocardial infarction patients in the 1990's—their risk factors, stratification and survival in Canada: the Canadian Assessment of Myocardial Infarction (CAMI) study, *J Am Coll Cardiol* 27:1119-1127, 1996.

50. Newby LK et al: Early discharge in the thrombolytic era: an analysis of criteria for uncomplicated infarctions from the GUSTO trial, *J Am Coll Cardiol* 27:625-632, 1996.

51. Chaitman BR et al: Impact of treatment strategy on predischarge exercise tests in the Thrombolysis in Myocardial Infarction (TIMI) II trial, *Am J Cardiol* 71:131-138, 1993.

52. Volpi A et al: Predictors of nonfatal reinfarction in survivals of myocardial infarction after thrombolysis. Results of the GISSI-2 database, *J Am Coll Cardiol* 24:608-615, 1994.

53. Valeur N et al: The prognostic value of pre-discharge exercise testing after myocardial infarction treated with either primary PCI or fibrinolysis: a DANAMI-2 sub-study, *Eur Heart J* 26(2):119-127, 2005.

54. Fletcher GF et al: American Heart Association exercise standards, *Circulation* 91:580-615, 1995.

55. US Department of Health and Human Services: *Clinical practice guideline #17: cardiac rehabilitation,* Agency for Health Care Policy and Research (AHCPR) pub no 96-0672, 1995 Washington, DC.

56. Wilke NA et al: Baltimore Therapeutic Equipment work simulator: energy expenditure of work activities in cardiac patients, *Arch Phys Med Rehabil* 74:419-424, 1993.

57. Sheldahl LM, Wilke NA, Tristani FE: Exercise prescription for return to work, *J Cardiopulm Rehabil* 5:567-575, 1985.

58. Balady GJ et al: American Heart Association scientific statement: cardiac rehabilitation programs, *Circulation* 90:1602-1610, 1994.

59. American College of Sports Medicine: *Guidelines for exercise testing and prescription,* Philadelphia, 1995, Williams & Wilkins.

9   Screening Apparently Healthy Individuals

Introduction

Definition of Screening

Screening can be defined as the presumptive identification of unrecognized disease by the utilization of procedures that can be applied rapidly. The relative value of techniques for identifying individuals who have asymptomatic or latent coronary heart disease (CHD) should be assessed to optimally and cost-effectively direct secondary preventive efforts toward those with disease.

Criteria for Selecting a Screening Procedure

Eight criteria have been proposed for the selection of a screening procedure:

1. The procedure is acceptable and appropriate.
2. The quantity or quality of life can be favorably altered.
3. The results of intervention outweigh any adverse effects.
4. The target disease has an asymptomatic period during which its outcome can be altered.
5. Acceptable treatments are available.
6. The prevalence and seriousness of the disease justify the costs of intervention.
7. The procedure is relatively easy and inexpensive.
8. Sufficient resources are available.

Guides for Deciding if Screening Should Be Performed

In addition, seven guides have been recommended for deciding whether a community screening program does more harm than good:

1. Has the program's effectiveness been demonstrated in a randomized trial?
2. If the program's effectiveness has been demonstrated in a randomized trial, are efficacious treatments available?
3. Does the current burden of suffering warrant screening?
4. Is there a good screening test?
5. Does the program reach those who could benefit from it?
6. Can the health care system cope with the screening program?
7. Will those who had a positive screening comply with subsequent advice and interventions?

> **Key Point:** The above list should be considered before implementing a screening program.

Screening Efficacy

These criteria will be considered and questions will be addressed relative to the exercise test in this chapter. However, true demonstration of the effectiveness of a screening technique requires randomizing the target population, with half receiving the screening technique, standardized action taken in response to the screening test results, and then outcomes assessed. For the screening technique to be effective, the screened group must have lower mortality or morbidity rates than a nonscreened group. Such a study has been completed for mammography but not for any cardiac testing modalities. The next best validation of efficacy is to demonstrate that the technique improves the discrimination of those asymptomatic individuals with higher risk for events over that possible with the available risk factors. Mathematical modeling makes it possible to determine how well a population will be classified if the characteristics of the testing method are known.

> **Key Point:** The proof of a preventive strategy requires a randomized trial of the screening technique resulting in a better outcome in those screened than in the control group.

Prevention of Coronary Artery Disease

Risk Factor Scores

Targeting asymptomatic individuals with early disease could facilitate the process of primary prevention of coronary heart disease. Thus it is advisable to evaluate screening methods for detection of coronary artery disease (CAD) before the occurrence of cardiac events. For a screening test to be worth the additional expense, it must add significantly to the ability of the standard risk factors to identify asymptomatic individuals with subclinical disease. The method with which the risk is estimated using established risk factors must also be considered for such a comparison. Simply adding risk factors, as recommended by JNC or NCEP, is not as accurate as using logistic regression equations such as those developed from the Framingham data.[1] In an asymptomatic population, the Framingham score calculates an estimate of the 5-year incidence of cardiovascular (CV) events using age, smoking, diabetes, standing systolic blood pressure, electrocardiographic–left ventricular hypertrophy (ECG-LVH), and the levels of high-density lipoprotein (HDL) and total cholesterol (TC).[2] The most recent version of the Framingham score removed ECG-LVH because its prevalence has declined with the improved treatment of blood pressure.[3]

The Framingham group evaluated its risk score, designed to estimate the 10-year risk of CHD. The score was assessed to see if it also predicted lifetime risk for CHD.[4] At 40 years old, in risk score tertiles 1, 2, and 3, respectively, the lifetime risks for CHD were 38%, 42%, and 51% for men and 12%, 25%, and 33% for women. At 80 years old, risks were 16%, 17%, and 39% for men and 13%, 22%, and 27% for women. The Framingham Risk Score stratified lifetime risk well for women at all ages. It performed less well in younger men but improved at older ages as remaining life expectancy approached 10 years. Lifetime risks contrasted sharply with shorter-term risks: at 40 years old, the 10-year risks of CHD in tertiles 1, 2, and 3, respectively, were 0%, 2%, and 12% for men and 0%, 0.7%, and 2% for women. The Framingham 10-year CHD risk prediction model discriminated short-term risk well for men and women. However, it may not identify subjects with low short-term but high lifetime risk for CHD, probably because of changes in risk factor status over time. The serial use of multivariate risk models is most likely the only way to reliably predict lifetime risk for CHD; the Framingham score can also be calculated yearly as a motivational tool to keep patients aware of their risk factor status.

Baseline levels of C-reactive protein (CRP) were evaluated among 27,939 apparently healthy women who were followed for incidence of myocardial infarction (MI), stroke, coronary revascularization, or CV death.[5] Cardiovascular risks increased linearly from the very lowest (referent) to the very highest levels of CRP from 1 to 8 times. After adjustment for Framingham Risk Score, these risks trended from 1 to 3 times. Of the total cohort, 15% had CRP < 0.50 mg/L, and 5% had CRP > 10 mg/L. Whether lowering CRP with statins and aspirin lowers risk has not been demonstrated, but this marker can be used along with the Framingham score to screen for CAD risk.

The SCORE project was initiated to develop a risk scoring system for use in the clinical management of CV risk in European clinical practice that would be more appropriate for Europeans than the American population–derived Framingham score (www.escardio.org/initiatives/prevention/SCORE+Risk+Charts.htm).[6] The project assembled a pool of data sets from 12 European cohorts, mainly carried out in general population settings. There were 205,178 persons (one third women) representing 2.7 million person-years of follow-up. Predictive value of the risk charts was examined by applying them to persons age 45 to 64 years; areas under ROC curves ranged from 0.71 to 0.84.

Data from two population studies (the Glostrup Population Studies, $n = 4757$, and the Framingham Heart Study, $n = 2562$) were used to examine three different levels of cross-validation.[7] CHD mortality rate was 515 per 100,000 person-years in Framingham and 311 per 100,000 person-years in Glostrup. The ROC areas were between 0.75 and 0.77 regardless of which risk score was used. The Framingham Risk Score significantly overestimated risk in the Glostrup sample, and the Glostrup risk score underestimated risk in the Framingham sample. Thus using a Framingham Risk Score on a Danish population led to a significant overestimation of coronary risk. The validity of risk scores developed from populations with different incidences of the disease should preferably be tested before their application.

Non–Exercise Test Measurements

Other non–exercise test measurements that have been recommended as screening techniques include the resting ECG, cardiac fluoroscopy, digital radiographic imaging, carotid ultrasound measurements of intimal thickening, the ankle-brachial index, and electron beam computed tomography (EBCT). Various add-on techniques have been recommended to improve the diagnostic characteristics of exercise ECG testing. These include ECG criteria, other exercise test responses, nuclear perfusion, cardiokymography (CKG), echocardiography, and the computerized application of Bayesian statistics.

> **Key Point:** Simple scores are effective in stratifying the risk for CAD in healthy populations and should be the first approach to screening.

Test Performance

To evaluate the value of any screening test, sensitivity, specificity, predictive value, and relative risk must be demonstrated. Though discussed in depth elsewhere, these terms are presented here briefly. *Sensitivity* is the percentage of times a test gives an abnormal response when those with disease are tested. *Specificity* is the percentage of times a test gives a normal response when those without disease are tested—a definition quite different from the conventional use of the word "specific." These two values are inversely related and are determined by the discriminant values or cutpoints chosen for the test that separate abnormals from normals and the intrinsic ability of the test to separate those with disease from those without disease. The *predictive value* of an abnormal test is the percentage of individuals with an abnormal test who have disease. The *relative risk* or odds ratio of an abnormal test response is the relative chance of having disease if the test is abnormal compared to having disease if the test is normal. The values for all these terms depend on the prevalence of disease in the population being tested.

A basic step in applying any testing procedure for the separation of normal subjects from patients with a disease is to determine a test value that best separates the two groups. One problem is that there is usually a considerable overlap of measurement values of a test in the groups with and without disease. Consider two bell-shaped normal distribution curves, one representing a normal population and the other representing a population with disease, with a certain amount of overlap of the two curves (see Figure 5-1). Along the vertical axis is the number of patients and along the horizontal axis could be the value for such measurements as Q-wave size, exercise-induced ST-segment depression, or troponin. The optimal test would be able to achieve the most marked separation of these two bell-shaped curves and minimize the overlap. Unfortunately, most tests have a considerable overlap of the range of measurements for the normal population and for those with heart disease. Therefore problems arise when a certain value is used to separate these two groups (i.e., Q-wave amplitude or width, 0.1 mV of ST-segment depression, < 5 METs exercise capacity, three ventricular beats). If the value is set far to the right (i.e., 0.2 mV of ST-segment depression) in order to identify nearly all the normal subjects as being free of disease, the test will have a high specificity. However, a substantial number of those with disease will be called "normal." If a value is chosen far to the left (i.e., 0.05 mV of ST-segment depression) so that nearly all those with disease are identified as being abnormal, giving the test a high sensitivity, many normal subjects will be identified as abnormal. If a cutpoint value is chosen that equally mislabels the normal subjects and those with disease, the test will have its highest predictive accuracy.

However, there may be reasons for wanting to adjust a test to have a relatively higher sensitivity or relatively higher specificity than possible when predictive accuracy is optimal. For instance, sensitivity should be highest in the emergency department and specificity highest when doing insurance examinations. Again, sensitivity and specificity are inversely related. That is, when sensitivity is the highest, specificity is the lowest, and vice versa. Any test has a range of inversely related sensitivities and specificities that can be chosen by selecting a certain discriminant or diagnostic value.

Key Point: Scores and tests to identify those with or those who will develop CAD events have characteristics that can be used to compare their discriminatory ability. When the prevalence of disease is known in a target population, simple mathematics can be used to determine the predictive value and ratio of true positives to false positives.

The Resting Electrocardiogram as a Screening Technique

As part of the Copenhagen City Heart Study, nearly 20,000 men and women, 20 years of age or older, had a resting 12-lead ECG performed.[8] The prevalence of all ECG findings of significance was very low below age 40 in men and age 50 in women. Rates for abnormalities increased with age and were higher for men than for women. A strong association between total mortality rate and major ST depression and T-wave abnormalities, Q-wave patterns, and left bundle branch block (LBBB) existed. The relative risk of

ST-segment depression was as high as 5 times, and some Q-wave abnormalities carried a relative risk of 3 times. Rose and colleagues[9] performed limb-lead ECGs on 8403 male civil servants ages 40 to 64 years. Q waves, left-axis deviation, ST depression, T-wave changes, ventricular conduction defects, and atrial fibrillation were related to mortality rate. Among the 6% of men with patterns suggesting ischemia, the subsequent CAD mortality rate was low (1% per year) but the risk ratio was 5 times.

As part of the Busselton City, Australia, Study, 2119 unselected subjects had an ECG and the Rose chest pain questionnaire.[10] Q-wave patterns had the highest risk ratio (3.7 times), whereas the other abnormalities had about a 2 times risk ratio. As part of the Manitoba Study, a cohort of 3983 men with a mean age of 30 years at entry were followed with annual examinations including ECGs since 1948.[11] LBBB had a 14 times risk for sudden death, and ST- and T-wave abnormalities, increased R wave, and premature ventricular contractions (PVCs) had relative risks as high as 5 times. In 2000 Framingham Study participants, the ECG had a sensitivity of 50% and a specificity of 90%.[12]

The independent contributions of baseline major and minor ECG abnormalities to subsequent 11-year risk of death were explored among 9643 white men and 7990 white women ages 40 to 64 years without definite prior CHD in the Chicago Heart Association Detection Project in Industry by Liao and colleagues.[13] Both major and minor ECG abnormalities were associated with an increased risk of death. The strength of these associations was greater in men than in women.

The aim of an Italian project was to determine the predictive power of ECG findings on 6-year mortality rate in asymptomatic subjects.[14] The strongest predictors of fatal events were Q-QS findings and blocks. Combinations of ECG findings were associated with relative risks over 3 times. The Reykjavik Study included 9139 men born in the years 1907 to 1934 followed up for 4 to 24 years.[15] After adjustment for other risk factors, ST-T changes had a risk ratio of 2 times for CAD events.

> **Key Point:** The routine resting ECG has limited sensitivity for screening asymptomatic individuals, but should be considered because it is frequently available.

Spatial QRS-T Wave Measurements

Numerous studies support the value of repolarization measures as determined by the spatial QRS-T angle as a tool for risk stratification (Figure 9-1).[16-18] Kors and colleagues[19] investigated the prognostic importance of the frontal T axis, using ECGs from 5781 men and women age 55 years and older from a prospective population-based study. Participants with an abnormal frontal plane T axis, defined as those in the range of 105° to 180° and -180° to -15° (11%), had an increased risk of cardiac events and death. Rautaharju and colleagues[20] focused on the spatial T-axis deviation in 4173 subjects considered free of CV disease. The prevalence of marked T-axis deviation was 12%. Adjusting for clinical risk factors and other ECG abnormalities, there was a nearly twofold excess risk of CV death and an approximately

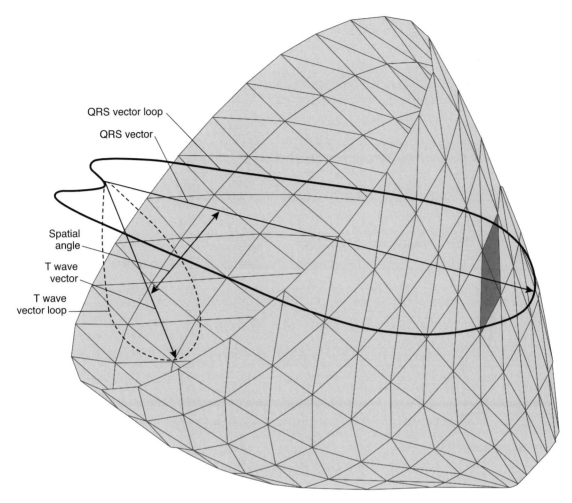

QRS vector loop

QRS vector

Spatial angle

T wave vector

T wave vector loop

FIGURE 9-1   *Illustration of QRS-T spatial angle.*

50% excess risk of CV and all-cause mortality for those with marked T-axis deviation. Investigators from the Netherlands demonstrated the spatial QRS-T angle to be a strong and independent predictor of cardiac death.[21] The 6134 men and women age 55 years and over in the prospective Rotterdam Study were categorized by spatial QRS-T angles. Abnormal angles independently predicted multiple cardiac endpoints, including sudden death, the latter with an impressive hazard ratio of 5.

Abnormalities on Serial Resting Electrocardiograms

As part of the Manitoba Study, a cohort of 3983 men with a mean age of 30 years at entry were followed with annual ECGs from 1948 to 1978.[22] There were 70 cases of sudden death in men without previous clinical manifestations of heart disease, and 50 of them had ECG abnormalities before sudden death. The frequencies of these abnormalities were 31% for major ST- and T-wave abnormalities, 16% for PVCs, 13% for LVH, and 7% for LBBB. The evolution of Q waves on serial ECGs was strongly associated with total and coronary disease mortality rates in the multiple risk factor intervention trial (MRFIT).[23] In assessing the value of serial ECGs, it is important that it is routine because symptoms often prompt an ECG and thus those with serial changes would be selected.

Summary of Outcome Prediction with the Electrocardiogram Studies

The outcome studies reviewed previously are summarized in Table 9-1, and the prevalence of ECG abnormalities for age groups by gender are illustrated in Figure 9-2.

> **Key Point:** Routine screening of asymptomatic individuals with the ECG is not indicated, but the ECG is ingrained as part of the health evaluation and thus is frequently available.

Angiographic Findings in Asymptomatic Men with Resting Electrocardiogram Abnormalities

Cardiac catheterization was used to evaluate 298 asymptomatic, apparently healthy aircrewmen with ECG abnormalities.[24] These men were identified from annual ECGs, and exercise tests were used to screen them for latent heart disease (Figure 9-3). Data from 27 additional symptomatic aircrewmen who underwent cardiac catheterization because of mild angina pectoris were also included. The men were grouped according to the major reason for cardiac catheterization. The order of groups by increasing prevalence of significant angiographic CAD was as follows: supraventricular tachycardia (14% prevalence of CAD), right bundle branch block (20%), left bundle branch block (24%), abnormal exercise-induced ST depression (31%), ventricular irritability (38%), probable infarct (56%), and angina (70%). Approximately 60% of the men were completely free of angiographic coronary disease. The ECG abnormalities studied had a poorer predictive value for CAD in asymptomatic, apparently healthy men than they do in a hospital or clinical population.

> **Key Point:** A reasonable hypothesis is that a first tier of serial screening with the resting ECG could identify a subpopulation that could be more effectively screened with another tier of testing (i.e., exercise testing).

Recommendations from the American College of Cardiology/American Heart Association Guidelines Regarding Exercise Testing as a Screening Procedure

The 1997 American College of Cardiology/American Heart Association (ACC/AHA) guidelines were updated in 2002 and had the following

TABLE 9-1   Outcome Studies Using the Resting ECG in Asymptomatic Individuals

Study	Population Size	Age (yr)	Q-Wave RR	ST Depression RR	LBBB RR	LVH RR	Atrial Fibulation RR	Duration	Endpoints
Copenhagen Heart Study[8]	20,000 men/ women	20-80	3x	5x	5x			4 yr	489 deaths
Rose (England)[9]	8403 men	40-64	2x	2x				5 yr	657 deaths
Busselton, Australia[10]	2119 men/ women	40-79	4x	2x	2x		2x	12 yr	
Italian RIFLE pooling project[14]	12,180 men; 10,373 women	30-69	10x	4x	4x		2x	6 yr	
Chicago Health Study[13]	9643 men; 7990 women	40-64	2x	2x	2x			11 yr	
British Regional Heart Study[76]	7735 men	40-59	2.5x	2x		2x			611 major CHD; 243 deaths
Italian HBP Study[77]	1717 hypertensives					4x		3.3 yr	159 major CHD; 33 deaths
MISAD (Diabetics)[78]	333 women, 592 men	40-65		10x					
Manitoba Study[79]	3983 men	30		5x	14x			30 yr	70 deaths
MRFIT trial[35]	2000 men	35-55	4x	2x				16 yr	

NOTE: The studies relied on visual analysis and have shown the predictive power of the ECG abnormalities for cardiovascular death and morbidity.
CHD, coronary heart disease; *LBBB*, left bundle branch block; *LVH*, left ventricular hypertrophy; *RR*, relative risk.

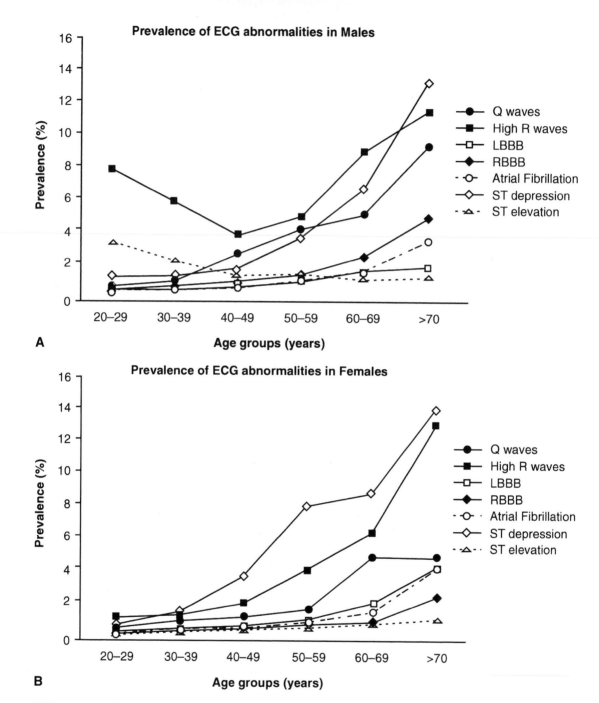

FIGURE 9-2 *Plots of prevalence of ECG abnormalities for age groups by gender.* **A,** *Males.* **B,** *Females.*

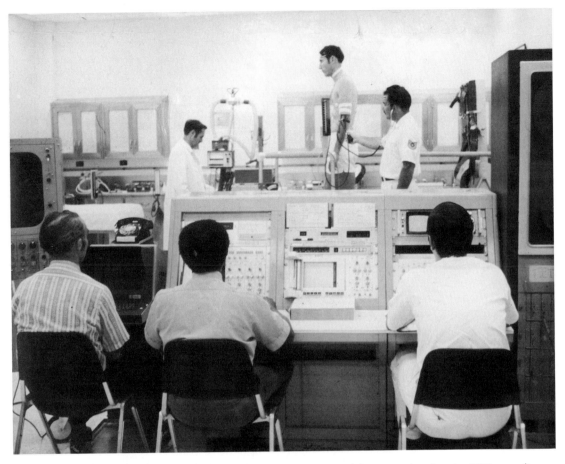

FIGURE 9-3 *Picture from 1972 of the USAFSAM exercise testing laboratory showing the ECG recording and expired gas analysis systems used for gathering the data for many of the early studies presented in this book. The console was acquired from NASA and the large digital tape drive (to the right) was used to record the ECG. The lab director was the treadmill subject in the photo.*

specific recommendations regarding this special application of the exercise test.[25]

Class I—Conditions for which there is evidence or general agreement that the standard exercise test is useful and helpful for screening asymptomatic individuals (definitely use)

None

Class IIa—Conditions for which there is conflicting evidence or a divergence of opinion that the standard exercise test is useful and helpful for screening but the weight of evidence for usefulness or efficacy is in favor of the exercise test (probably use)

Evaluation of asymptomatic diabetics who plan to start vigorous exercise (evidence level: C)

Class IIb—Conditions for which there is conflicting evidence or a divergence of opinion that the standard exercise test is useful and helpful for screening asymptomatic individuals but the usefulness/efficacy is less well established (maybe use)

1. Evaluation of individuals with multiple risk factors as a guide to risk factor reduction
2. Evaluation of asymptomatic men > 45 years old and women > 55 years old who (a) plan to start vigorous exercise (especially if sedentary), (b) are involved in occupations where impairment may affect public safety, or (c) are at high risk of CAD due to other diseases (such as peripheral vascular disease and chronic renal disease)

Class III—Conditions for which there is evidence or general agreement that the standard exercise test is not useful and helpful for screening and in some cases may be harmful (do not use)

Routine screening of asymptomatic men or women

Multiple risk factors defined by hypercholesterolemia (> 240 mg/dl), hypertension (systolic blood pressure [SBP] > 140 mm Hg or diastolic blood pressure [DBP] > 90 mm Hg), smoking, diabetes, and family history of heart attack or sudden cardiac death in a first-degree relative < 60 years old. An alternative approach might be to select individuals with a Framingham Risk Score consistent with at least a moderate risk of a >2% chance of serious cardiac events within 5 years.

Logic for the Guidelines

The purpose of screening for possible CAD in individuals without known CAD is either to prolong the individual's life or improve its quality because of early detection of disease. In asymptomatic individuals with severe CAD, data from the CASS and ACIP studies suggest that revascularization may prolong life. The detection of ischemia may identify individuals for risk factor modification. Although risk factor reduction should be attempted in all individuals, the identification of exercise capacity less than expected for age or those at increased risk may motivate individuals to be more compliant with risk factor modification.

The predictions of MI and death are considered the most important endpoints of screening in asymptomatic individuals. In general, the relative risk of a subsequent event is increased in individuals with an abnormal exercise test, although the absolute risk of a cardiac event in an asymptomatic individual remains low. The annual rate of MI and death in such individuals is only approximately 1%, even if ST-segment changes are associated with risk factors. A positive exercise test is more predictive of later development of angina than the occurrence of a major event. Even when angina is taken into account, fewer individuals with a positive test suffer cardiac events than those individuals with a normal test. Unfortunately, those with abnormal tests can suffer from being labeled as being "at risk of CAD."

General population screening programs—for example, those attempting to identify young individuals with early disease—have the limitation that severe CAD that requires intervention in asymptomatic individuals is exceedingly rare. Although the physical risks of exercise testing are negligible, false-positive test results usually cause anxiety, and have serious consequences related to work and insurance. For these reasons, the use of exercise testing in healthy, asymptomatic persons is not recommended.

Selected individuals with multiple risk factors for CAD are at greater absolute risk for subsequent MI and death. Screening may be potentially helpful in those individuals who are at least at moderate subsequent risk (> 2% annual risk of death or nonfatal MI). Such individuals may be identified from the available data in asymptomatic individuals from the Framingham study (point system chart). These criteria could be used to stratify the highest-risk individuals for CAD screening. Alternatively, screening may be performed in individuals with multiple risk factors. For these purposes, risk factors should be very strictly defined. Attempts to extend screening to individuals with lower degrees of risk, and fewer risk factors, are not recommended, because they are unlikely to improve individual outcome.

Key Point: In the majority of asymptomatic people, screening with any test or test add-on is more likely to yield false positives than true positives. This is the mathematical reality because of the limited discriminatory characteristics of all of the available tests.

Follow-Up Studies That Have Used a Screening Exercise Test

Next we discuss the follow-up studies that used maximal or near-maximal exercise testing to screen asymptomatic individuals for latent CHD. The populations in these studies were tested and followed for the CHD endpoints of angina, acute MI, and sudden death. Later, distinction will be made as to the results of these studies by the endpoints used, and they will be divided into two groups: angina included as an endpoint (Table 9-2) and "hard" endpoints (Table 9-3). Table 9-4 lists the endpoints in all of the studies for comparison. As we will see later, the controversy over whether or not, in the absence of conventional risk factors, exercise testing provides additional prognostic information has been resolved in the affirmative. Another concern is whether the knowledge of having an abnormal exercise test makes an individual more likely to report angina.

Bruce and McDonough[26] studied 221 clinically normal men in Seattle, 35 to 82 years of age. A CB5 bipolar lead was used, and 0.1 mV or more of ST-segment depression was the criterion for an abnormal response. Ten percent of the subjects had abnormal ST-segment responses to the symptom-limited maximal treadmill test. Aronow and colleagues[27] tested 100 normal men in Los Angeles, ages 38 to 64 years, and followed them for 5 years. In these apparently healthy men, an abnormal exercise ECG was associated with the development of CAD over the subsequent 5 years. Cumming and colleagues[28] reported their 3-year follow-up for CHD endpoints in 510 asymptomatic men 40 to 65 years of age. Twelve percent had an initial abnormal response to a bicycle exercise test. Subjects with an abnormal response had a higher prevalence of hypertension and hypercholesterolemia. It is notable that these

TABLE 9-2   Screening Studies That Included Angina as an Endpoint

Study	Number	Years Followed	Incidence of CHD (%)	Sensitivity (%)	Specificity (%)	Positive Predictive Value (%)	Risk Ratio
Bruce[26]	221	5	2.3	60	91	14	14×
Aronow[27]	100	5	9.0	67	92	46	14×
Cumming[28]	510	3	4.7	58	90	25	10×
Froelicher[29]	1390	6	3.3	61	92	20	14×
Allen[31]	356	5	9.6	41	79	17	2.4×
Manca[30]	947	5	5.0	67	84	18	10×
	508 (women)	5	1.6	88	73	5	15×
MacIntyre[33]	578	8	6.9	16	97	26	4×
McHenry[34]	916	13	7.1	14	98	39	6×
			Averages*	**48**	**90**	**26**	**9×**

*Averages do not include women.
CHD, coronary heart disease.

TABLE 9-3   Four Screening Studies with Hard Endpoints Only (Not Angina)

Study	Number	Years Followed	Incidence of CHD (%)	Sensitivity (%)	Specificity (%)	Positive Predictive Value (%)	Risk Ratio
Seattle Heart Watch[32]	2365	6	2.0	30	91	5	3.5×
MRFIT (SI) (UC)[35]	6217	6-8	1.7	17	88	2.2	1.4×
	6205		1.9	34	88	5.2	3.7×
LRC (Gordon)[37]	3630	8	2.2	28	96	12	6×
(Ekelund)	3806	7	1.8	29	95	7	5×
			Averages	**27**	**91**	**6**	**4×**

LRC, Lipid Research Clinics Coronary Primary Prevention Trial; *MRFIT,* Multiple Risk Factor Intervention Trial; *SI,* special intervention group; *UC,* usual care group.

TABLE 9-4   Events Used as Endpoints for Follow-up Studies

Study	Number	Events	Total Deaths	Cardiovascular Deaths	MI	CABS	AP
Aronow[27]	100	9	3	3	4	1	1
Bruce[26]	221	5	NR	1	1		3
Cumming[28]	510	26	5	3	8		13
McHenry[34]	916	65	8	8	26		30
MacIntyre[33]	548	38	NR	10	16	6	6
Allen[31]	888	48	NR	?	?	NR	?
Froelicher[29]	1390	65	47	25	82	35	11
Seattle Heart Watch[32]	2365	65	47	25	82	35	11
MRFIT (SI)[35]	6427	265	115	NR	NR	NR	NR
(UC)[36]	6438	260	124	NR	NR	NR	NR
LRC[37]	3630	NR	151	75	NR	NR	NR

AP, angina pectoris; *CABS,* coronary bypass surgery; *MI,* myocardial infarction; *MRFIT,* Multiple Risk Factor Intervention Trial; *NR,* not reported; *SI,* special intervention group, *?,* used as endpoint.

and other studies suggest that 10% to 12% of apparently healthy middle-aged individuals will have an abnormal exercise ECG.

At USAFSAM (see Figure 9-3), 1390 asymptomatic men 20 to 54 years of age who did not have any of the known causes for false-positive treadmill tests were screened for latent CHD by maximal treadmill testing and followed for a mean of 6.3 years.[29] In Italy, Manca and colleagues[30] studied 947 men and 508 women who were referred for exercise testing because of atypical chest pain. Eighteen percent of the men and 28% of the women had an abnormal electrocardiographic response. The endpoints for coronary disease were MI or sudden death, and there was a mean follow-up of 5.2 years. The overall incidence of coronary disease was 5% in the men and 1.6% in the women. The sensitivity was 67% in the men versus 88% in the women. The specificity of the test in the men was 84% versus 73% in the women. The predictive value of a positive test was 18% in men, but only 5% in women. Men with positive tests had a relative risk of 10 for developing clinical manifestations of coronary heart disease; the relative risk for women with positive tests was 15.

Allen and colleagues[31] reported a 5-year follow-up of 888 asymptomatic men and women. There was a 1.1% incidence of CHD per year, including angina pectoris, but 10% were lost to follow-up. Only 2 of 221 men 40 years old or younger developed heart disease endpoints. These results contrast with those of the USAFSAM study of 563 men 30 to 39 years old that found a 1.4% incidence of coronary disease. The exercise ECG was found to have 50% sensitivity, 95% specificity, 13% predictive value, and a risk ratio of 17. Allen and colleagues concluded that the exercise test was only of value in men older than 40 years old. Of the 311 women whom Allen and colleagues followed, 10 developed CHD. Incomplete follow-up and the low incidence of coronary disease endpoints in women and in men younger than 40 years old are limitations of this study.

Bruce and colleagues[32] reported a 6-year follow-up of 2365 clinically healthy men (mean age 45 years) who were exercise tested as part of the Seattle Heart Watch. Conventional risk factors were assessed at the time of the initial examination in a subset of the population. Forty-seven men (2%) experienced CHD morbidity or mortality. Only when the sum of risk factors in an individual were assessed did conventional risk factors become statistically significant in relation to the event rate. Four variables from treadmill testing were predictive:

1. Exercise duration less than 6 METs
2. 0.1 mV of ST depression during recovery
3. Greater than 10% heart rate impairment
4. Chest pain at maximal exertion

The ST-segment criteria had a sensitivity of 30%, a specificity of 89%, a predictive value of 5.3%, and a risk ratio of 3.3. Angina and exercise duration each had sensitivities of about 6%. Heart rate impairment had a sensitivity of 19% and was comparable to ST-segment depression for the other parameters.

TABLE 9-5 Performance of Exercise Test Variables and Risk Factors in Detecting Asymptomatic Coronary Artery Disease

Study	Abnormal Response	Sensitivity (%)	Specificity (%)	Predictive (%)	Risk Ratio
Allen[31]	ST depression	41	79	17	2
	METs <6	27	96	43	6
	ST depression and METs<6	24	99	71	11
Bruce[32]	ST depression	30	91	5	4
	Angina during test	6	99	15	8
	METs <6	6	99	19	10
	HRI	19	93	7	4
	≥1 RF and ≥2 Ex RP	19	—	46	*18*
Uhl[43]	≥0.3mV ST	36	79	38	2
	METs <8	46	92	67	4
	Persistent ST depression 28	87	43	6	
	≥1 RF and ≥2 Ex RP	55	86	84	*4*

The striking finding is the increase in risk ratio when conventional risk factors are considered with the exercise test responses, as well as the importance of exercise capacity, in these three screening studies.
Ex RP, exercise risk predictor; *HRI*, heart rate impairment; *RF*, risk factor.

Table 9-5 summarizes the performance of the exercise test predictors and conventional risk factors. The presence of two or more of the exercise test predictors identified men in all age groups who were at increased risk. Furthermore, it was found that in the presence of one or more conventional risk factors, as the prevalence of exertional risk predictors rose from none to any three, the relative risk rose from 1 to 30. The group that had one or more conventional risk factors and two or more exertional risk predictors was found to have the highest 5-year probability of primary CHD. The most striking finding was the increase in risk ratio when conventional risk factors are considered with the exercise test responses, as well as the importance of exercise capacity in these three screening studies.

Maximal exercise tests were performed on 548 fit, healthy middle-aged former aviators at the Naval Aerospace Medical Laboratory.[33] Criteria for coronary disease after an 8-year follow-up were sudden death, MI, coronary artery bypass surgery, or angina. The predictive value of the test was not significantly greater in those with the cardinal risk factors. An abnormal ST response generated a higher risk ratio than the risk factors.

McHenry and colleagues[34] reported the results of an 8- to 15-year follow-up of 916 apparently healthy men between ages 27 and 55 who underwent serial medical and exercise test evaluations. In 1968, the Indiana University School of Medicine entered into an agreement with the Indiana State Police Department to provide employees with periodic medical evaluations, including treadmill tests. During the initial evaluation, there were 23 subjects with an abnormal ST-segment response. They concluded that an abnormal ST-segment response to exercise predicted angina pectoris but not other coronary events. Sensitivity/specificity calculations from their data are shown in Table 9-2.

They found that serial testing did not improve the predictive value of the test and that angina was the main cardiac event predicted. Sudden death was actually more common in the individuals with normal test results. The USAFSAM study also had angina as its most common endpoint, both supporting the concept that the knowledge of an abnormal exercise test makes an individual more likely to report angina. McHenry and colleagues also performed serial exercise tests on 900 presumably healthy men and identified 14 men with labile ST-T changes with standing or hyperventilation at rest along with abnormal ST-segment depression during exercise. At the 7-year follow-up, none had manifested a coronary event. In 24 men with exercise-induced ST changes but no labile ST-T wave phenomena before exercise, 10 (42%) had a coronary event.

The Multiple Risk Factor Intervention Trial (MRFIT), a primary prevention trial, examined the effect of a special intervention (SI) program to reduce cholesterol, high blood pressure, and cigarette smoking in men 35 to 57 years old.[35] Half of the 12,866 participants were randomly assigned to usual care (UC) in the community. During a 6- to 8-year follow-up, the CAD mortality rate was 7% lower in the SI than in the UC group, a nonsignificant difference. A prior subgroup hypothesis proposed that men with an abnormal exercise ECG would particularly benefit from intervention. An abnormal ST integral measured by computer of -16 mV/sec was observed in 12.5% of the men at baseline and was associated with a threefold risk of CAD death within the UC group. In the subgroup with a normal ECG, there were no significant SI-UC differences in the CAD mortality rate. In contrast, there was a 57% lower death rate among men in the SI group with an abnormal test compared with men in the UC group. The relative risks (SI/UC) in these two strata were significantly different. These findings suggest that men with elevated risk factors who have an abnormal exercise ECG benefit from risk factor reduction. This study is the largest and probably the most reliable for demonstrating the predictive accuracy of exercise testing in an asymptomatic population because only cardiac deaths were considered the endpoint as opposed to angina in most of the other studies.

Rautaharju and colleagues[36] presented the prognostic value of the exercise ECG in the 6438 UC men of MRFIT in relation to fatal and nonfatal CHD events, resting ECG abnormalities, and CHD risk factors. An abnormal response to exercise, defined as an ST depression integral of -16 uV-s or more, was observed in 12.2% of the men. There was a fourfold increase in 7-year coronary mortality rate among men with an abnormal response to exercise. Gordon and colleagues[37] presented one of many interesting analyses of the Lipid Research Clinics Mortality Follow-up Study. More than 3600 white men, from 30 to 79 years old and without a history of MI, underwent submaximal treadmill tests as part of their baseline evaluation. Cumulative CV mortality rate was 11.9% (22 of 185) over a mean 8 year follow-up among men with a positive exercise test versus 1.2% (36 of 2993) among men with a negative test. Three quarters (43) of these deaths were due to CHD. The age-adjusted relative risk for CV mortality associated with a positive exercise test was 5 times. CV mortality rates were especially elevated among the 82 men whose exercise tests were judged "strongly" positive based on degree and timing of the ST response (the relative risk was 16 before and 5 after age adjustment). An abnormal exercise test was a stronger predictor of CV death than were conventional risk factors, having an impact on risk of CV death equivalent to being 17 years older.

Ekelund and colleagues[38] attempted to predict CHD morbidity and mortality rates in hypercholesterolemic men from an exercise test performed as part of the Lipid Research Clinics Coronary Primary Prevention Trial. To study whether the test was more predictive for hypercholesterolemic men (i.e., thus increasing the pretest probability for disease), data from 3806 asymptomatic men were analyzed. During the 7- to 10-year follow-up period, the CV mortality rate was 7% in men with an abnormal test and 1% in men with a negative test. As part of the Baltimore Longitudinal Study of Aging, serial exercise tests were performed at two to four intervals in 726 male and female volunteers, ages 22 to 84 years.[39] Over a mean overall follow-up of 7 years, coronary events occurred in 34 of 178 (19%) of those with an abnormal ST response to exercise versus 30 of 548 (5.5%) in those with a normal response. Angina pectoris was the most common coronary event. Among individuals with an abnormal ST-segment response, the incidence of events was virtually identical between those with an initially abnormal response and those who converted from a normal to an abnormal response, about 20% in both. Conversion from a normal to an abnormal exercise ST-segment response was associated with a prognosis similar to an initially abnormal response.

Gordon and colleagues[40] analyzed smoking, physical activity, and other predictors of endurance and heart rate response to exercise in asymptomatic hypercholesterolemic men. The association of known coronary risk factors with progressive submaximal treadmill exercise test performance was studied in 6238 asymptomatic white 34- to 60-year-old hypercholesterolemic men screened between 1973 and 1976 for the Lipid Research Clinics Coronary Primary Prevention Trial. Cigarette smoking and habitual physical inactivity were each associated with a doubling of the rate of symptom-related discontinuation of the exercise test; the tests of sedentary smokers were discontinued at four times the rate observed for active nonsmokers. Smaller increases in heart rate were observed during exercise testing in physically active men and in smokers than in their sedentary and nonsmoking counterparts. Thus smoking, like habitual physical activity, reduced the heart rate required to sustain a given external workload. However, the heart rates of smokers tended to remain elevated after exercise, whereas those of physically active men returned more rapidly toward resting levels. Age, Quetelet index, and low plasma levels of HDL cholesterol were also strong predictors of decreased exercise capacity, and resting heart rate and blood pressure levels were significant predictors of the heart rate response.

Endpoint Considerations in the Screening Studies

The Seattle Heart Watch was the first study that reported quite different results from previous studies including those of Bruce's earlier findings. The explanation became apparent considering the endpoints used.

The earlier studies all considered angina pectoris as one of the cardiac events or endpoints. In the Seattle Heart Watch, the angina endpoint had to be associated with a hospital admission diagnosis of angina, making it a more definite cardiac endpoint. The other studies considered only hard endpoints such as death or MI and not angina.

When the studies are separated by those that used angina as an endpoint (see Table 9-2), the average sensitivity was 50%, predictive value was 26%, and risk ratio was 9 times. This means that 26%, or one out of four with ST depression, would have a cardiac event including angina during approximately 5 years of follow-up. However, when the studies that used only hard endpoints were considered (see Table 9-3), much poorer results were obtained. The sensitivity was 27% and the predictive value was 6%. Only 6%, or 1 out of 17 with ST-segment depression, would have a hard endpoint during follow-up. Rather than 1 cardiac event out of 4 with ST-segment depression, it turns out to be 1 out of 17. This means that 16 out of 17 abnormal responses are false positives. This must be considered because these studies are being cited as showing the dangers of silent ischemia. Silent ischemia induced by exercise testing in apparently healthy men is not as predictive of a poor outcome as once thought. The earlier, better results can be explained by the cardiac concerns caused by an abnormal exercise test. Individuals with abnormal tests would be more likely to report chest pain and doctors would be more likely to diagnose it as angina given the exercise test results.

CV mortality should be the ideal endpoint, but it is usually determined by death certificates. Although death certificates have their limitations, in general they classify those with accidental, gastrointestinal, pulmonary, and cancer deaths accurately so that the remaining deaths are most likely to be of CV causes. This endpoint is more appropriate for a test for CV disease and when screening for CV risk. Whereas all-cause mortality is a more important endpoint for intervention studies, CV mortality is more appropriate for evaluating a CV test.

Key Point: The earlier screening studies all considered angina pectoris as one of the cardiac endpoints, but more recent studies considered only hard endpoints such as death or MI and not angina. When the studies are separated by those that included angina as an outcome endpoint (see Table 9-2), the average sensitivity was 50%, predictive value was 26%, and risk ratio was 9 times. However, when the studies that used only hard endpoints were considered (see Table 9-3), much poorer results were obtained: The sensitivity was 27% and the predictive value was 6%. Subject knowledge of an abnormal test most likely led to reporting any chest pain as angina, thus falsely creating CV endpoints.

Exercise Testing and Coronary Angiography in Asymptomatic Populations

In the United States Air Force Medical Corps (USAFMC), we used cardiac catheterization to evaluate 111 asymptomatic men with abnormal exercise test–induced ST depression. Only one third of the subjects had at least one lesion causing 50% or greater lumenal narrowing of a major coronary artery. Resting mild ST-segment depression that appears on serial ECGs and persists during exercise increases the predictive value of an abnormal exercise test. Borer and colleagues[41] reported angiographic findings in 11 asymptomatic individuals with hyperlipidemia and an abnormal exercise test. Only 37% were found to have coronary artery occlusions.

Barnard and colleagues[42] used near-maximal treadmill testing to screen randomly selected Los Angeles firefighters. Ten percent had abnormal exercise-induced ST depression despite few risk factors for coronary disease. Six men with an abnormal exercise test elected to undergo cardiac catheterization. One had severe three-vessel disease, and another had a 50% obstruction of the left circumflex coronary artery. The other four men had normal studies.

Uhl and colleagues[43] reported their findings in 255 asymptomatic men with exercise-induced ST depression who underwent coronary angiography over a 7-year period at the USAFSAM. None of the clinical or ECG variables were able to detect those with significant disease. The three exercise test responses with high likelihood ratio were (1) at least 0.3 mV of depression, (2) persistence of ST depression 6 minutes after exercise, and (3) an estimated oxygen uptake of less than 9 METs. However, because of their low sensitivity and predictive value, it was necessary to combine them with risk factors. A combination of any risk factor and two exercise responses was highly predictive (89%) but insensitive (39%) for any coronary disease. However, this combination had a sensitivity of 55% and a predictive value of 84% for two- or three-vessel disease.

Erikssen and colleagues[44] reported angiographic findings in 105 men ages 40 to 59 years of a working population with one or more of the following criteria: (1) a questionnaire for angina pectoris positive on interview or either (2) typical angina or (3) ST depression as responses to a near-maximal bicycle test. The exercise test had a predictive value of 84% if a slowly ascending ST segment was included. The higher predictive value in this study may be due to the older age of the population and inclusion of men with angina. Of the 36 who were found to have normal coronary arteries, a 7-year follow-up revealed that 3 died of sudden death, 4 received a diagnosis of cardiomyopathy, and 1 had developed aortic valve disease.[45] They had a relative decline in their physical performance over the follow-up period.

Kemp and colleagues[46] evaluated 7-year survival in patients having normal or near-normal coronary angiograms using data from the CASS registry of 21,487 consecutive coronary angiograms taken in 15 clinical sites. Of these, 4051 angiograms were normal or near normal, and the patients had normal left ventricular function as judged by absence of a history of congestive heart failure, no reported segmental wall motion abnormality, and an ejection fraction of at least 50%; 3136 angiograms were entirely normal, and the remaining 915 revealed mild disease with less than 50% stenosis in one or more segments. Of the total number, 843 patients had exercise tests, and of these, 195 had abnormal ST depression. The 7-year survival rate was 96% for the patients with a normal angiogram and 92% for those whose study revealed mild disease. The authors noted that the ECG response to exercise was not a predictive variable. This is in contrast to the 7-year follow-up study of only 36 apparently healthy middle-aged men with a positive exercise test and normal coronary angiograms reported by Erikssen. Erikssen concluded that patients with abnormal exercise tests could not be assured of a good prognosis on the basis of a normal coronary angiogram. The CASS data did not support this conclusion. There were 195 subjects with abnormal ST-segment depression, and Kemp and colleagues were unable to show any predictive value of even marked amounts of depression. If exercise-induced ST-segment depression is due to ischemia in patients with normal coronaries, it is not related to a disease process that has an impact on mortality rate over 7 years of follow-up. In general, these angiographic studies confirm the low predictive value of an abnormal exercise test response similar to that found in the epidemiologic studies of populations with a low prevalence of CHD.

> **Key Point:** Subjects with false-positive exercise tests (i.e., normal angiograms) have a good prognosis.

Techniques to Improve Screening

Numerous techniques have been recommended to improve the sensitivity and specificity of exercise testing. Various computerized criteria for ischemia have been proposed, as well as new standard visual ST criteria. In addition, there are ancillary techniques that could possibly improve the discriminating power of the exercise test. These methods are listed in Table 9-6.

Electrocardiographic Criteria

Hollenberg and colleagues[47] have applied their computerized treadmill score in an asymptomatic Army population with success. Okin and colleagues[48] compared the ST/HR index and the heart rate–recovery loop with standard electrocardiographic criteria for prediction of CHD events in

TABLE 9-6 Ancillary Techniques That Have Been Used to Screen for Asymptomatic Coronary Heart Disease

Nuclear perfusion imaging
Intimal thickening of the carotid arteries
Imaging coronary artery calcification with cardiac fluoroscopy or electron beam computed tomography
Cardiokymography
Total cholesterol/high-density lipoprotein ratio, conventional risk factors
ECG gated chest x-ray before and after exercise
Computerized multifactorial risk prediction using Bayesian statistics
Holter monitoring (Table 9-7)
Digital subtraction angiography with intravenous injection of contrast medium to visualize the coronary arteries
Echocardiography
Biomarkers

TABLE 9-7   Holter Study of Hedblad Reporting Results of Screening in Both Asymptomatic and Symptomatic Population

History of CAD	ST Depression on Holter	Number	MI/Deaths	Risk Ratio
Yes	No	34	2 (5.9%)	2.6×
	Yes	19	7 (39%)	16×
No	No	262	6 (2.3%)	1×
	Yes	79	8 (10.8%)	4.4×

From Hedblad B: *Eur Heart J* 10:149-158, 1989.
CAD, Coronary artery disease = previous MI or positive Rose qestionnaire result; *MI,* myocardial infarction.

3168 asymptomatic men and women in the Framingham Offspring Study who underwent treadmill testing. These individuals were free of clinical and ECG evidence of heart disease. After a mean follow-up of 4.3 years, there were 65 new CHD events: 4 sudden deaths, 24 new MIs, and 37 new cases of angina pectoris. When a Cox proportional hazards model with adjustment for age and sex was used, an abnormal exercise ECG by standard criteria (> 0.1 mV of horizontal or downsloping ST-segment depression) was not predictive of new CHD events. In contrast, stratification according to the presence or absence of an abnormal ST/HR index (> 1.6 uV/beat/min) and an abnormal (counterclockwise) rate-recovery loop was associated with CHD event risk and separated subjects into three groups with varying risks of coronary events: high risk, when both tests were abnormal (relative risk 4 times); intermediate risk, when either the ST/HR index or the rate-recovery loop was abnormal (relative risk, 2 times); and low risk, when both tests were negative. After multivariate adjustment for age, sex, smoking, total cholesterol (TC) level, fasting glucose level, DBP, and ECG-LVH, the combined ST/HR index and rate-recovery loop criteria remained predictive of coronary events. The problem with this study is that actual visual interpretation of the exercise ECGs was not available and the computer criteria were too rigorous. To match visual analysis, the computer measurement threshold must be set at 0.75 mm of depression and 1 mV/sec slope because the eye flattens out the ST slope and rounds off depression. The results obtained did not justify screening asymptomatic individuals because of the high false-positive rate. Angina was included as an endpoint and this is a problem, as previously noted.

Exercise-Induced Dysrhythmias

Studies in asymptomatic subjects have evaluated exercise-induced ventricular premature beats for detecting coronary disease. In a USAFSAM study of 1390 men, only 39 men (2.1%) of the population developed "ominous" dysrhythmias. The risk ratio of developing coronary disease over 6 years of follow-up with these dysrhythmias was 3 times; however, the predictive value was only 10% and sensitivity only 7%. Controversy exists regarding the meaning of exercise test–associated PVCs because they appear to predict later risk than other responses and no preventive or therapeutic strategy has been developed for them. Exercise-induced premature atrial contractions (PACs) appear to be benign except that they are associated with increased risk for atrial fibrillation.

Exercise Test Add-ons

The most popular add-ons to the exercise test in clinical practice are nuclear perfusion and echocardiography. It has generally been concluded that the slightly enhanced test characteristics do not have that much of an impact for screening over the standard exercise test.[49,50] However, either test can be the first means of evaluating a patient with an abnormal ST response thought to be a false positive. We usually advise that whatever procedure is favored and performed best at the patient's point of evaluation should be used.

Multivariable Prediction Techniques with Exercise Testing for Screening

Angiographic Multivariable Prediction Studies

At the USAFSAM, fasting lipids were measured in 572 asymptomatic aircrewmen.[51] Of these, 132 had an abnormal treadmill test and underwent coronary angiography. Coronary disease (defined as a lesion of 50% or greater diameter narrowing) was found in 16, with the rest having minimal or no CAD ($N = 102$). The 14 men with minimal CAD had TC-HDL ratios that differed from the normals ($P < 0.001$). Two of the 16 with angiographic CAD had TC-HDL ratios of less than 6, whereas 4 of the 102 angiographic normal subjects had a ratio of greater than 6 times. Only 42 of 440 (9.5%) with a normal treadmill test had a TC-HDL ratio greater than 6; 87% of those with CHD had TC-HDL ratios greater than 6. This ratio generated a risk of 172. A limitation of this study is that true sensitivity cannot be determined because only those with an abnormal treadmill test underwent coronary angiography.

Also at the USAFSAM, 255 totally asymptomatic men underwent cardiac catheterization because of at least 0.1 mV of ST depression. Sixty-five men had at least 50% coronary artery narrowing.[52] Thus the predictive value of ST-segment changes was only 24%. However, 41 men had no abnormal risk factors, and the odds ratio was over 3:1 with hypercholesterolemia alone or the presence of three risk factors. The presence of at least one risk factor and two or more exercise variables identified as predictive (including 0.3 mV of ST depression early, persistent ST depression after exercise, or exercise duration under 10 minutes) identified over half the cases of two- or three-vessel disease with a predictive value of 84%.

Recent Follow-up Multivariable Prediction Studies

Whereas some of the earlier screening studies applied multivariate approaches to prediction, recent studies have applied modern statistical techniques in an attempt to improve screening characteristics. From the Cooper Clinic comes the largest screening study of the exercise test to predict CV death in a self-selected population of asymptomatic men.[53] It was a prospective study performed between 1970 and 1989, with an average follow-up of 8.4 years. Their were 25,927 healthy men, 20 to 82 years of age at baseline (mean 43 years) who were free of CV disease and who were evaluated in the Cooper preventive medicine clinic (i.e., self-selected and willing to pay). During follow-up there were 612 deaths from all causes and 158 deaths from CV causes. The sensitivity of an abnormal exercise test to predict coronary death was 61%. The age-adjusted relative risk of an abnormal exercise test for CV death was 21 times in those with no risk factors, 27 times in those with one risk factor, 54 times in those with two risk factors, and 80 times in those with three or more factors. This elegant study, summarized in Table 9-8, supports the remarkable risk generated by the standard exercise test as found in the earlier studies, but it adds support to the additive value of considering risk factors.

At the Cleveland Clinic, the validity for prediction of all-cause mortality of the Framingham Risk Score and the European global scoring system Systematic Coronary Risk Evaluation (SCORE) was evaluated.[54] This was done in asymptomatic individuals evaluated in a clinical setting including an exercise test. A prospective cohort of 3554 asymptomatic adults between 50 and 75 years old who underwent exercise testing as part of an executive health program between October 1990 and December 2002 were followed up for a mean of 8 years. Global risk was calculated using the Framingham Risk Score and the European SCORE. The primary endpoint was all-cause mortality; there were 114 deaths. The c-index, which corresponds to area under the curve (AUC) for range of characteristics (ROC), and the Akaike Information Criteria found that the European SCORE was superior to the Framingham Risk Score in estimating global mortality risk. In a multivariable model, independent predictors of death were a higher SCORE (relative risk [RR], 1.07), impaired functional capacity (RR, 3), and an abnormal heart rate recovery (RR, 1.6). ST-segment depression did not predict mortality. Among patients in the highest tertile from the SCORE, an abnormal exercise test, defined as either impaired functional capacity or an abnormal heart rate recovery, identified a mortality risk of more than 1% per year. We hope that

TABLE 9-8   Results of the Cooper Clinic Screening Study Using Exercise Testing and Conventional Risk Factors

Testing Results	Age-Adjusted Relative Risk for CV Death
Abnormal ETI ST depression only	21×
Abnormal ETI ST depression plus one risk factor	27×
Abnormal ETI ST depression plus two risk factors	54×
Abnormal ETI ST depression plus three risk factors	80×

CV, cardiovascular; ETI, exercise test–induced.

our friends at Cleveland will repeat this analysis using CV event data, which is a more appropriate endpoint for a study attempting to evaluate means of predicting CV risk.

Using Framingham data, Balady and colleagues[55] evaluated the usefulness of exercise testing in asymptomatic persons in predicting CHD events over and above the Framingham Risk Score. Included were 3043 members of the Framingham Heart Study offspring cohort without CHD (1431 men and 1612 women; mean age 45 ± 9 years) who were followed for 18 years. The risk of developing CHD was evaluated considering three exercise test variables: (1) ST-segment depression of 1 mm or greater, (2) failure to achieve target heart rate of 85% predicted maximum, and (3) exercise capacity. In multivariable analyses that adjusted for age and Framingham risk score, among men, ST-segment depression or failure to achieve target heart rate doubled CHD risk, whereas a greater exercise capacity predicted lower CHD risk. Although similar hazard ratios were seen in women, those results were not statistically significant. Among men with 10-year predicted risk greater than 20%, failure to reach target heart rate and ST-segment depression more than doubled the risk of an event, and each MET increment in exercise capacity reduced risk by 13%. In this random sample of asymptomatic men, ST-segment depression, failure to reach target heart rate, and exercise capacity provided additional prognostic information in age-adjusted and Framingham Risk Score–adjusted models, particularly among those in the highest risk group (10-year predicted CHD risk of > 20%).

Erikssen and colleagues[56] recently compared the accuracy of CV risk assessment based on classical risk factors with the addition of multiple exercise test parameters. In 1972–1975, 2014 apparently healthy men 40 to 60 years old had a symptom-limited exercise test during a CV survey. Their average maximal heart rate was 162 beats per minutes and their average SBP at a submaximal load of 100 watts was 180 mm Hg. The prognostic exercise test variables included the ST response, elevated submaximal SBP (> 1 SD [25 mm Hg] above the norm), and exercise capacity. There were 300 CV deaths during 26 years of follow-up. Compared to Cox regression models solely including classical risk factors (CRF), models also including multiple exercise test parameters (CRF + ExTest) were clearly superior. Risk scores were computed based on the models. CRF and CRF + ExTest risk scores often differed markedly; CRF + ExTest scores were generally most reliable in both the high- and low-risk range. In smokers with elevated cholesterol (n = 470), the CRF and CRF + ExTest models identified 67 versus 110 men at the highest CV risk level according to European guidelines (34% vs. 32% CV mortality). This study demonstrated that integration of multiple exercise test parameters and conventional risk factors can improve CV risk assessment substantially—especially in smokers with high cholesterol. This same group later asked whether reasons for terminating an exercise test might influence long-term mortality rate in this population of healthy men.[57] The following reasons for test termination were noted: impaired breathing, lower limb fatigue, exhaustion (i.e., combined lower limb fatigue and impaired breathing), high heart rate, abnormal blood pressure response, arrhythmias, increasing chest pain during exercise, marked ST depression

TABLE 9-9   Three Contemporary Screening Studies That Considered Multiple Exercise Test Response and Risk Factors Together with 8-Year or More Follow-up for Hard Endpoints

Study	Sample size	Years of Follow-up
Cooper Clinic	26,000 men	8
Norway	2,000 men	26
Framingham	3,000 men	18

during the test, and refusal to continue. When adjusting for age, men who stopped exercising exclusively because of impaired breathing ($n = 178$) had twice the risk of dying from CHD or from any cause, and a 3.5-fold increased risk of dying from pulmonary causes compared with men having described exhaustion as the reason for stopping ($n = 1376$). After adjustment for age, smoking, total serum cholesterol, fasting blood glucose, systolic blood pressure, and physical fitness, impaired breathing remained significantly associated with an increased risk of dying from CHD, pulmonary disease, or any cause. The authors concluded that healthy men who stop bicycle exercising only because of impaired breathing have high long-term CHD, pulmonary, and total mortality rates that must be addressed.

These three important contemporary studies are summarized in Table 9-9.

Computer Probability Estimates

Diamond and Forrester[58] performed a literature review to estimate pretest likelihood of disease by age, sex, symptoms, and the Framingham risk equation. In addition, they have considered the sensitivity and specificity of four diagnostic tests (the exercise test, CKG, nuclear perfusion, and cardiac fluoroscopy) and applied Bayes's theorem. CADENZA is the acronym for the computer program that calculates these estimates. The biggest weakness of this approach is that the sensitivities and specificities of the secondary tests are not certain, and it is uncertain how they interact because of similar inadequacies.

Exercise Testing for Special Screening Purposes

Exercise Testing for Exercise Programs

The optimal exercise prescription, based on a percentage of an individual's maximal heart rate or oxygen consumption (50% to 80%) or to exceed the ventilatory threshold, can only be developed after performing an exercise test. The best way to assess the risk of an adverse reaction during exercise is to observe the individual during exercise. The level of exercise training then can be set at a level below that at which adverse responses or symptoms occur. Some individuals motivated by popular misconceptions about the benefits of exercise may disregard their natural "warning systems" and push themselves into dangerous levels of ischemia.

An individual with a good exercise capacity and only 0.I mV of ST-segment depression at maximal exercise has a relatively low risk of CV events over the next several years compared to an individual with marked ST-segment depression at a low heart rate or systolic blood pressure. Most individuals with an abnormal test can safely participate in an exercise program if the intensity level of the exercise at which the response occurs is considered. Such patients can be followed with risk factor modification rather than being excluded from exercise or their livelihood.

Siscovick and colleagues[59] determined whether the exercise ECG predicted acute cardiac events during moderate or strenuous physical activity among 3617 asymptomatic, hypercholesterolemic men (age range, 35 to 59 years) who were followed in the Coronary Primary Prevention Trial. Submaximal exercise test results were obtained at entry and at annual follow-up visits in years 2 through 7. ST-segment depression or elevation was considered to be an abnormal result. The cumulative incidence of activity-related acute cardiac events was 2% during a mean follow-up period of 7 years. The risk was increased 2.6-fold in the presence of clinically silent, exercise-induced ST-segment changes at entry after adjustment for 11 other potential risk factors. Of 62 men who experienced an activity-related event, 11 had an abnormal test result at entry (sensitivity, 18%). The specificity of the entry exercise test was 92%. The sensitivity and specificity were similar when the length of follow-up was restricted to 1 year after testing. For a newly abnormal test result on a follow-up visit, the sensitivity was 24% and the specificity was 85%; for any abnormal test result during the study (six tests per subject), the sensitivity was 37% and the specificity was 79%. The authors concluded that the test was not sensitive when used to predict the occurrence of activity-related events among asymptomatic, hypercholesterolemic men. For this reason, the utility of the exercise test to assess the safety of physical activity among asymptomatic men at risk of CHD appeared limited.

> **Key Point:** The hypothetical need to obtain clearance by exercise testing should not impede efforts for most people to become more active; however, those desirous of reaching higher levels of fitness using exercise training should be considered for testing.

Military Fitness

U.S. Army Program to Screen for Coronary Artery Disease
The U.S. Army evaluated a program of serial testing to detect latent CHD. Screening was considered necessary before initiating a mandatory exercise program for all personnel older than 40 years. The screening tests were applied in a sequential manner in an attempt to eliminate low-risk patients from further testing and to enhance the pretest likelihood of disease in the remaining subset. Initial history, physical examination, and rest ECGs were performed on 285 men and 2 women over 40 years old (mean age 44). A fasting biochemical profile was obtained and a risk factor index based on the Framingham database was calculated. All subjects underwent maximal

exercise testing. All were encouraged to exercise to exhaustion, and the average METs was 10 (range 7 to 18). CKGs were performed before and after exercise. A risk factor index over 5 was considered abnormal. An abnormal ST-segment response occurred in 4 men and an "abnormal nondiagnostic" response, defined as upsloping ST changes, occurred in 15 men. Six men had frequent exercise-induced PVCs. These 26 men underwent cardiac fluoroscopy and nuclear perfusion. Seven men had abnormal nuclear perfusion findings, six underwent cardiac catheterization, and one died of an MI. One man with a low risk index and normal treadmill test, CKG, and fluoroscopic findings had an MI after 6 months of follow-up. No patient had coronary calcification. An abnormal ST-segment response was insensitive and not highly predictive of coronary disease. CKG had 63% sensitivity, 74% specificity, and a predictive value of 50%, and was the most accurate individual test. Risk factor analysis alone was not predictive, and screening accuracy improved only when there were two or more risk factors and an abnormal CKG.

Zoltick and colleagues[60] reported preliminary results with application of the United States Army Cardiovascular Screening Program. A two-tier, staged approach was initiated for a CV screening program for all active duty Army personnel over 40 years of age. Criteria for primary CV screen failure included any one of the following abnormalities: (1) Framingham risk index > 5%; (2) abnormal CV history or examination; (3) abnormal ECG; and (4) fasting blood sugar > 115 mg/dl. Failure of the primary screen requires a secondary screening test, which includes an internal medicine or cardiology consultation and a maximum treadmill test and/or further sequential follow-up. During the follow-up, recommendations were made for risk factor modification and exercise programs. Between June 1981 and August 1983, 42,752 individuals were screened. Of these, 23,428 (55%) cleared the primary screen, 7279 (17%) cleared the secondary screen, and 1040 (2.4%) did not pass the secondary screen. Hopefully, the long-term results of this important study will be published soon.

The ability of atherosclerosis imaging to overcome limitations of clinical risk screening with coronary risk factors is being explored in a study called the Prospective Army Coronary Calcium (PACC) Project. The goals of the PACC Project are to determine the utility of EBCT for the detection of coronary calcium as a screening test for CAD and as an intervention for risk factor modification among young, asymptomatic, active-duty personnel undergoing the U.S. Army's Cardiovascular Screening Program.[61] Three study designs will be used to address the objectives of this investigation: (1) a cross-sectional study of 2000 unselected, consecutive participants to determine the prevalence and extent of coronary calcification in the 40- to 50-year-old Army population; (2) a randomized, controlled trial with a 2×2 factorial design involving 1000 participants to assess the impact of EBCT information on several dimensions of patient behavior, with and without intensive risk factor case management; and (3) a prospective cohort study of 2000 participants followed for at least 5 years to establish the relation between coronary calcification and CV events in an unselected, "low-risk" (by conventional standards) Army population. From these aims, data from the PACC Project support that subclinical coronary calcium is prevalent in asymptomatic individuals, even those with optimal risk factor profiles.[62] In the PACC Project, 22.4% of asymptomatic men have identifiable foci of subclinical atherosclerosis. Emerging data from this study show that, after adjusting for coronary risk factor levels and family history, this finding is associated with a ninefold risk of coronary events over the following 5 years, compared to those with no detectable coronary artery calcium.[63]

Flying Fitness

Unfortunately, politics and economics are two of the strongest factors influencing the use of exercise testing in subjects with flying responsibilities.[64] The pool of available pilots is obviously an important national resource. If many pilots are available, society is more likely to be stricter with regulations regarding flying standards. Clearly, physicians must be concerned with public safety. Allowing an individual with an increased health risk to take responsibility for many other peoples' lives could result in a tragedy. The presence of a backup pilot and the impact of modern technology on flying do not lessen the stresses of this occupation. There are numerous situations of very high stress, such as takeoffs and landings, where it might not be possible for other cockpit personnel to take over control of the aircraft, and a disaster might not be averted if the key pilot were to have a cardiac event. In general, pilots are a highly motivated, intelligent group of men and women who feel a high level of responsibility for the performance of their work. Flying is their livelihood, however, and most of them love it so dearly that they may conceal medical information that could endanger their flying status. In addition, the stress of work often leaves them unable to maintain a healthy lifestyle. The stress of altering one's circadian cycle and trying to navigate in and out of today's busy airports leaves many of them overweight, deconditioned, and smoking heavily. Whenever possible, health professionals should recommend that these men and women have the full benefits of modern preventive medicine, including the periodic assessment of exercise capacity, response to stress, and the probability of coronary atherosclerosis.

EBCT for Screening Asymptomatic Subjects

Atherosclerotic calcification is an organized, regulated process similar to bone formation that occurs only when other aspects of atherosclerosis are also present. Nonhepatic Gla-containing proteins such as osteocalcin, which are actively involved in the transport of calcium out of vessel walls, are suspected to have key roles in the pathogenesis of coronary calcification. Osteopontin, which is involved in bone mineralization, is in calcified atherosclerotic lesions. Calcification is an active process and not simply a passive precipitation of calcium phosphate crystals. Although calcification is found more frequently in advanced lesions, it may also occur in small amounts in earlier lesions, which appear in the second and third decades of life. Histopathologic investigation has shown that plaques with microscopic evidence of mineralization are larger and associated with larger coronary arteries than plaques or arteries without calcification. The relation of arterial calcification to the probability of plaque rupture is unknown. Although the amount of coronary calcium correlates with the amount of atherosclerosis in different individuals and to a lesser extent in segments of the coronary tree in the same individuals, it is not known if the quantity of calcification tracks the quantity of atherosclerosis over time in the same individuals. Epidemiologic evidence and postmortem studies show that the prevalence of coronary calcium deposits in a given decade of life is 10 to 100 times higher than the expected 10-year incidence of CHD events for individuals of the same age. This disparity is less evident and symptomatic in the elderly than in the young and asymptomatic.

Though some excellent studies have been performed,[65,66] insufficient data exist to determine whether the relation between coronary calcium and CHD risk warrants the use of calcium screening in low-risk, asymptomatic subjects. As mentioned earlier, experience from the studies using exercise testing suggests that hard endpoints must be used but not interventions when evaluating a test. The ACC/AHA recommendations state that EBCT is a research tool and is not recommended for screening for CAD.[67] EBCT researchers should examine the experience of workers in the exercise test arena and avoid the same mistakes. The rules of Feinstein should be considered in evaluating this exciting new procedure.

The societal question to be answered: Is this modest gain in risk prediction worth the cost of this test? But an even more basic question: Is this test better than the available tests, such as exercise testing? The available data do not suggest that this is so. The test characteristics of exercise test scores exceed EBCT.

Does Screening Motivate Patients to Alter Their Risk?

Exercise testing may prove to have value in asymptomatic populations other than for screening. Bruce and colleagues[68] examined the motivational effects of maximal exercise testing for modifying risk factors and health habits. A questionnaire was sent to nearly 3000 men 35 to 65 years of age who had undergone symptom-limited treadmill testing at least 1 year earlier. Individuals were asked if the treadmill test motivated them to stop smoking (if already a smoker), increase daily exercise, purposely lose weight, reduce the amount of dietary fat, or take medication for hypertension. There was a 69% response to this questionnaire, and 63% of the responders indicated that they had modified one or more risk factors and health habits and that they attributed this change to the exercise test. In fact, a greater percentage of patients with decreased exercise capacity, compared with normal subjects, reported a modification of risk factors or health habits.

The Army Cardiology Research group studied the effects of incorporating EBCT as a motivational factor into a CV screening program in the context of either intensive case management (ICM) or usual care by assessing its impact over 1 year on a composite measure of projected risk.[69] The investigators performed a randomized controlled trial with a 2 × 2 factorial design and 1 year of follow-up involving a consecutive sample of 450 asymptomatic active-duty U.S. Army personnel ages 39 to 45 years old. All were scheduled to undergo a periodic Army-mandated physical examination between January 1999 and March 2001 (mean age, 42 years; 79% male; 66 [15%] had coronary calcification; predicted 10-year coronary risk was 6%). Patients were randomly assigned to one of four intervention arms: EBCT results provided in the setting of either ICM (n = 111) or usual care (n = 119) or EBCT results withheld in the setting of either ICM (n = 124) or usual care (n = 96). The primary outcome measure was change in a composite measure of risk, the 10-year Framingham Risk Score (FRS). Comparing the groups who received EBCT results with those who did not, the mean absolute risk change in 10-year FRS was +0.30 versus +0.36. Comparing the groups who received ICM with those who received usual care, the mean absolute risk change in 10-year FRS was -0.06 versus +0.74. Improvement or stabilization of cardiovascular risk was noted in 157 patients (40%). In multivariable analyses predicting change in FRS, after controlling for knowledge of coronary calcification, motivation for change, and multiple psychologic variables, only the number of risk factors (odds ratio, 1:4 for each additional risk factor) and receipt of ICM (odds ratio, 1:6) were associated with improved or stabilized projected risk. Using coronary calcification screening to motivate patients to make evidence-based changes in risk factors was not associated with improvement in modifiable cardiovascular risk at 1 year. Case management was superior to usual care in the management of risk factors.

> **Key Point:** There are limited data demonstrating that a screening test can be used to motivate people to achieve a healthy life style. Thus health care providers are encouraged to focus on motivating patients toward healthy lifestyles in traditional ways, such as education and managed care.

Summary

Screening has become a controversial topic because of the remarkable efficacy of the statins even in asymptomatic individuals.[70] We now have agents that can cut the risk of cardiac events almost in half. The first step in screening asymptomatic individuals for preclinical coronary disease should be using global risk factor equations such as the Framingham score. This is available as nomograms that are easily applied by health care professionals or it can be calculated as part of a computerized patient record. Additional testing procedures with promise include the simple ankle-brachial index (particularly in the elderly), C-reactive protein, carotid ultrasound measurements of intimal thickening, and the resting ECG (particularly spatial QRS-T wave angle). Despite the promotional concept of atherosclerotic burden, EBCT does not have test characteristics superior to the standard exercise test. If any screening test could be used to determine the need for statin therapy and not affect insurance or occupational status, this would be helpful. However, a screening test should not lead to more procedures.

True demonstration of the effectiveness of a screening technique requires randomizing the target population, with one half receiving the screening technique; standardized action taken in response to the screening test results; and then outcomes assessed. For the screening technique to be effective, the screened group must have a lower mortality or morbidity rate (or both). Such a study has been completed for mammography but not for any cardiac testing modalities. The next best validation of efficacy is to demonstrate that the technique improves the discrimination of those asymptomatic individuals with higher risk for events over that possible with the available risk factors. Mathematical modeling makes it possible to determine how well a population will be classified if the characteristics of the testing method are known.

Several well-designed follow-up studies and one angiographic study from the CASS population (where 195 individuals with abnormal exercise-induced ST depression and normal coronary angiograms were followed for 7 years) have improved our understanding of the application of exercise testing as a screening tool. No increased incidence of cardiac events was found; therefore the concerns raised by Erikssen's findings in 36 subjects that they were still at increased risk have not been substantiated.

The later follow-up studies (MRFIT, Seattle Heart Watch, Lipid Research Clinics, and Indiana State police) have shown different results compared to prior studies, mainly because hard cardiac endpoints rather than angina were required. The first 10 prospective studies of exercise testing in asymptomatic individuals included angina as a cardiac disease endpoint. This led to a bias for individuals with abnormal tests to subsequently report angina or to be diagnosed as having angina. When only hard endpoints (death or MI) were used, as in the MRFIT, Lipid Research Clinics, Indiana State Police, or Seattle Heart Watch studies, the results were less encouraging. The test could only identify one third of the patients with hard events, and 95% of abnormal responders were false positives; that is, they did not die or have an MI. The predictive value of the abnormal maximal exercise ECG ranged from 5% to 46% in the studies reviewed. However, in the studies using appropriate endpoints (other than angina pectoris), only 5% of the abnormal responders developed CHD over the follow-up period. Thus more than 90% of the abnormal responders were false positives. In reality, the exercise test's characteristics as a screening test probably lie in between the results of studies using hard or soft endpoints because some of the subjects who develop chest pain have angina and coronary disease. The sensitivity is probably between 30% and 50% (at a specificity of 90%), but the critical limitation is the predictive value (and risk ratio), which depends on the prevalence of disease (which is low in the asymptomatic population).

Some of these individuals have coronary disease that has yet to manifest itself, but angiographic studies have supported this high false-positive rate when using the exercise test in asymptomatic populations. Moreover, the CASS study indicates that such individuals have a good prognosis. In a second Lipid Research Clinics study, only patients with elevated cholesterol levels were considered, yet only a 6% positive prediction value was found. If the test is to be used to screen, it should be done in groups with a higher estimated prevalence of disease using the Framingham score and not just one risk factor. The iatrogenic problems resulting from screening must be considered. Hopefully, using a threshold from the Framingham score would be more successful in identifying asymptomatic individuals who should be tested.

Some individuals who eventually develop coronary disease will change on retesting from a normal to an abnormal response. However, studies by both McHenry and Fleg have reported that a change from a negative to a positive test is no more predictive than is an initially abnormal test. One individual has even been reported who changed from a normal to an abnormal test but was free of angiographically significant disease.[71] In most circumstances an add-on imaging modality (echo or nuclear) should be the first choice in evaluating asymptomatic individuals with an abnormal exercise test.

The concept that there is a motivational impact through screening for CAD is not evidence based. Of the two available studies, one was positive for exercise testing and one negative for EBCT. Further research in this area is needed.

Although the risk of an abnormal exercise test is apparent from these studies, the iatrogenic problems resulting from screening must be considered (i.e., employment, insurance, etc.). The recent U.S. Preventive Services Task Force (USPSTF) statement states that "false positive tests are common among asymptomatic adults, especially women, and may lead to unnecessary diagnostic testing, over treatment and labeling." This statement summarizes the current USPSTF recommendations on screening for CHD and the supporting scientific evidence and updates the 1996 recommendations on this topic. The complete information on which this statement is based, including evidence tables and references, is available in the background article and the systematic evidence review, available through the USPSTF Web site (www.preventiveservices.ahrq.gov) and through the National Guideline Clearinghouse (www.guideline.gov).[72] In the majority of asymptomatic people, screening with any test or test add-on is more likely to yield false positives than true positives. This is the mathematical reality associated with all of the available tests.

Three recent studies (see Table 9-9) lead to the logical conclusion that exercise testing should be part of the preventive health recommendations for screening healthy, asymptomatic individuals along with risk factor assessment. The following reasons justify this conclusion:

1. These three contemporary studies have demonstrated incremental risk ratios for the synergistic combination of the standard exercise test and risk factors.
2. Other modalities without the documented favorable test characteristics of the exercise test are currently being promoted for screening.
3. Physical inactivity has reached epidemic proportions, and what better way to make our patients conscious of their deconditioning than having them do an exercise test that can also "clear them" for exercise?
4. Each 1 MET increase in exercise capacity equates to a 10% to 25% improvement in survival in all populations studied,[73] as well a 5% decline in health care costs.[74]

The additional risk classification power documented by the data from Norway (2000 men, 26-year follow-up), the Cooper Clinic (26,000 men, 8-year follow-up), and Framingham (3000 men, 18-year follow-up) provides convincing evidence that the exercise test should be added to the screening process. Furthermore, exercise capacity itself has substantial prognostic predictive power. Given the emerging epidemic of physical inactivity, including the exercise test in the screening process sends a strong message to our patients that we consider their exercise status as important.

If screening could be performed in a logical way with test results helping to make decisions regarding therapies rather than leading to invasive interventions, insurance problems, or occupational problems, the recent results summarized in this chapter could be applied to preventive medicine policy. Because of the inherent difficulties, few preventive medicine recommendations are based on randomized trials demonstrating improved outcomes but rely on reasonable assumptions from available evidence. There is now enough evidence to consider recommending a routine exercise test every 5 years for men over 40 and women over 50 years of age, especially if one of the potential benefits is the adoption of an active lifestyle.[80]

References

1. Grover SA, Coupal L, Hu XP: Identifying adults at increased risk of coronary disease. How well do the current cholesterol guidelines work? *JAMA* 274(10):801-806, 1995.
2. Anderson P: An updated risk factor profile, *Circulation* 83:356-362, 1991.
3. Wilson PW et al: Prediction of coronary heart disease using risk factor categories, *Circulation* 97(18):1837-1847, 1998.
4. Lloyd-Jones DM et al: Framingham Risk Score and prediction of lifetime risk for coronary heart disease, *Am J Cardiol* 94(1):20-24, 2004.
5. Ridker PM, Cook N: Clinical usefulness of very high and very low levels of C-reactive protein across the full range of Framingham Risk Scores, *Circulation* 109(16):1955-1999, 2004.
6. Conroy RM et al: Estimation of ten-year risk of fatal cardiovascular disease in Europe: the SCORE project, *Eur Heart J* 24(11):987-1003, 2003.
7. Thomsen TF, McGee D, Davidsen M, Jorgensen T: A cross-validation of risk scores for coronary heart disease mortality based on data from the Glostrup Population Studies and Framingham Heart Study, *Int J Epidemiol* 31(4):817-822, 2002.
8. Ostor E et al: Electrocardiographic findings and their association with mortality in the Copenhagen City Heart Study, *Eur Heart J* 2:317-328, 1981.
9. Rose G, Baxter PJ, Reid DD, McCartney P: Prevalence and prognosis of electrocardiogram findings in middle-aged men, *Br Heart J* 15:636-643, 1978.
10. Cullen K, Stenhouse NS, Wearne KL, Cumpston GN: Electrocardiograms and 13 year cardiovascular mortality in Busselton study, *Br Heart J* 47:209-212, 1982.

11. Rabkin SW, Mathewson FAL, Tate RB: The electrocardiogram in apparently healthy men and the risk of sudden death, *Br Heart J* 47:546-552, 1982.

12. Dawber TR, Kannel WB, Love DE, Streeper RB: The Framingham Study, *Circulation* 5:559-566, 1952.

13. Liao Y et al: Major and minor electrocardiographic abnormalities and risk of death from coronary heart disease, cardiovascular diseases and all causes in men and women, *J Am Coll Cardiol* 12:1494-1500, 1988.

14. Menotti A, Seccareccia F: Electrocardiographic Minnesota code findings predicting short-term mortality in asymptomatic subjects. The Italian RIFLE Pooling Project (risk factors and life expectancy), *G Ital Cardiol* 27(1):40-49, 1997.

15. Sigurdsson E, Sigfusson N, Sigvaldason H, Thorgeirsson G: Silent ST-T changes in an epidemiologic cohort study—a marker of hypertension or coronary heart disease, or both: the Reykjavik study, *J Am Coll Cardiol* 27(5):1140-1147, 1996.

16. Kors JA, van Herpen G, van Bemmel JH: QT dispersion as an attribute of T-loop morphology, *Circulation* 99(11):1458-1463, 1999.

17. Lee KW, Kligfield P, Dower GE, Okin PM: QT dispersion, T-wave projection, and heterogeneity of repolarization in patients with coronary artery disease, *Am J Cardiol* 87(2):148-151, 2001.

18. Okin PM et al: Principal component analysis of the T wave and prediction of cardiovascular mortality in American Indians: the Strong Heart Study, *Circulation* 105(6):714-719, 2002.

19. Kors JA et al: T axis as an indicator of risk of cardiac events in elderly people, *Lancet* 352(9128):601-605, 1998.

20. Rautaharju PM et al: Usefulness of T-axis deviation as an independent risk indicator for incident cardiac events in older men and women free from coronary heart disease (the Cardiovascular Health Study), *Am J Cardiol* 88(2):118-123, 2001.

21. Kardys I et al: Spatial QRS-T angle predicts cardiac death in a general population, *Eur Heart J* 24(14):1357-1364, 2003.

22. Rabkin SW, Mathewson FAL, Tate RB: The electrocardiogram in apparently healthy men and the risk of sudden death, *Br Heart J* 47:546-552, 1982.

23. Crow RS et al: Prognostic associations of Minnesota code serial electrocardiographic change classification with coronary heart disease mortality in the Multiple Risk Factor Intervention Trial, *Am J Cardiol* 80(2):138-144, 1997.

24. Froelicher VF et al: Angiographic findings in asymptomatic aircrewmen with electrocardiographic abnormalities, *Am J Cardiol* 39:32-39, 1977.

25. Gibbons RJ et al: ACC/AHA 2002 guideline update for exercise testing: summary article: a report of the American College of Cardiology/American Heart Association Task Force on Practice Guidelines (Committee to Update the 1997 Exercise Testing Guidelines), *Circulation* 106(14):1883-1892, 2002.

26. Bruce RA, McDonough JR: Stress testing in screening for cardiovascular disease, *Bull N Y Acad Med* 45:1288-1295, 1969.

27. Aronow WS, Cassidy J: Five year follow-up of double Master's test, maximal treadmill stress test, and resting and postexercise apexcardiogram in asymptomatic persons, *Circulation* 52:616-622, 1975.
28. Cumming GR et al: Electrocardiographic changes during exercise in asymptomatic men: 3-year follow-up, *Can Med Assoc J* 112:578-585, 1975.
29. Froelicher VF et al: An epidemiological study of asymptomatic men screened with exercise testing for latent coronary heart disease, *Am J Cardiol* 34:770-779, 1975.
30. Manca C et al: Multivariate analysis of exercise ST depression and coronary risk factors in asymptomatic men, *Eur Heart J* 3:2-8, 1982.
31. Allen WH, Aronow WS, Goodman P, Stinson P: Five-year follow-up of maximal treadmill stress test in asymptomatic men and women, *Circulation* 62:522-531, 1980.
32. Bruce RA, Fisher LD, Hossack KF: Validation of exercise-enhanced risk assessment of coronary heart disease events: longitudinal changes in incidence in Seattle community practice, *J Am Coll Cardiol* 5:875-881, 1985.
33. MacIntyre NR et al: Eight-year follow-up of exercise electrocardiograms in healthy, middle-aged aviators, *Aviat Space Environ Med* 52:256-259, 1981.
34. McHenry PL, O'Donnell J, Morris SN, Jordan JJ: The abnormal exercise electrocardiogram in apparently healthy men: a predictor of angina pectoris as an initial coronary event during long-term follow-up, *Circulation* 70:547-551, 1984.
35. Multiple Risk Factor Intervention Research Group: Exercise electrocardiogram and coronary heart disease mortality in the multiple risk factor intervention trial, *Am J Cardiol* 55:16-24, 1985.
36. Rautaharju PM et al: Prognostic value of exercise electrocardiogram in men at high risk of future coronary heart disease: multiple risk factor intervention trial experience, *J Am Coll Cardiol* 8:1-10, 1986.
37. Gordon DL et al: Predictive value of the exercise tolerance test for mortality in North American men: the Lipid Research Clinics Mortality Follow-Up Study, *Circulation* 74:252-261, 1986.
38. Ekelund LG et al: Coronary heart disease morbidity and mortality in hypercholesterolemic men predicted from an exercise test: the Lipid Research Clinics Coronary Primary Prevention Trial, *J Am Coll Cardiol* 14:556-563, 1989.
39. Josephson RA et al: Can serial exercise testing improve the prediction of coronary events in asymptomatic individuals? *Circulation* 81:20-24, 1990.
40. Gordon DJ et al: Smoking, physical activity, and other predictors of endurance and heart rate response to exercise in asymptomatic hypercholesterolemic men, *Am J Epidemiol* 125:587-600, 1987.
41. Borer JS et al: Limitations of the electrocardiographic response to exercise in predicting coronary artery disease, *N Engl J Med* 193:367-375, 1975.
42. Barnard RJ, Gardner GW, Diaco NV, Kattus AA: Near-maximal ECG stress testing and coronary artery disease risk factor analysis in Los Angeles City fire fighters, *J Occup Med* 18:818-827, 1975.
43. Uhl GS et al: Predictive implications of clinical and exercise variables in detecting significant coronary artery disease in asymptomatic men, *J Cardiac Rehabil* 4:245-252, 1984.

44. Erikssen J, Enge I, Forfang K, Storstein O: False positive diagnostic tests and coronary angiographic findings in 105 presumably healthy males, *Circulation* 54:371-376, 1976.

45. Erikssen J, Dale J, Rottwelt K, Myhre E: False suspicion of coronary heart disease: A 7 year follow-up study of 36 apparently healthy middle-aged men, *Circulation* 68:490-497, 1983.

46. Kemp HG, Kronmal RA, Vlietstra RE, Frye RL: Seven year survival of patients with normal and near normal coronary arteriograms: a CASS registry study, *J Am Coll Cardiol* 7:479-483, 1986.

47. Hollenberg M et al: Comparison of a quantitative treadmill exercise score with standard electrocardiographic criteria in screening asymptomatic young men for coronary artery disease, *N Engl J Med* 313(10):600-606, 1985.

48. Okin PM, Anderson KM, Levy D, Kligfield P: Heart rate adjustment of exercise-induced ST-segment depression. Improved risk stratification in the Framingham Offspring Study, *Circulation* 83:866-874, 1991.

49. Fleg JL et al: Prevalence and prognostic significance of exercise-induced silent myocardial ischemia detected by thallium scintigraphy and electrocardiography in asymptomatic volunteers, *Circulation* 81:428-436, 1990.

50. Uhl GS, Kay TN, Hickman JR: Computer-enhanced thallium-scintigrams in asymptomatic men with abnormal exercise tests, *Am J Cardiol* 48:1037-1046, 1981.

51. Uhl GS, Troxler RG, Hickman JR, Clark D: Angiographic correlation of coronary artery disease with high density lipoprotein cholesterol in asymptomatic men, *Am J Cardiol* 48:903-911, 1981.

52. Uhl GS et al: Predictive implications of clinical and exercise variables in detecting significant coronary artery disease in asymptomatic men, *J Cardiac Rehabil* 4:245-252, 1984.

53. Gibbons LW et al: Maximal exercise test as a predictor of risk for mortality from coronary heart disease in asymptomatic men, *Am J Cardiol* 86(1):53-58, 2000.

54. Aktas MK et al: Global risk scores and exercise testing for predicting all-cause mortality in a preventive medicine program, *JAMA* 292(12): 1462-1468, 2004.

55. Balady GJ et al: Usefulness of exercise testing in the prediction of coronary disease risk among asymptomatic persons as a function of the Framingham Risk Score, *Circulation* 110:1920-1925, 2004.

56. Erikssen G et al: Exercise testing of healthy men in a new perspective: from diagnosis to prognosis, *Eur Heart J* 25(11):978-986, 2004.

57. Bodegard J et al: Reasons for terminating an exercise test provide independent prognostic information: 2014 apparently healthy men followed for 26 years, *Eur Heart J* 26(14):1394-1401, 2005.

58. Diamond GA, Forrester JS: Analysis of probability as an aid in the clinical diagnosis of coronary artery disease, *N Engl J Med* 300: 1350-1359, 1979.

59. Siscovick DS et al: Sensitivity of exercise electrocardiography for acute cardiac events during moderate and strenuous physical activity, *Arch Intern Med* 151:325-330, 1991.

60. Zoltick JM, McAllister HA, Bedynek JL: The United States Army Cardiovascular Screening Program, *J Cardiac Rehabil* 4:530-535, 1984.

61. O'Malley PG et al: Rationale and design of the Prospective Army Coronary Calcium (PACC) study: utility of electron beam computed tomography as a screening test for coronary artery disease and as an intervention for risk factor modification among young, asymptomatic, active-duty United States Army personnel, *Am Heart J* 137(5):932-941, 1999.

62. Taylor AJ et al: Do conventional risk factors predict subclinical coronary artery disease? Results from the Prospective Army Coronary Calcium Project, *Am Heart J* 141(3):463-468, 2001.

63. Taylor AJ et al: The independent prognostic value of coronary calcium over measured cardiovascular risk factors in an asymptomatic male screening population: 5 year outcomes in the Prospective Army Coronary Calcium Project, *J Am Coll Cardiol* 46:807-814, 2005.

64. Bruce RA, Fisher LD: Clinical medicine: exercise-enhanced risk factors for coronary heart disease vs. age as criteria for mandatory retirement of healthy pilots, *Aviation, Space, and Environmental Magazine* 58:792-798, 1987.

65. Shaw LJ et al: Prognostic value of cardiac risk factors and coronary artery calcium screening for all-cause mortality, *Radiology* 228(3):826-833, 2003.

66. Greenland P et al: Coronary artery calcium score combined with Framingham score for risk prediction in asymptomatic individuals, *JAMA* 291(2):210-215, 2004.

67. O'Rourke RA et al: American College of Cardiology/American Heart Association Expert Consensus Document on electron-beam computed tomography for the diagnosis and prognosis of coronary artery disease, *J Am Coll Cardiol* 36(1):326-340, 2000, and *Circulation* 102(1):126-140, 2000.

68. Bruce RA, DeRouen TA, Hossack KF: Pilot study examining the motivational effects of maximal exercise testing to modify risk factors and health habits, *Cardiology* 66:111, 1980.

69. O'Malley PG, Feuerstein IM, Taylor AJ: Impact of electron beam tomography, with or without case management, on motivation, behavioral change, and cardiovascular risk profile: a randomized controlled trial, *JAMA* 289(17):2215-2223, 2003.

70. Downs JR et al: Primary prevention of acute coronary events with lovastatin in men and women with average cholesterol levels: results of AFCAPS/TexCAPS. Air Force/Texas Coronary Atherosclerosis Prevention Study, *JAMA* 279:1615-1622, 1998.

71. Thompson AJ, Froelicher VF: Normal coronary angiography in an aircrewman with serial test changes, *Aviation Space Environmental Med* 46:69-73, 1975.

72. U.S. Preventive Services Task Force: Screening for coronary heart disease: recommendation statement, *Ann Intern Med* 140(7):569-572, 2004.

73. Myers J et al: Fitness versus physical activity patterns in predicting mortality in men, *Am J Med* 117(12):912-918, 2004.
74. Weiss JP, Froelicher VF, Myers JN, Heidenreich PA: Health-care costs and exercise capacity, *Chest* 126(2):608-613, 2004.
75. DiPietro L, Kohl HW III, Barlow CE, Blair SN: Improvements in cardiorespiratory fitness attenuate age-related weight gain in healthy men and women: the Aerobics Center Longitudinal Study, *Int J Obes Relat Metab Disord* 22(1):55-62, 1998.
76. Wincup PH et al: Resting electrocardiogram and risk of coronary heart disease in middle-aged British men, *J Cardiovasc Risk* 2:533-543, 1995.
77. Verdecchia P et al: Prognostic value of a new electrocardiographic method for diagnosis of left ventricular hypertrophy in essential hypertension, *J Am Coll Cardiol* 31:383-390, 1998.
78. Milan Study on Atherosclerosis and Diabetes (MiSAD) Group: Prevalence of unrecognized silent myocardial ischemia and its association with atherosclerotic risk factors in noninsulin-dependent diabetes mellitus, *Am J Cardiol* 79:134-139, 1997.
79. Mathewson FA, Manfreda J, Tate RB, Cuddy TE: The University of Manitoba Follow-up Study—an investigation of cardiovascular disease with 35 years of follow-up (1948-1983), *Can J Cardiol* 3:378-382, 1987.
80. Froelicher VF: Screening with the exercise test: time for a guideline change? *Eur Heart J* 26:1353-1354.

10   Case Examples

Case One: Failure of CABS and PCI to Normalize Exercise-Induced ST Depression

This patient is a 65-year-old man with hypertension, hyperlipidemia, status post four-vessel coronary artery bypass surgery (CABS) 2/03. Surgery included two left internal mammary artery grafts and three saphenous vein grafts (LIMA-D1, SVG-LAD, SVG-OM, SVG-PDA). He did well until 2 years later when he began to experience chest tightness and SOB at reproducible levels of exertion.

On 5/05 he underwent an exercise test with similar chest pain and 1.5 mm of ST depression at maximal exercise.

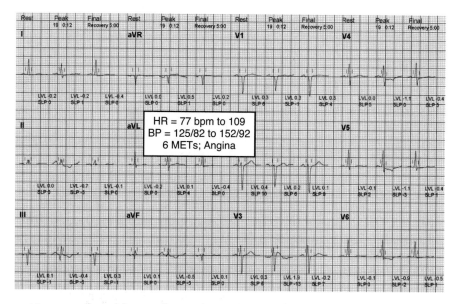

HR = 77 bpm to 109
BP = 125/82 to 152/92
6 METs; Angina

He was referred for cardiac catheterization, which showed the following results:

1. Left main coronary artery is a moderate-sized vessel that trifurcates into left anterior descending artery, ramus intermedius artery, and left circumflex artery. The distal left main coronary artery (LMCA) has a filling defect due to calcified plaque.
2. Left anterior descending is totally occluded after a large septal branch and small diagonal artery. The first diagonal (D1) has a high-grade proximal lesion.
3. Left circumflex is a moderate-sized vessel that gives rise to two obtuse marginal arteries, the second of which has a high-grade ostial lesion.

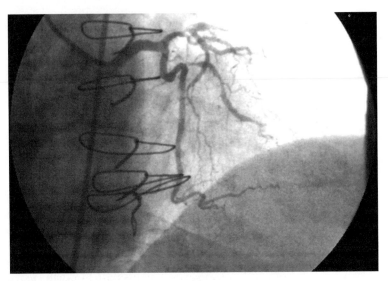

4. Right coronary artery is a moderate-sized dominant vessel that has mild diffuse disease and supplies an RV continuation branch and PLV. The PDA is occluded at its takeoff.

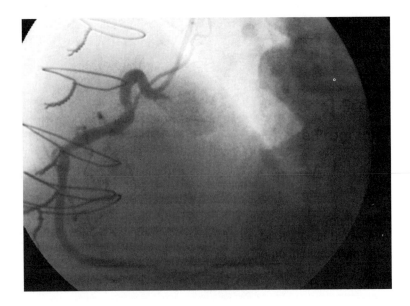

5. The LIMA to the second diagonal (D2) is a moderate-sized patent vessel with normal distal anastomosis. The D2 vessel has a high-grade (80%) lesion just distal to the LIMA anastomosis and is a small-caliber vessel distally. There is limited backfilling to the left anterior descending artery (LAD).

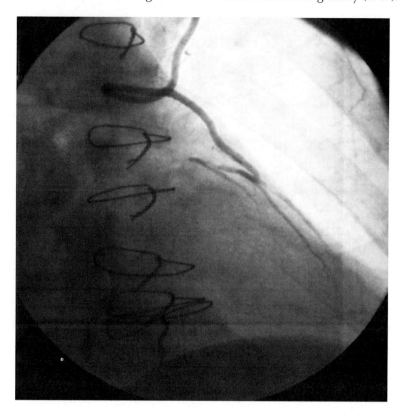

6. The saphenous venous graft (SVG) to the LAD is a smaller graft with moderate diffuse disease and a moderate (50%) ostial narrowing.

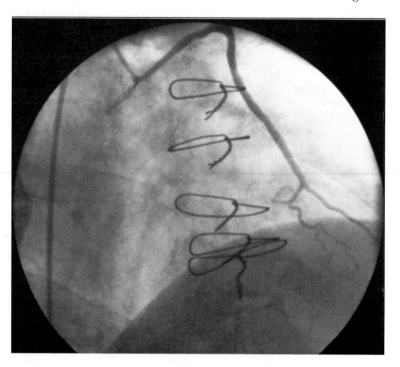

7. SVG to obtuse marginal (OM) is patent.
8. SVG to posterior descending artery (PDA) is a moderate-sized graft with 80% ostial-proximal narrowing.

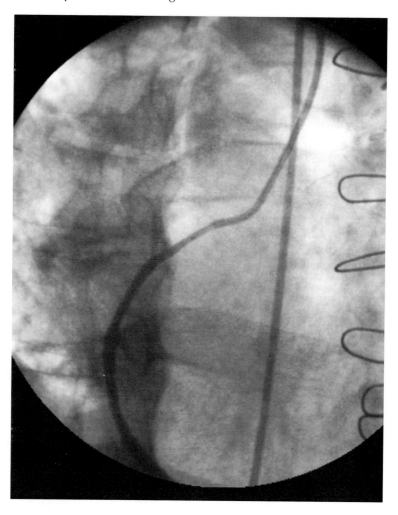

A successful PCI of the ostial SVG-RCA was performed with good angiographic result and improved flow into a now moderate-sized PDA with limited collaterals to the left.

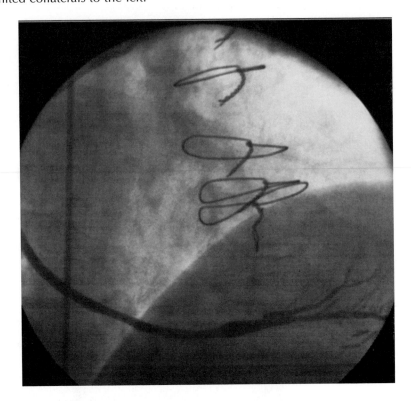

A repeat treadmill test was performed 1 month later.

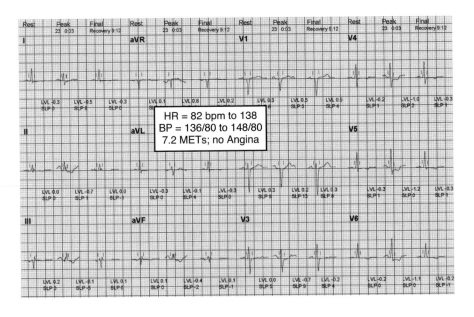

HR = 82 bpm to 138
BP = 136/80 to 148/80
7.2 METs; no Angina

He was on beta blockers for both tests. A stent in the SVG to the RCA relieved the angina and increased exercise capacity by 1 MET and maximal HR by 30 beats/min but did not normalize the exercise-induced ST-segment depression.

Commentary

Although dramatic improvements in exercise test–induced ST depression can be seen (per later examples), sometimes both PCI and CABS do not do so. Although the angina disappeared, the ST depression remained. Perhaps ischemia was relieved, but this could be a placebo effect. Nuclear imaging was not decisive in clarifying this issue.

Case Two: False-Positive ST Depression

This is a 68-year-old gentleman with HBP and hyperlipidemia; he had endocarditis on 7/03/04, with severe mitral regurgitation that led to mitral valve repair and myotomy/myectomy on 9/10/04 and DDDR pacemaker placement at another hospital. He also had a cardiac catheterization that showed nonocclusive disease that did not require bypass surgery along with the valvular surgery.

The patient wanted to defer management of his cardiovascular care primarily to his private physician but also wanted to continue to follow up with the VA cardiology group and to continue to receive his medications through the VA. Though asymptomatic, he requested a treadmill test before entering an exercise program.

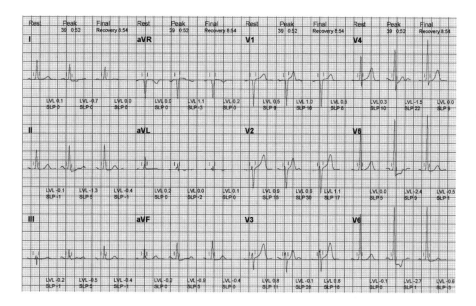

His private physician decided that this was a false-positive ST response and allowed him to enter a gym-based exercise program without monitoring.

Commentary

His lack of symptoms and normal cath support, this being a false-positive (FP) ST response, and the myocardial stress of his valvular lesion could account for the FP ST response. However, he could have ruptured a plaque since or had a coronary embolus during the surgery. We would have performed a nuclear stress study as well.

Case Three: Left Main Obstruction

This patient is a 69-year-old man with hypertension, hyperlipidemia, and a stroke '01 without residual defects; he is 153 lb and 66 inches tall. He was referred for a treadmill test because of the recent onset of SOB with exertion. He had been able to polka 5 nights/week, 4 hours/night without symptoms but noted DOE within 3 minutes of polka starting 1 week ago. An echo showed normal LV function and mild mitral regurgitation (MR).

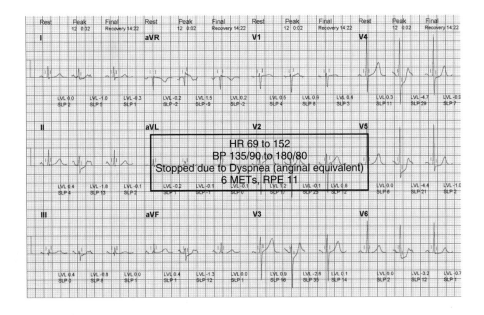

HR 69 to 152
BP 135/90 to 180/80
Stopped due to Dyspnea (anginal equivalent)
6 METs, RPE 11

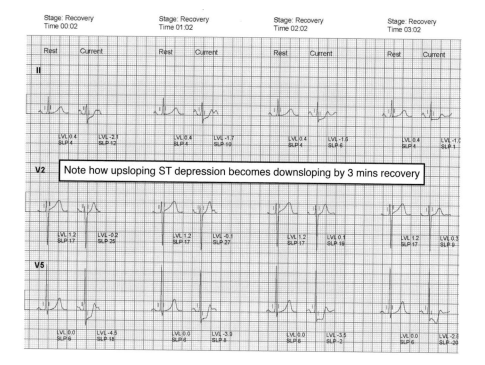

Stage: Recovery Time 00:02	Stage: Recovery Time 01:02	Stage: Recovery Time 02:02	Stage: Recovery Time 03:02

| Rest | Current | Rest | Current | Rest | Current | Rest | Current |

II

| LVL 0.4 SLP 4 | LVL -2.1 SLP 12 | LVL 0.4 SLP 4 | LVL -1.7 SLP 10 | LVL 0.4 SLP 4 | LVL -1.6 SLP 6 | LVL 0.4 SLP 4 | LVL -1.0 SLP 1 |

V2

Note how upsloping ST depression becomes downsloping by 3 mins recovery

| LVL 1.2 SLP 17 | LVL -0.2 SLP 25 | LVL 1.2 SLP 17 | LVL -0.1 SLP 27 | LVL 1.2 SLP 17 | LVL 0.1 SLP 19 | LVL 1.2 SLP 17 | LVL 0.3 SLP 9 |

V5

| LVL 0.0 SLP 6 | LVL -4.5 SLP 18 | LVL 0.0 SLP 6 | LVL -3.9 SLP 8 | LVL 0.0 SLP 6 | LVL -3.5 SLP -2 | LVL 0.0 SLP 6 | LVL -2.8 SLP -20 |

He was taken directly to the cath lab from the exercise lab on 1/10/2006 with the following findings:

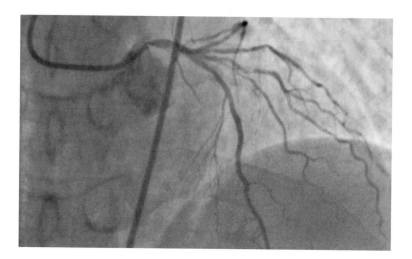

The left main coronary artery is of intermediate length and bifurcates into the LAD and left circumflex. There is 95% ostial left main narrowing, with moderate diffuse disease afterward. There was a ventricularized waveform on engagement of the left main coronary artery. The left anterior descending is a moderate-sized vessel that gives off a moderate-sized diagonal branch. There is 60% proximal LAD stenosis, followed by the diagonal with 80%

ostial stenosis. The distal LAD does not have significant angiographic disease. The left circumflex is a moderate-sized vessel that gives rise to an obtuse marginal branch. There is a 60% lesion in the mid-obtuse marginal.

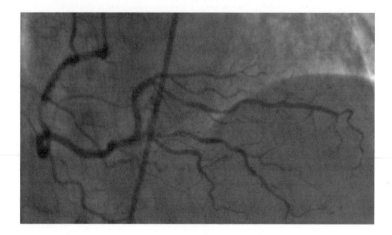

The right coronary artery is a large dominant vessel that supplies the PDA and PLV. There is a 70% mid-RCA lesion and moderate (60%) stenoses in the bifurcating PDA and PLV vessels.

He underwent CABS.

Commentary

This patient is interesting for several reasons. First, he presented with an anginal equivalent of dyspnea on exertion. Second, his treadmill responses are surprising because his SBP did not drop during exercise and his most abnormal ST depression occurred at 3 minutes of recovery. In fact, the depression during exercise was all upsloping, though it was suspicious for ischemia because of the depth and ST depression area.

Case Four: Exertional Hypotension

This patient is a 55-year-old man with a history of hypertension, hyperlipidemia, prostate cancer, and sleep apnea. He came into clinic on 10/3/05 for follow-up of his multiple medical issues. The main issue was the new onset of exertional chest tightness. For 2 months he noticed that when he walked up stairs, especially if he carried something or if he rushed, he experienced tightness in his chest, a heaviness that radiated into his left arm. He denied associated dyspnea, but there were occasions when he panted and gasped for breath as he rushed to catch a train, whereas 6 months ago he did that with no difficulty. He noted that he is somewhat diaphoretic when he has chest tightness.

He was taking simvastatin, losartan, and aspirin.

A nuclear medicine study was performed 10/05. He was given technetium 99m tetrofosmin 7.6 mCi IV at rest and 23.4 mCi IV during exercise. Myocardial perfusion images were acquired in the prone position 40 minutes after injection of the radiopharmaceutical at rest. The patient returned later in the day for the exercise part of the study.

The baseline ECG was normal. The resting heart rate and blood pressure were 56 beats/min and 109/74 mm Hg. He was tested using a treadmill ramp protocol for 8 minutes and 45 seconds to a maximum workload of 9.5 METs before stopping because of chest pain and ST-segment changes. The peak heart rate and blood pressure were 160 beats/min and 93/54 mm Hg. The patient began to have midsternal chest pressure 3 minutes after starting exercise and developed exertional hypotension.

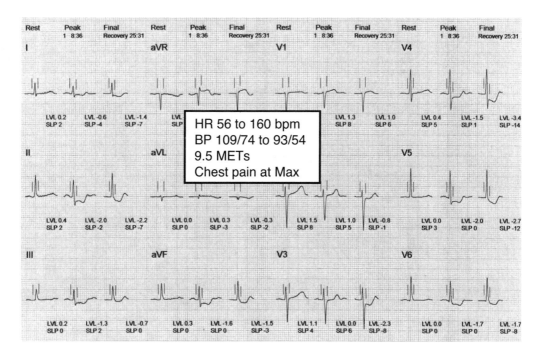

The ECG showed 2 mm of ST-segment depression in the inferior and lateral precordial leads. The patient continued to have chest pain after exercise was stopped. The ECG showed atrial fibrillation with 3 mm of downsloping ST-segment depression in the inferior and lateral precordial leads. The patient was given 0.4 mg of nitroglycerin sublingually, as well as oxygen by nasal cannula. The patient's chest pain subsided, although it never resolved entirely, and the ST depression persisted long into the recovery period.

Myocardial perfusion images were acquired in the prone position minutes after injection of the radiopharmaceutical. The patient was transferred to the Emergency Department, and Cardiology consultation was requested for acute coronary syndrome.

Findings

The images acquired following exercise showed a large area of moderately severe hypoperfusion involving the anterior wall, apex, septum, and lateral wall, areas supplied by the left anterior descending and left circumflex coronary arteries, or the left main coronary artery. All of the perfusion abnormalities were reversible when compared with the images obtained at rest. Only the inferior wall appeared relatively well perfused. The resting left ventricular ejection fraction was 18%, but an echo the next day revealed a normal EF and LV dimensions. The erroneous EF with nuclear imaging could be explained by the atrial fibrillation in recovery, but we often see EF errors with the perfusion gating.

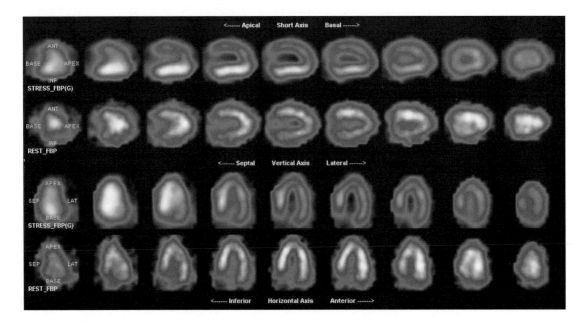

Emergent cardiac catheterization

Hemodynamics: RA 5, RV 27/6, PA 26/10, PCW 10, Fick CO 5.3, CI 2.8

Angiography:

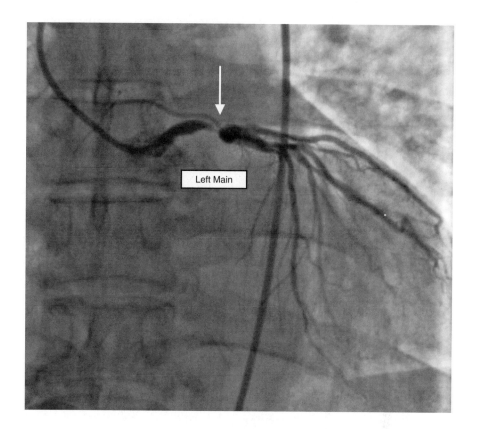

Left Main

1. The left main coronary artery is a moderate-sized vessel that trifurcates into the left anterior descending artery, the ramus, and the left circumflex artery. There is an 80% distal LM narrowing.
2. Left anterior descending artery is a small, branching vessel that reaches the apex of the heart and gives origin to one significant diagonal artery. The artery has no significant disease.
3. The left circumflex is a small, branching vessel that gives rise to two obtuse marginal arteries. The artery has no significant disease.
4. The right coronary artery is a dominant vessel that gives rise to the PDA and two PLs. The RCA is normal, but there is a moderate, 40% lesion in the proximal PDA.

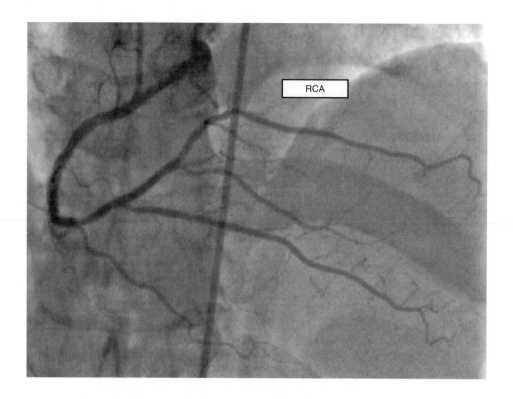

Assessment/Plan
Start heparin drip and continue aspirin. CT surgery contacted for urgent bypass surgery.

Coronary artery bypass grafting with two vessels with saphenous vein graft to the LAD and saphenous vein graft to the obtuse marginal was performed on cardiopulmonary bypass on 10/29/05.

Commentary

Exertional hypotension, angina, and marked ST depression are common with LM disease. Having reasonable perfusion via the RCA obviated some of his ischemic risk. Exertional hypotension is perhaps the only marker for increased risk for cardiac arrest during exercise testing.

Case Five: ST Depression with Persantine

This patient is a 57-year-old man with diabetes and coronary artery disease who had shortness of breath and chest discomfort for the last 6 months whenever walking up a hill. He walks approximately two blocks before he has symptoms.

Medical History
1. Hypertension.
2. Hyperlipidemia.
3. Type 2 diabetes since 1985.
4. Obesity.
5. Erectile dysfunction.
6. Vertebral artery insufficiency with CVA treated with Aggrenox.
7. MRA shows occlusion of the left vertebral artery and high-grade stenosis of the right vertebral artery. He had a full recovery from his stroke.

Nuclear Study
Pharmacologic stress myocardial perfusion scintigraphy examination was performed 12/17/04. Tc99m tetrofosmin 8.6 mCi IV was injected in the morning and 25.9 mCi IV in the afternoon. Myocardial perfusion images were acquired in the prone position 45 minutes following injection at rest. The patient returned later in the day for the second part of the examination. Resting heart rate and blood pressure were 92 beats/min and 138/74 mm Hg. 60 mg of Persantine was infused intravenously over 4 minutes. Additionally, the patient walked on a treadmill at 1 mph at 5.1% grade. The patient reported mild throat discomfort but no significant chest pain. At 10 minutes, the heart rate and blood pressure were 110 beats/min and 128/69 mm Hg. A postinfusion ECG demonstrated 2.5 mm of ST-segment depression in V5-V6. A second dose was injected intravenously 10 minutes after beginning the infusion of Persantine. Additional myocardial perfusion images were acquired in the prone position 60 minutes later.

Impression
1. Probable moderate-sized inferobasal inferior wall infarct (area typically supplied by the RCA) with likely inferoapical peri-infarct ischemia of moderate extent and severity.

2. Inferobasal hypokinesis with otherwise normal wall motion and EF of 41%; however, the echo showed normal EF greater than 55% with mild LVH with hypokinesis of the basal inferior wall.

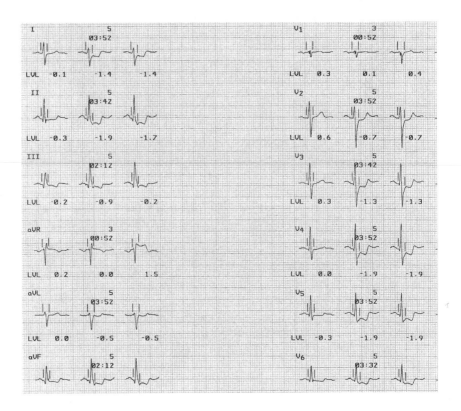

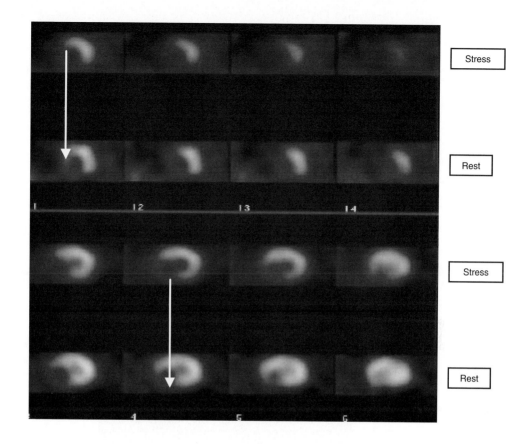

Cardiac catheter was performed on 3/9/05 and showed severe three-vessel coronary artery disease, 100% right coronary lesion. He had 80% proximal stenosis at origin of first D1 in his LAD ("widow maker") with reconstitution of his PDA of the collaterals from the left. He also had an anomalous left circumflex with significant disease.

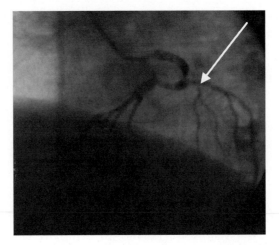

Proximal LAD lesion

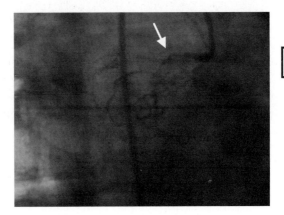

RCA – total occlusion

He was admitted for CABS at the end of 3/05 and received two vein grafts (OM and PDA) and a LIMA to the LAD.

A follow-up treadmill test was performed on 9/4/05:

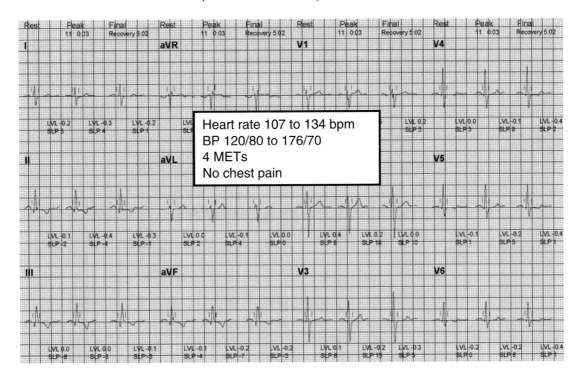

Heart rate 107 to 134 bpm
BP 120/80 to 176/70
4 METs
No chest pain

Commentary

The significance of ECG changes with Persantine is uncertain because the mechanism of ischemia is due to steal rather than limited flow. Nonetheless, the changes are striking between before and after coronary artery bypass surgery.

Case Six: Abnormal Screening Treadmill Test

This patient is a 39-year-old active male who is 69 inches tall and 165 lb. He underwent a treadmill exercise ECG test (ramp protocol) and gas exchange (CPX) on 5/23/05 for a policeman fitness test to evaluate exercise capacity. (10 METs is a requirement for the VA Police.)

Current Medications
The patient is not taking any cardiac medications.

Medical History
The patient has no chest pain, angina, or other symptoms. The patient has no history of dysrhythmias or cardiac disease. No other medical problems are noted. No history of noncardiac problems was noted.

Risk Factors

The patient has never smoked. The patient is 4 lb over the average appropriate body mass index (BMI = 24.4). The patient has a history of high cholesterol with a current level reported at 221 mg/dl. HDL level was somewhat low at 47 mg/dl (normal ≥55 mg/dl); in addition, the LDL level was high at 144 mg/dl (normal <100 mg/dl). Triglycerides level was slightly elevated at 148 mg/dl (≥100 mg/dl). No other risk factors are noted.

The Framingham-1 Score estimated a 5-year incidence of cardiovascular events (angina, MI, or death) of <1% (as expected for age and gender).

Cardiac Events and Interventions

No previous myocardial infarction, symptoms, or testing reported.

Baseline pretest heart rate was within normal limits at 78 beats/min. Pretest baseline BP was within normal limits at 120/80 mm Hg and rose to 220 mm Hg at peak exercise.

Resting ECG

No resting QRS-conduction defects were observed, but voltage criteria for LVH were present with no ST depression and there was marked early repolarization.

Symptoms

No noncardiac test-limiting conditions for this patient were noted, and the test was terminated due to general fatigue without angina during exercise or recovery.

Hemodynamic Response

The patient achieved 15 estimated METs and 13.5 measured METs (from gas analysis) at a perceived exertion level of 17 out of 20 on the Borg scale. The heart rate was 78 beats/min at baseline and rose 112 beats/min to 190 beats/min at maximal exercise. The 2-minute recovery heart rate was 136 beats/min and dropped 54 beats/min from maximal exercise. The systolic BP was 120 mm Hg at baseline and rose 100 mm Hg to 220 mm Hg at maximal exercise.

Exercise ECG

At maximal exercise the ST segments showed 1 mm of horizontal ST depression in the inferior and lateral leads. In recovery the ST segments showed no depression. No significant dysrhythmias occurred in response to exercise. No bundle branch blocks or conduction defects were present at rest or developed during exercise.

Complications

No complications occurred during this test.

The Duke Score (METs, ST depression, and exercise angina) of 13 estimates an annual cardiovascular mortality rate of 0.7%.

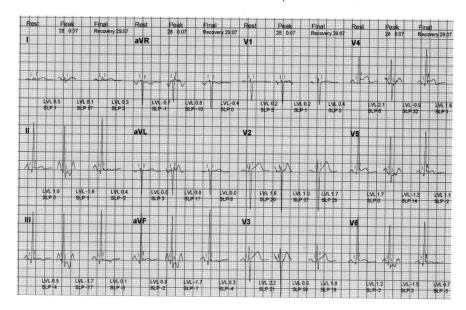

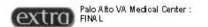

Palo Alto VA Medical Center :
FINAL

Test Patient 06   Tested: January 01, 2006 at 12:00 PDT
SSN: N/A
Male Caucasian Age: 29 (DOB: 1975-01-01)
Height: 69 in.   Weight: 165 lbs.   BMI: 24.4

Imaging: None
Encounter Type: Out-Patient: General Consult
Treadmill : Ramp : ECG and Gas Exchange (CPX)
1°: General Exercise Capacity
2°: None

Comments: Exercise capacity for job.
Supervising HCP: Not Available   Referring MD: Not Available   Technician: Not Available   Reviewer: Vic Froelicher (Confirmed)

RISK FACTORS
Non-Modifiable :   Male
Modifiable: HiChol, Low HDL, HiLDL, HiTRIGL
Healthful: Non-smoker ... Active Lifestyle ... Only 3.7 lbs over ideal weight
Fram-1: 5yr @ 0.3% (1.3x) Fram-2: [2yr @ 0.3% (1.3x); 4yr @ 0.7% (1.3x)]

MEDICAL HISTORY SUMMARY
- No Medical Problems or History Reported -

CARDIOVASCULAR EXERCISE TEST SUMMARY

• Resting ECG: ABNORMAL
LVH
Marked early repolarization.

• Any CAD: LOW

Prediction	Scores	Cutoffs
Pre-Test (Morise):	LOW: 4 / 16	L:≤8 H:≥16
Post-Test (Froelicher):	LOW: 11 / 95	L:≤39 H:≥61

• Severe CAD: LOW

Prediction	Scores	Cutoffs
Pre-Test (Morise %):	LOW: 1%	L:≤15 H:≥40
Post-Test (Froelicher):	LOW: 11 / 105	L:≤54 H:≥76

• Post-Test CV Prognosis: LOW RISK (GOOD)
(cf: Age, Gender, Race)

Prediction	Natl @0.1% ... (Expected: <2% or <2s)
Duke:	LOW: 13.0: 0.7% 6.6x
VA/Froelicher:	LOW: 15.0: 0.6% 6.0x

• Post-Test All-Cause Mortality: LOW RISK (GOOD)

Prediction	Scores	Cutoffs
VA/Froelicher Score %:	LOW: 0 / 5 (1x)	L:≤1 H:≥3
HR Recovery Score:	LOW: -100 (1x)	L:≤20 H:≥25
HR Recovery:	LOW: -54 bpm	L:≤-22 H:≥-17

• Exercise ECG: NORMAL
ST depression during exercise mainly in inferior leads that clears in recovery.

Hemodynamics	Findings	Normal Values
Baseline HR	78	60-89 bpm
Peak Exer HR(ABL:HRR)	190 (112)	≥162 bpm
Target HR (% Reached)	191 (99%)	≥85% Target HR
1min Recovery HR (ΔPK)	155 (-35)	
2min Recovery HR (ΔPK)	136 (-54)	≤168 bpm (≤-22)
Estimated HRR (CI)	113 (0.99)	CI≥0.80
Baseline SBP/DBP	120 / 80	<130/85 mmHg
Peak Exercise SBP/DBP	220 / 90 BOR	<220/110 mmHg
SBP Rise ΔBL	100	Δ~20 mmHg
Max SBP Reached (ΔPK)	220 (0)	Δ<10 mmHg
2min Recovery SBP (%PK)	190 (86%) ABN	<220 mmHg (≤79%)

Exercise Capacity		
Exercise Duration	09:00	(-Per Protocol-)
Borg (6-20)	17	(-Per Patient-)
Estimated METs (%Pred)	15.00 (110%)	≥10.18 METS (≥75%)

ECG Response		
Baseline ST	0	(-Per ACC/AHA-)
Peak Exer ST(ΔBL) m	1 (1) T	(-Per ACC/AHA-)
Recovery ST(ΔBL) m	0 (0) T	(-Per ACC/AHA-)
ST-Depr Regions	Inf	No Depression
ST-Elev Regions	-None-	No Elevation

Findings and Recommendations

• No abnormal ST-Depression occurred during test
• No Angina occurred (No Hx Angina)
• Exertional Hypertension and Poor SBP Recovery
• Good Functional Capacity

• LOW Risk for Any CAD
• CV Prognosis: LOW Risk (GOOD)
• All-Cause Mortality: LOW Risk (GOOD Prognosis)
• Limitations: None
• Reasons Stopped: Fatigue (typical endpoint)
• Complications: None

• Recommend: Reduce risk factors (see below). Monitor blood-pressure and consider anti-HTN treatment. Refer also to cardiopulmonary stress test results.

• Modifiable Risk Factors: Maintain active lifestyle. Maintain current weight. Lessen risks from hyperlipidemia with appropriate healthy diet and regular exercise. Consider treatment with statins and niacin.
• Base interpretation of findings and recommendations in the context of the patient's young age, medical history, co-morbidities, current activity level and lifestyle.

• Reviewer's Comments: abnormal

Test Patient 06
SSN: N/A

Male Caucasian (Age at Test: 29) (DOB: 1975-01-01) Height 69 in. 165lbs. (BMI: 24.42)
Tested: January 01, 2005 at 12:00 PDT Treadmill : Ramp Both ECG and CPX

CARDIOPULMONARY EXERCISE TEST SUMMARY

Resting Pulmonary Function Test Results		
--- Spirometry ---		
FVC:	5.15	Liters
Predicted FVC (%Pred):	0.00 (0%)	
FEV-1:	0.00	Liters
Predicted FEV-1 (%Pred):	0.00 (0%)	
FEV-1/FVC:	0	%
Predicted FEV-1/FVC (%Pred):	0 (0%)	
Estimated MVV:	0	Liters / min

Exercise Cardiopulmonary Test Results		
Measured METs:	13.5	
Predicted (%-Pred):	15.3 (88%)	
Workload:	334	Watts
Measured Peak VO2:	47.3	ml / Kg / min
Predicted (%-Pred):	53.6 (88%)	
Ventilatory Threshold:	77	% (10.3 METs)
Minute Ventilation (VE):	96.7	Liters / min
(Estimated VE):	(0.0)	
VE/VCO2 Slope:	0.15	
RER (RQ):	1.19	
Arterial O2 Saturation:	92	%

Pretest Spirometry Findings:

Cardiopulmonary Exercise Test Findings:
• The measured peak VO2 was 47.3 ml/kg/min (METs = 13.5) and is 88% of expected from the Wasserman equation (53.6 ml/kg/min for a subject within normal weight limits).
• The estimated peak arterial O2 saturation of 92% was within low-normal limits (Normal is > 90% at peak exercise).
… Breathing reserve is not available. …
• The ventilatory threshold (VT) of 76% of peak VO2 was well above normal (Normal is > 40% of peak VO2).
• The VE/VCO2 slope was normal at 0.15 (Normal < 0.30).

CONCLUSIONS:
• … (No Resting Spirometry Testing results are available) …
• The patient's measured exercise capacity (88%) was within normal limits for age, gender and weight with no significant cardiac or pulmonary limitation to exercise indicated.

CT Angio

Because his pretest probability was so low, it was decided that going to invasive testing directly was inappropriate. Rather than nuclear perfusion or echo exercise testing, ultrafast 64-slice CT was available and so it was recommended for this patient:

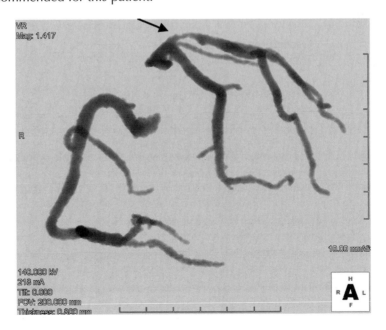

The ultrafast 64-slice CT revealed that the patient had a proximal high-grade lesion in the LAD.

Commentary

There was no ST depression at rest, and the ST elevation (early repolarization) is quite normal in an athletic young man. The voltage criteria for LVH also is common and not associated with increased risk when there is no ST depression. The ST depression was only present at maximal exercise and disappeared immediately on stopping the test. These surprising results in a patient we felt would be a false positive led us to consider that ultrafast CT will eventually be the best test in such patients. Unfortunately, with current technology, it is equivalent to 300 chest x-rays, and a large bolus of contrast media is required. Clinically significant CAD is unusual (particularly as a cause of death) in individuals younger than 40 years old without familial hyperlipidemia. The critical risk factor for MI in younger males is cigarette smoking.

Case Seven: Pre-/Post-CABG

This patient is a 59-year-old active Caucasian man who is 65 inches tall and 145 lb and who works for the post office. He was seen in general medical clinic on 11/24/04, complaining of exertional chest pain when using his treadmill at home. The chest pain only occurred when he increased to a high intensity, and it subsided when he stopped. On 12/9/04, he underwent an exercise test with abnormal ST depression during exercise and recovery. He achieved an exercise capacity and maximal heart rate appropriate for his age (12 METs, MHR 155, 2 min HR drop 56, resting SBP 160, which rose to 165 mm Hg).

Current Medications
The patient is taking antihypertensives, ASA, and a statin.

Medical History
The patient has chest pain, most likely angina as described above.

Risk Factors
The patient has never smoked but has high blood pressure. The patient is 3 lb over the average appropriate body mass index (BMI = 24.2). The patient has a history of high cholesterol, and HDL was low at 31 mg/dl.

Cardiac Events and Interventions
None

Resting ECG

The resting ECG is normal, so there is a 95% probability of a normal ejection fraction (later confirmed).

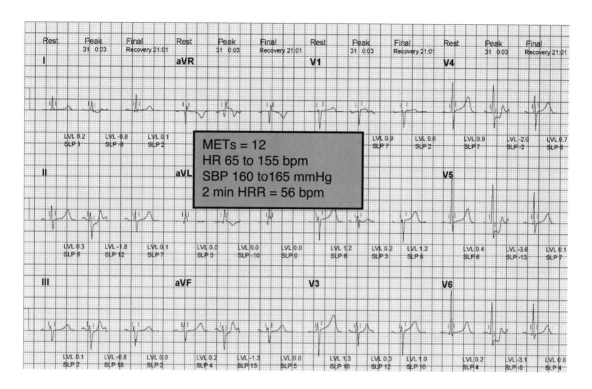

METs = 12
HR 65 to 155 bpm
SBP 160 to165 mmHg
2 min HRR = 56 bpm

The exercise response is normal.

Palo Alto VA Medical Center :
FINAL

Generated: January 01, 2006 @ 12:00 pm (PDT)

Test Patient 03   Tested: Jan 01, 2006 at 12:00 PDT
SSN: N/A
Male Caucasian Age: 58 (DOB: 1946-01-01)
Height: 65 in. Weight: 157 lbs. BMI: 26.2

Imaging: None
Encounter Type: Out-Patient: General Consult
Treadmill : Ramp : ECG and Gas Exchange (CPX)
1°: Signs/Symptoms of CAD or Risk-Factors
2°: None

Comments:
Supervising HCP: Not Available   Referring MD: Not Available   Technician: Not Available   Reviewer: Vic Froelicher (Confirmed)

RISK FACTORS
Non-Modifiable :   Male (Age>50)
Modifiable: HiChol, Low HDL, HiLDL, HTN
Healthful: Non-smoker ... Active Lifestyle ... Only 8.1 lbs over ideal weight
Fram-1: 5yr @ 6.9 % (1.9x) Fram-2: [2yr @ 1.7 % (1.9x); 4yr @ 4.2 % (1.8x)]

MEDICAL HISTORY SUMMARY
Typical Angina
Beta-Blocker

CARDIOVASCULAR EXERCISE TEST SUMMARY

- Resting ECG: NORMAL
(A 95 % probability of a normal ejection-fraction is estimated)

- Any CAD: HIGH

Prediction	Score :	Cutoffs
Pre-Test (Morise):	HIGH: 16 / 18	L:≤8 H:≥16
Post-Test (Froelicher):	HIGH: 73 / 95	L:≤39 H:≥61

- Severe CAD: INTERMEDIATE

Prediction	Score :	Cutoffs
Pre-Test (Morise %):	LOW: 12%	L:≤15 H:≥40
Post-Test (Froelicher):	INT: 73 / 105	L:≤54 H:≥76

- Post-Test CV Prognosis: INTERMEDIATE RISK (GUARDED)
Reasons: METs, ST-depr, SBP response (cf: Age, Gender, Race)

Prediction	Natl @ 1.2% ... (Expected: <2% or <2 :)		
Duke:	HI: -10.2:	4.0%	3.4x
VA/Froelicher:	INT: 3.5:	3.1%	2.6x

- Post-Test All-Cause Mortality: LOW RISK (GOOD)

Prediction	Score :	Cutoffs
VA:Froelicher Score %:	LOW: 0.75 (1x)	L:≤1 H:≥3
HR Recovery Score:	LOW: -46 (1x)	L:≤20 H:≥25
HR Recovery:	LOW: -56 bpm	L:≤-22 H:≥-17

- Exercise ECG: ABNORMAL
ST-Depr (Exer+Recov),
Dysrhythmias: Occasional PVCs

Hemodynamics	Findings		Normal Values
Baseline HR	53	BO R↓	60-89 bpm
Peak Exer HR(ΔBL:HRR)	155 (102)		≥137 bpm
Target HR (%Reached)	162 (95%)		≥85% Target HR
1min Recovery HR (ΔPK)	112 (-43)		
2min Recovery HR (ΔPK)	99 (-56)		≤133 bpm (≤-22)
Estimated HRR (CI)	109 (0.94)		CI≥0.80
Baseline SBP/DBP	160 / 100	ABN	<130/85 mmHg
Peak Exercise SBP/DBP	165 / 100		<220/110 mmHg
SBP Rise ΔBL	5	BOR	Δ>20 mmHg
Max SBP Reached (ΔPK)	165 (0)		Δ<10 mmHg
2min Recovery SBP (%PK)	140 (85%)	BOR	<220 mmHg (≤79%)

Exercise Capacity			
Exercise Duration	10:12		(-Per Protocol-)
Borg (6-20)	19		(-Per Patient-)
Estimated METs (%Pred)	11.50 (127%)		≥6.79 METS (≥75%)

ECG Response			
Baseline ST	0		(-Per ACC/AHA-)
Peak Exer ST(ΔBL) m	4 (4) ↓	ABN	(-Per ACC/AHA-)
Recovery ST(ΔBL) m	2 (2) ↓	ABN	(-Per ACC/AHA-)
ST-Depr Regions	Lat	ABN	No Depression
ST-Elev Regions	-None-		No Elevation

Findings and Recommendations

- ST-Depression occurred during Exercise and Recovery
- Exercise-Induced Occasional PVCs
- No Angina occurred (Hx Angina)
- Baseline Bradycardia and Hypertension
- Exertional Hypotension and Poor SBP Recovery
- Good Functional Capacity

- HIGH Risk for Any CAD and INTERMEDIATE Risk for Severe CAD
- CV Prognosis: INTERMEDIATE Risk (GUARDED)
- All-Cause Mortality: LOW Risk (GOOD Prognosis)
- Limitations: None
- Reasons Stopped: Fatigue (typical endpoint)
- Complications: None

- HEMO-Notes: Exertional hypotension may be due to ischemia (ST-depression). Beta-Blockers can blunt SBP reponses and make ischemia painless.
- Recommend: Reduce risk factors (see below). Monitor blood-pressure and consider anti-HTN treatment. Refer also to cardiopulmonary stress test results.

- Modifiable Risk Factors: Maintain active lifestyle. Maintain current weight. Lessen risks from hyperlipidemia and hypertension with appropriate healthy diet and regular exercise. Consider treatment with statins, niacin and anti-HTN medication.
- Base interpretation of findings and recommendations in the context of the patient's older age, medical history, co-morbidities, current activity level and lifestyle.

- Reviewer's Comments: Very Abnormal.

12/10/2004 Cardiac Catheterization

1. Left main coronary artery shows no significant disease.
2. Left anterior descending is a moderate-sized vessel that reaches around the apex of the heart and gives rise to a branching diagonal artery. It has high-grade ostial disease and high-grade disease just after the first septal branch. There is diffuse disease in the remainder of the LAD. The branching diagonal also has diffuse disease.
3. Left circumflex is a moderate-sized vessel that gives rise to two obtuse marginal arteries. There is a high-grade proximal stenosis in the large first obtuse marginal artery.

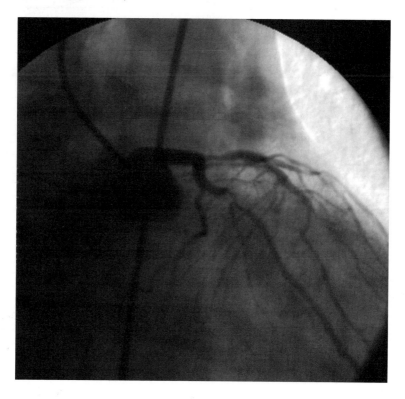

4. Large dominant right coronary artery supplying the PDA and PLV both with high-grade disease.

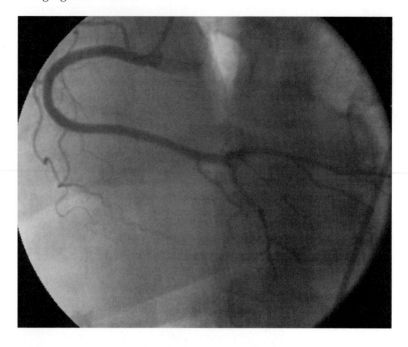

Conclusions
1. Severe three-vessel coronary artery disease.
2. Normal LV function.

Coronary Artery Bypass Surgery

The patient underwent two-vessel CABS, left internal mammary artery (LIMA) to LAD and SVG to OM on 12/20/04. His hospital course was uneventful and he was discharged 12/27/04 to home. Follow-up echo showed normal LV function.

Repeat Treadmill Test
- He underwent a follow-up treadmill test (ramp protocol) with gas exchange on 5/3/05. The primary reason for performing this exercise test was to evaluate completeness of revascularization after CABS 5 months ago.
- ST segments exhibited no depression during exercise and no depression in recovery.
- Exertional hypotension occurred (systolic BP failed to rise more than 20 mm Hg from baseline to peak exercise) with baseline systolic BP of 140 mm Hg and an SBP of 185 mm Hg at peak exercise (change = 5 mm Hg).
- Both the exercise capacity and maximal heart rate were normal for his age.

Resting ECG

The resting ECG is normal, consistent with a normal ejection fraction.

Limitations to Exercise

No noncardiac test-limiting conditions for this patient were noted.

Exercise Response

The test was terminated due to general fatigue, which is a typical endpoint.

Chest Pain

No angina occurred during exercise or recovery.

Hemodynamic Response

The patient achieved 9.9 estimated METs and 6.7 measured METs (from gas analysis) at a perceived exertion level of 17 of 20 on the Borg scale. The heart rate was 65 beats/min at baseline and rose 71 beats/min to 136 beats/min at maximal exercise. The 2-minute recovery heart rate dropped 62 beats/min from maximal exercise. The systolic BP was 140 mm Hg at baseline and rose 45 mm Hg to 185 mm Hg at maximal exercise.

Exercise ECG

The baseline ECG shows no ST depression. At maximal exercise or in recovery the ST segments showed no depression. No significant dysrhythmias occurred.

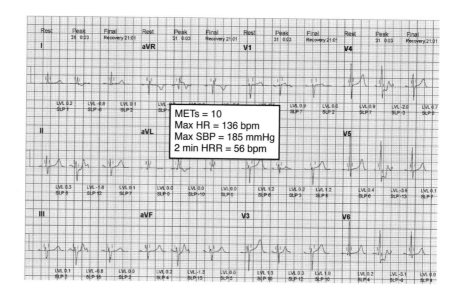

No bundle branch blocks or conduction defects were present at rest or developed during exercise.

Commentary

There had been no intervention that corrected abnormal ST depression and treated angina pectoris as well as coronary artery bypass surgery until the advent of drug-eluting stents. Comparison of the average tracings before and after the procedure is dramatic. The use of an LIMA is always preferred although no randomized trial data exist. Clinical experience and follow-up suggest that an arterial conduit lasts longer than the 10-year average before repeat revascularization is needed. Also, flow volumes appear to be superior to venous grafts.

This patient is interesting because exercise capacity was not altered. His prognosis was good even before the CABS based on his normal exercise capacity (>10 METs) but hopefully his quality of life was improved with the disappearance of angina.

Case Eight: Pre-/Post-PCI

This patient is a 66-year-old athletic Caucasian male outpatient who is 72 inches tall and 180 lb and who underwent a treadmill test using a ramp protocol with gas exchange on 4/25/05. The primary reason for performing this exercise test was to evaluate him for possible angina and elevated risk factors.

Current Medications
The patient is taking beta blocker, calcium antagonist, and statins.

Medical History
The patient has reported typical angina. No history of cardiac diseases, myocardial infarction, bypass surgery, PCI, or cardiac catheterization reported. No other medical problems except hypertension.

Risk Factors
The patient is currently not smoking and admits to only 3 pack-years of smoking. The patient is 4 lb over the average appropriate body mass index (BMI = 24.5). The patient has a history of high cholesterol (>200 mg/dl) with a current level reported at 165 mg/dl and high blood pressure. HDL level

was somewhat low at 50 mg/dl with a normal LDL level of 97 mg/dl. Triglycerides level was 91 and within normal limits. The Framingham Score estimates a 5-year incidence of cardiovascular events (angina, MI, or death) of 6% (as expected for age and gender).

Exercise Test Information

Resting ECG
No resting QRS-conduction defects were observed. The resting ECG is normal, so there is a 95% probability of a normal ejection fraction.

Limitations to Exercise
No noncardiac test-limiting conditions.

Exercise Response
The test was terminated due to angina.

Hemodynamic Response
The patient achieved 8 estimated and measured METs at a perceived exertion level of 13 of 20 on the Borg scale. The heart rate was 54 beats/min at baseline and raised 78 beats/min to 132 beats/min at maximal exercise. The 2-minute recovery heart rate was 88 beats/min and dropped 44 beats/min from maximal exercise. The systolic BP was 148 mm Hg at baseline and raised 32 mm Hg to 180 mm Hg at maximal exercise. Based on age from a male veteran population, the patient achieved normal exercise capacity and maximal heart rate.

Exercise ECG
The baseline ECG showed no ST depression. At maximal exercise the ST segments showed 4 mm of horizontal depression in the lateral and anterior leads. In recovery the ST segments showed 2 mm of downsloping depression in the lateral and anterior leads. There were occasional PVCs (<6/min).

Complications
No complications occurred during this test.

Results
The Duke Treadmill Score of –21.6 estimates an annual cardiovascular mortality rate of 10.1%. (This represents 4 times the age-expected mortality rate.) This indicates that the patient is at high risk with a poor prognosis.

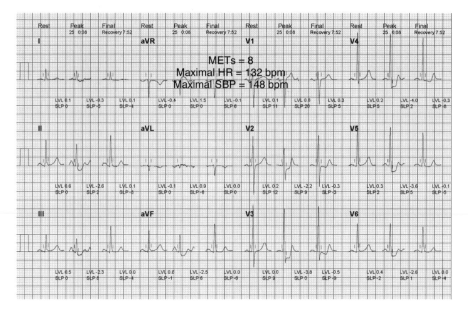

He underwent a cardiac cath on 5/25/05 with the following findings: Severe mid-LAD stenosis.

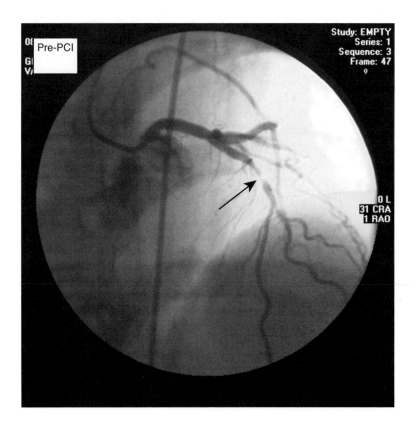

After successful PCI of mid-LAD artery with Taxus stent placement, there was no residual stenosis and TIMI-3 flow.

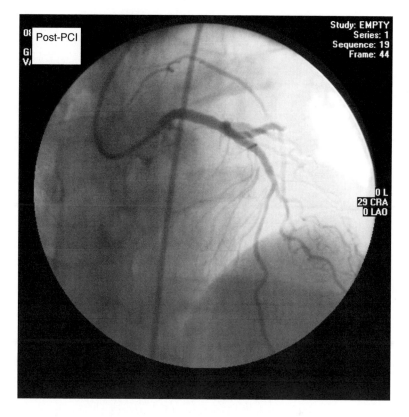

He was retested on 8/26/05:

Baseline HR 73, peak exercise HR 148, 2-minute recovery HR 98 (–50), baseline BP 136/72, peak exercise 176/70, exercise duration 9 minutes, Borg (6-20) 19, 12 METs (152% predicted). No abnormal ST depression or angina occurred, and the test was stopped due to fatigue.

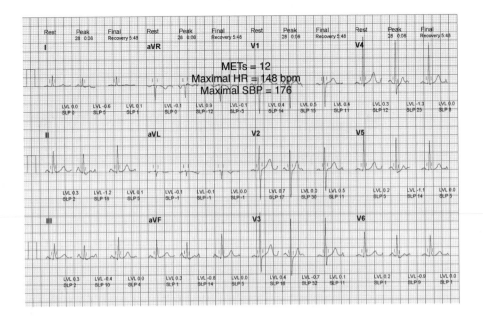

Commentary

This is not an isolated "best" case; we often see such dramatic results since PCI has evolved to the current level of technology. It is interesting to appreciate that Grunzig insisted on pre- and post-PTCA exercise testing for nonacute cases but that this concept was not widely adapted in clinical practice. In one of the few studies in which patients were tested while off of medications pre- and post-PTCA, Atwood and I found that there often was residual ST depression, particularly late in recovery. Before drug-eluting stents, it could be argued that a PTCA put patients at higher risk of an event than with medical management given the 30% reocclusion rate and frequent need for CABS or repeat of the procedure. Now those concerns do not exist, and it is difficult to justify not intervening in even low-risk patients with known ischemic lesions.

Case Nine: Exercise-Induced ST Elevation

The patient is a 62-year-old man with HTN, DM, s/p liver transplant in 1994 for hepatitis C. He had no heart disease symptoms until late 8/05 when he developed chest pain at rest. He has a negative family history and has not smoked for 20 years. His total cholesterol was 200. Admitted 8/23/05 for chest pain, he ruled out for an MI and was scheduled for a stress perfusion study on 8/31/05. He continued to have accelerating angina acute coronary syndrome (ACS). During the nuclear perfusion study, he exercised to 9.5 METs, his heart rate rose from 46 to 122 beats/min, and SBP dropped from 129 to 108 mm Hg at maximal exercise. He developed 7/10 chest pain with transient 3 mm ST elevation in V3-V4, and several 3 beat runs of ventricular tachycardia (VT).

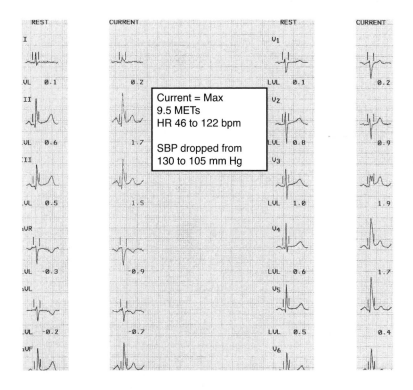

Current = Max
9.5 METs
HR 46 to 122 bpm

SBP dropped from
130 to 105 mm Hg

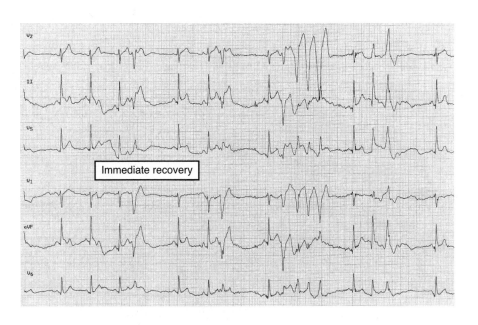

Immediate recovery

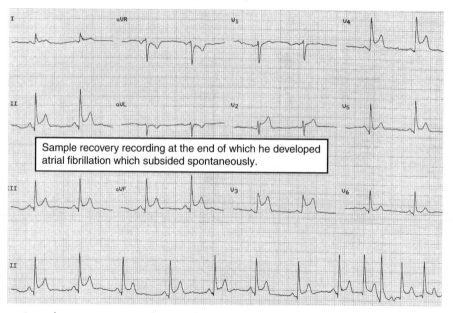

Sample recovery recording at the end of which he developed atrial fibrillation, which subsided spontaneously.

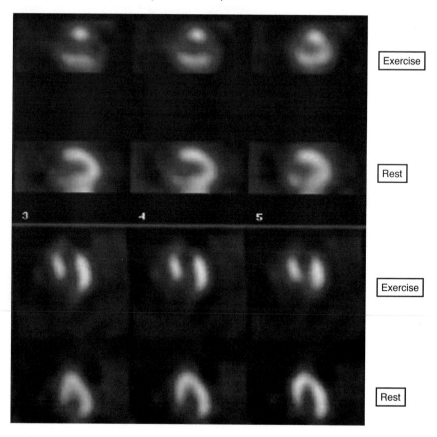

The perfusion scan above showed a large area of reperfusion in anterior/apical walls. EF was normal.

He underwent cardiac cath on 9/1/05, which showed the following:

1. The left main coronary artery is a moderate-sized vessel free of disease that bifurcates into the left anterior descending artery and the left circumflex artery.
2. The left anterior descending artery is a moderate-sized vessel that reaches the apex of the heart and gives rise to two diagonal arteries. The artery had a 70% smooth proximal lesion.
3. The left circumflex is a small codominant vessel free of significant disease.
4. The right coronary artery is a codominant vessel that supplies the PDA. The artery has no significant disease.

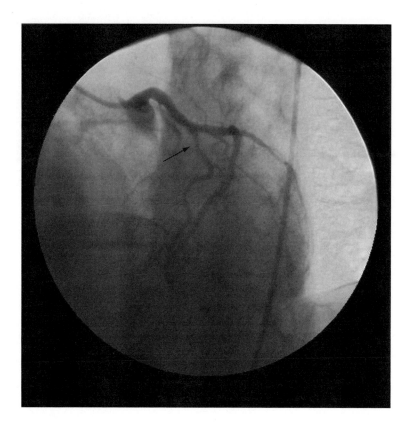

Repeat angio of left system after percutaneous coronary intervention: successful Taxus stent deployment in the mid-LAD.

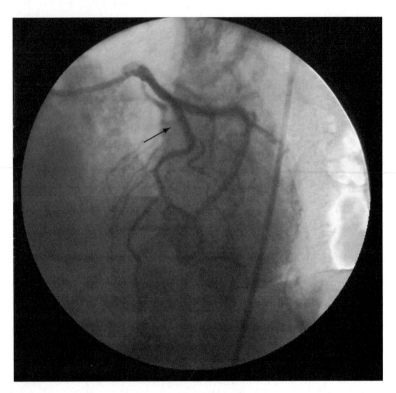

The patient is doing well since stent placement, remaining free of chest pain.

Commentary

Exercise test–induced ST elevation can occur due to spasm around a tight lesion such as this one. Elevation localizes to the area of ischemia and points to the involved vessel. It is frequently associated with VT and other arrhythmias, as well as hemodynamic abnormalities. Serial troponins had been negative in this patient, which is the reason he had a careful treadmill test instead of going straight to cath; also, some of his physicians considered the chest pain atypical.

Case Ten: ST Depression and Ventricular Tachycardia

This patient is a 46-year-old fireman who presented with chest pain early in summer but had a normal treadmill test with excellent exercise capacity. He weighs 160 lb and is 68 inches tall. His history is as follows: total cholesterol 208, LDL 138, HDL 59, no DM or HBP, no cigarettes or drinking, negative family history, no drug history.

He went on vacation with his family and passed out while riding an exercise cycle at Disneyland. He reported chest pain, then woke up on the floor; his wife called 911 but he refused to go to the emergency department.

He had follow-up studies on 6/25/04. His resting ECG and echo were totally normal. An exercise perfusion scan was normal, no chest pain during the test. He reached 13 METs, heart rate rose from 60 to 184 beats/min, 114/80 to 200/100 mm Hg, 2 min recovery HR 141 (drop of 43), terminated due to fatigue.

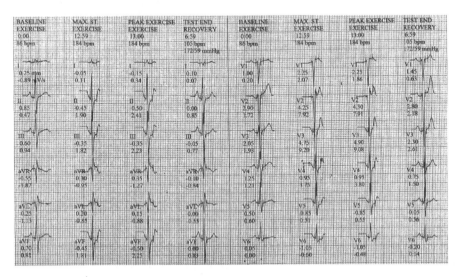

These averages demonstrate the normal resting ECG and abnormal ST depression at maximal exercise with rapid return to normal in recovery.

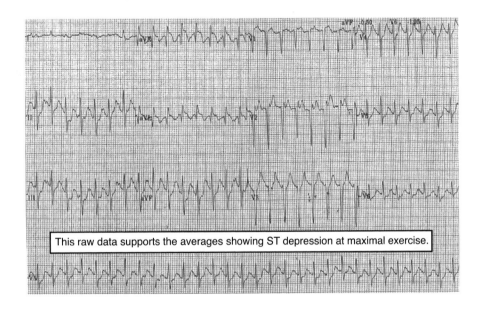

This raw data supports the averages showing ST depression at maximal exercise.

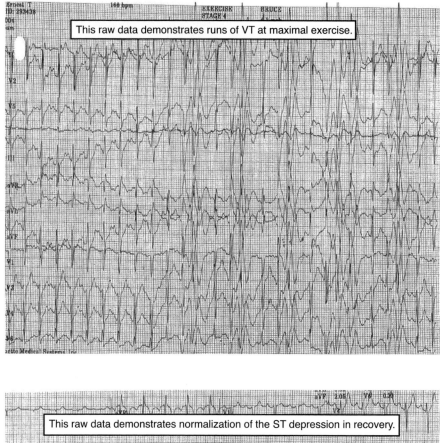

This raw data demonstrates runs of VT at maximal exercise.

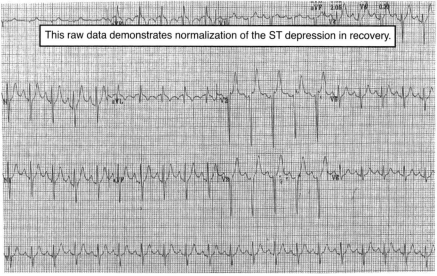

This raw data demonstrates normalization of the ST depression in recovery.

He died suddenly while vacationing at Yosemite on 8/11/04. No autopsy was performed.

Commentary

This is a sad case to consider because he was followed so closely by his physicians. In retrospect it is easy to say that too much weight was put on the normal scan and that the ST depression and VT should have led to an emergent cath. Most likely he died due to VT induced by ischemia, which could have been prevented by a PCI. While ischemic VT is more likely to be associated with ST elevation, when it is seen with ST depression it cannot be disregarded. Our understanding of this outcome would have been enhanced by actually seeing the perfusion scan and an autopsy.

Index

Page numbers followed by f refer to figures; page numbers followed by t refer to tables

Systolic blood pressure, 25, 181
  automated devices for measuring, 75
  excessive rise in,during peak exercise, 79
  failure of, 81
  heart rate and, 74, 112

T

T-wave amplitude, 90
Thallium, an isotopic analog of potassium, 44
Thermal head printers, 33
Three-lead vectorcardiographic approach, 31
Transmural ischemia with ST-segment elevation, 126
Transplant recipients, exercise testing and selection of, 215
Treadmill exercise
  bicycle ergometer versus, 35
  change in heart rate during, 55
  hemodynamic responses of, 65f
Treadmill score, steps to derive prognostic, 179
Treadmill test
  abnormal screening, 319–321
  with angina pectoris, 91
  electrocardiographic response to, 87
  indications for, 21
  reproducibility of, 131–132
12-lead ECG, 23

U

U-wave, changes in, 91
United States Air Force Medical Corps (USAFMC), 88, 279
United States Air Force School of Aerospace Medicine (USAFSAM), 38, 57, 64, 69f
Univariate analysis, Kaplan-Meier survival curves for, 176
U.S. Preventive Services Task Force (USPSTF), 293
USAFMC Normal Aircrewmen Study, 88–90

V

Vasoregulatory abnormalities, 111
Vasoregulatory asthenia, 111
VCO_2, major purpose of, 6
VE/VCO_2 slope, 220, 231
Venous oxygen content, determinants of, 10–11

Venous pressure
  determinant of ventricular filling, 8
  factors affecting, 8
Ventilatory gas exchange responses, 43–44
Ventilatory oxygen
  consumption, 2t
  oxygen uptake, 1
Ventricular function and exercise capacity, discrepancy between, 56
Ventricular function, resting and exercise performance, relationship between, 55
Ventricular pressure, left and end-diastolic volume, 3
Ventricular tachycardia
  exercise-induced, 127f–128f
  nonsustained, 129
Ventriculograms with gated perfusion scans, 45
Veterans Administration (VA) Health Care System, 18
Veterans Affairs Coronary Artery Bypass Surgery Study, 201t
Veterans Affairs Medical Centers Score (VAMCS), 252
Veterans Specific Activity Questionnaire (VSAQ), 39, 40t, 54
VO_2, 223
  on age, gender, activity status, and disease states, 58
  measurement of, 224
  plateau in, 71
VO_2 max
  defined by Fick principle, 6
  factors on, 53

W

Waveform, processing, 30
Weber classifications, 51
Wilson's central terminal, use of, 29
Wolfe-Parkinson-White syndrome (WPW), 43, 109
Women's Ischemia Syndrome Evaluation (WISE) study, 189
Work, definition of, 3
Workup bias, effect of, on follow-up prognostic studies, 182

Z

Z-fold paper, 33